Atlas of the Supraaortic Craniocervical Arterial Variations

Akira Uchino

Atlas of the Supraaortic Craniocervical Arterial Variations

MR and CT Angiography

Springer

Akira Uchino
Department of Radiology
Saitama Sekishinkai Hospital
Sayama, Saitama, Japan

ISBN 978-981-16-6802-9 ISBN 978-981-16-6803-6 (eBook)
https://doi.org/10.1007/978-981-16-6803-6

This Springer imprint is published by the registered company Springer Nature Singapore Pte Ltd.
The registered company address is: 152 Beach Road, #21-01/04 Gateway East, Singapore 189721, Singapore

Preface

I am a diagnostic neuroradiologist who has worked in Japan for more than 40 years. I am interested in supra-aortic craniocervical arterial variations and vascular malformations. Using catheter angiography, MR angiography, and CT angiography, I have experienced numerous cases of arterial variations, and I have published many papers reporting arterial variations, mainly in Springer Journals, such as *Surgical and Radiologic Anatomy*, *Neuroradiology*, and *European Radiology*.

Several great textbooks describing the normal variations of the supra-aortic craniocervical region have already been published. These textbooks usually contain embryology, normal anatomy, and variations of the brain, skull, artery, and vein. The presented figures of arterial variations were mainly obtained using catheter angiography. In this concise atlas, I describe only arterial variations with figures obtained by MR and/or CT angiography.

This concise atlas presents 208 cases of various variations of the supra-aortic craniocervical arteries detected by MR and/or CT angiography. Improved MR and CT angiographic image quality permits the incidental detection of even small anomalous arterial branches. Although the arterial variations may have limited clinical significance, their correct diagnosis during MR and CT angiographic image interpretation is important for interventional neuroradiologists as well as neurosurgeons and otorhinolaryngologists, who must be familiar with arterial variations to prevent complications during surgery. By referring to this textbook, I believe that readers will be able to easily identify arterial variations and make a correct diagnosis during image interpretation.

I am grateful to the doctors who sent me figures of extremely rare arterial variations. I also thank Dr. Yuji Numaguchi who recommended that I publish a textbook in English. I dedicate this book to my wife, Machiko, my daughters, Akemi, Hiromi, and Yoshimi, and my grandchildren, Ryoma, Tomoki, Yuri, Emiri, and Shunya.

Akira Uchino, M.D., Ph.D.

Acknowledgments

Thirty-nine figures were reprinted with permission from the following textbook published in Japanese.

- Extra- and Intracranial Arterial Variations: MRA and CTA
- First Edition
- By Akira Uchino, MD, PhD
- © 2015 by KANEHARA & Co, LTD, Tokyo
- ISBN 978-4-307-07097-3

Figures 1.1, 1.19, 2.10, 3.8, 3.10, 3.15, 3.18, 3.19, 3.20, 3.21, 4.3, 4.5, 5.5, 5.8, 5.13, 5.18, 5.21, 6.2, 6.7, 7.3, 7.5, 7.7, 7.9, 7.18, 7.19, 7.20, 7.23, 8.3, 8.17, 9.4, 9.10, 9.15, 9.23, 9.24, 9.33, 9.34, 10.6, 10.11, and 11.3

The following 17 figures were supplied by doctors in Japan

- Fig. 1.22 (Dr. Tomoki Kaneko)
- Fig. 2.1 (Dr. Kiyotaka Liu)
- Fig. 2.3 (Dr. Takashi Yamamoto)
- Fig. 3.5 (Drs. Toshiyuki Ohuchida and Yaeko Kanamiya)
- Fig. 3.9 (Dr. Noriharu Yanagimachi)
- Fig. 3.13 (Dr. Koji Yamashita)
- Fig. 3.14 (Dr. Naomi Fujiwara)
- Fig. 3.19 (Dr. Hideki Sato)
- Fig. 3.20 (Dr. Morio Nagahata)
- Fig. 3.25 (Dr. Yuji Numaguchi)
- Fig. 5.8 (Dr. Harushi Mori)
- Fig. 5.27 (Dr. Kazufumi Kikuchi)
- Fig. 5.29 (Dr. Takashi Yoshiura)
- Fig. 9.10 (Dr. Kanehiro Hasuo)
- Fig. 10.6 (Dr. Maki Umino)
- Fig. 11.6 (Dr. Shinichi Kan)
- Fig. 11.11 (Dr. Takashi Okazaki)

About the Book

This book presents numerous figures of various variations of the supra-aortic arteries detected by MR and CT angiography. Improved both MR and CT angiographic image quality permits incidental detection of even small anomalous arterial branches. Although the cerebral arterial variations may have limited clinical significance, their correct diagnosis during MR and CT angiographic image interpretation is important to interventional neuroradiologists as well as both neurosurgeons and otorhinolaryngologists, who must be familiar with arterial variations to prevent complications during surgery. Readers can easily identify arterial variations and make a correct diagnosis during image interpretation using this textbook.

Contents

About the Author

Akira Uchino, M.D., Ph.D., is Chief Radiologist of Saitama Sekishinkai Hospital and Visiting Professor of Saitama Medical University, Saitama, Japan. He graduated from Kyushu University Faculty of Medicine. He completed a radiology residency and neuroradiology fellowship at Kyushu University Hospital. He is a Board-Certified Diagnostic Radiologist of Japan Radiological Society, and Honorary Member of Japanese Society of Neuroradiology. He was a Councilor of Japan Radiological Society, Japanese Society of Neuroradiology, Japanese Society for Magnetic Resonance in Medicine, and Japanese Society of Interventional Radiology. He was an Associate Member of the European Society of Neuroradiology, the American Society of Neuroradiology, and the Radiological Society of North America. His clinical and research interests include craniocervical arterial variations. He has published numerous papers mainly in Springer Journals.

List of Abbreviations

AA	Aortic arch
ACA	Anterior cerebral artery
AChA	Anterior choroidal artery
ACoA	Anterior communicating artery
AICA	Anterior inferior cerebellar artery
A-P	Antero-posterior
AI-PS	Anteroinferior-posterosuperior
APA	Ascending pharyngeal artery
AS-PI	Anterosuperior-posteroinferior
BA	Basilar artery
BCT	Brachiocephalic trunk
BPAS	Basiparallel anatomic scanning
CCA	Common carotid artery
CT	Computed tomography
CW	Circle of Willis
ECA	External carotid artery
FLAIR	Fluid-attenuated inversion recovery
FM	Foramen magnum
FS	Foramen spinosum
HC	Hypoglossal canal
ICA	Internal carotid artery
ID	Infundibular dilatation
I-S	Infero-superior
JF	Jugular foramen
LAO	Left anterior oblique
LPO	Left posterior oblique
MCA	Middle cerebral artery
MIP	Maximum-intensity-projection
MMA	Middle meningeal artery
MR	Magnetic resonance
OphA	Ophthalmic artery
P-A	Postero-anterior
PCA	Posterior cerebral artery
PCoA	Posterior communicating artery
PHA	Persistent hypoglossal artery
PICA	Posterior inferior cerebellar artery
POA	Persistent otic artery

PPOA	Persistent primitive olfactory artery
PSA	Persistent stapedial artery
PTA	Persistent trigeminal artery
RAO	Right anterior oblique
RPO	Right posterior oblique
SA	Subclavian artery
SCA	Superior cerebellar artery
S-I	Supero-inferior
TF	Transverse foramen
TOF	Time-of-flight
VA	Vertebral artery
VBJ	Vertebrobasilar junction
VR	Volume-rendering

Branching Variations from the Aortic Arch and Aortic Arch Anomaly

1

Abstract

This chapter includes (1) Left common carotid artery origin variations, (2) Left vertebral artery origin variations, (3) Right vertebral artery origin variations, (4) Right subclavian artery origin variations and associated arterial variations, and (5) Aortic arch anomaly and related variations. There are 20 figures and 2 illustrations.

Before catheterization of the branches arising from the aortic arch, these variations should be recognized to reduce both examination time and catheterization failure.

Keywords

Aortic arch · Brachiocephalic trunk · Common carotid artery · Subclavian artery · Vertebral artery

1.1 Left Common Carotid Artery (CCA) Origin Variations

1.1.1 Left CCA Arising from the Brachiocephalic Trunk (BCT)

The left CCA is usually a second branch of the aortic arch (AA) that arises between the BCT and left subclavian artery (SA). Relatively frequently, it also arises from the BCT (Fig. 1.1). In patients with a left CCA of BCT origin, transfemoral catheterization into the left CCA is sometimes

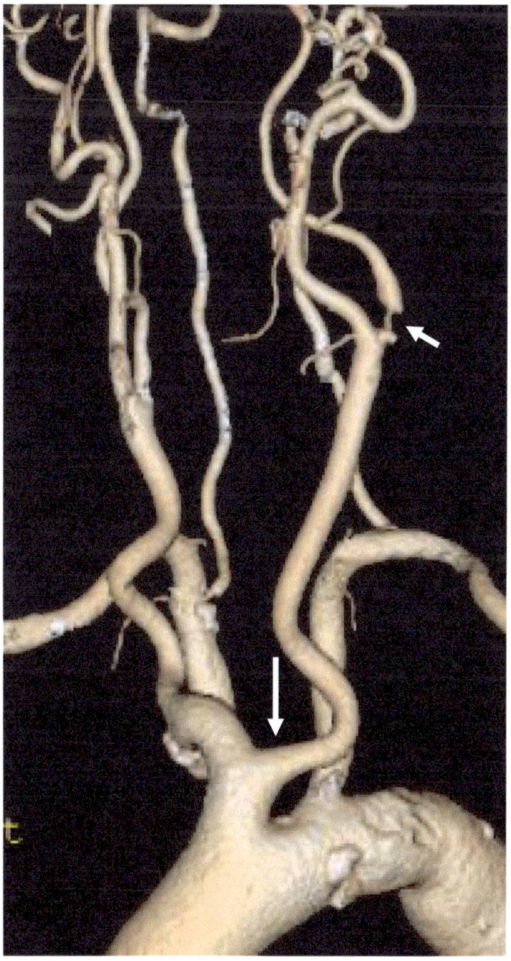

Fig. 1.1 Slightly LAO projection of CT angiography shows severe stenosis of the left ICA at its origin (*short arrow*). The left CCA arises from the BCT (*long arrow*). The stenotic lesion of this patient was successfully treated by stenting using a right transradial approach

A. Uchino, *Atlas of the Supraaortic Craniocervical Arterial Variations*,
https://doi.org/10.1007/978-981-16-6803-6_1

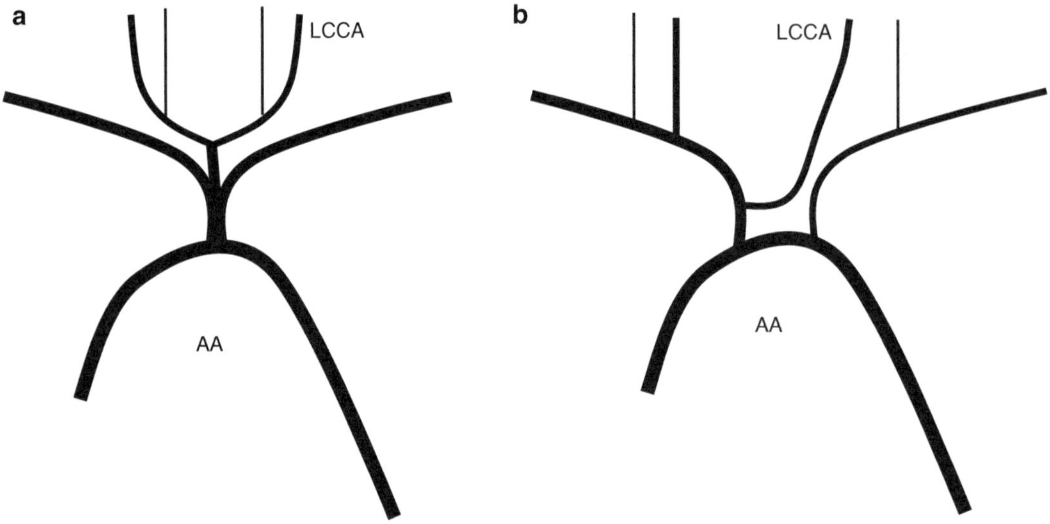

Fig. 1.2 Schematic illustrations of (**a**) true bovine AA and (**b**) this variation. *AA* aortic arch, *LCCA* left common carotid artery

difficult, and a right transradial or transbrachial approach may be recommended.

The prevalence of this variation was reported to be 7.8% [1] and 6.0% [2]. This variation has been termed "bovine AA," but this name is inaccurate because cattle have a single BCT that originates from the AA, which eventually splits into the bilateral SAs and a bicarotid trunk (Fig. 1.2) [3].

1.1.2 Common Origin of the Left CCA with BCT

The left CCA relatively frequently shares a common origin with the BCT (Fig. 1.3). The prevalence of this variation was reported to be 19.6% [1] and 5.5% [2]. However, other papers describing the left CCA origin variation included both types (Sects. 1.1.1 and 1.1.2) together. In patients with a left CCA of common origin with the BCT, transfemoral catheterization into the left CCA is not difficult. Therefore, these two types of left CCA origin variation should be diagnosed correctly without confusion.

If this variation is associated with an aberrant right subclavian artery (SA), it forms a bicarotid trunk (Sect. 1.4.2) (Fig. 1.17). In some papers, however, the term "bicarotid trunk" is used for all variations of both Sects. 1.1.1 and 1.1.2 [4].

1.1.3 Bilateral Brachiocephalic Trunks

Extremely rarely, the left CCA and left SA have a common origin, creating bilateral BCTs (Figs. 1.4 and 1.5) [1]. Both patients presented here have left SA that arises at an extremely proximal point. Thus, this variation can be regarded as a left SA origin variation rather than a left CCA origin variation. Its prevalence is unknown. The bilateral BCTs are very rarely seen in humans but are very commonly seen and "normal" in some of the mammalian species [5].

1.2 Left Vertebral Artery (VA) Origin Variations

1.2.1 Direct Origin of the Left VA from the Aortic Arch (AA) Proximal to the Left Subclavian Artery (SA)

The left VA usually arises from the proximal left SA; however, it relatively frequently arises from the AA, between the left CCA and left SA (Fig. 1.6). Its prevalence on CT angiography was reported to be approximately 4% [6]. The prevalence of this variation in Caucasians was reported

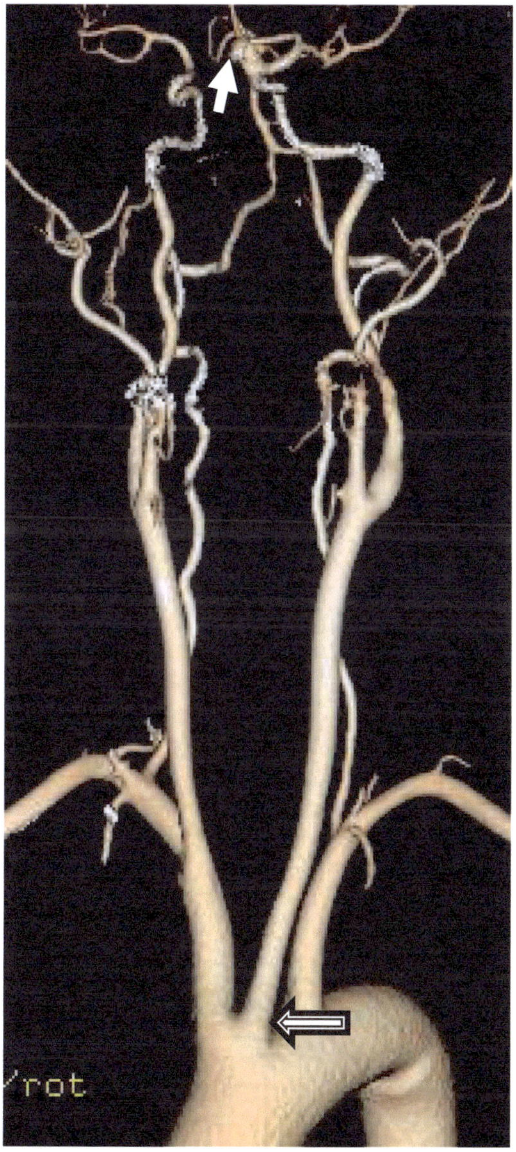

Fig. 1.3 Slightly LAO projection of CT angiography shows a common origin of the BCT and left CCA (*long arrow*). There is a large left paraclinoid ICA aneurysm (*short arrow*). The aneurysm of this patient was successfully treated by coil embolization using a transfemoral approach

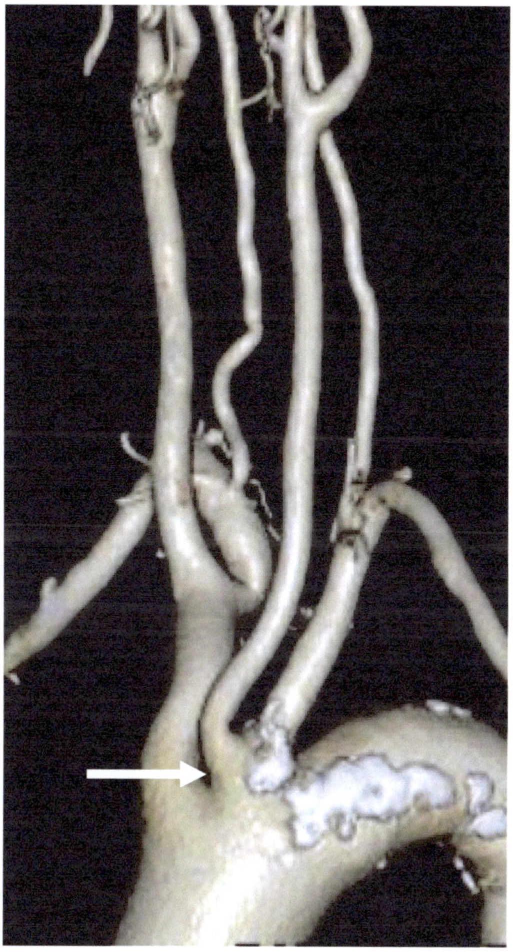

Fig. 1.4 LAO projection of CT angiography shows a common origin of the left CCA and left SA, forming bilateral BCTs (*arrow*)

The direct origin left VA is usually slightly small in caliber, and enters the fifth, fourth, or third transverse foramen (TF), not the sixth TF [6]. Before catheterization to the left VA, this common variation should be recognized to reduce both the examination time and catheterization failure.

to be 4.2–6.1% [1, 7, 8]. According to the double aortic arch model (Fig. 1.7), this variation is formed when the left sixth segmental artery persists instead of the seventh. Rarely, the left VA shares a common origin with the left SA (Fig. 1.8). This may be a variant of left VA of direct AA origin.

1.2.2 Duplicate Origin of the Left VA

The left VA extremely rarely arises from both the AA and the normal point of the left SA, forming the duplicate (dual, double) origin of the left VA [9]. These two arteries fuse at the level of C5 TF (Fig. 1.9) [6]. Duplicate origin of the left VA is

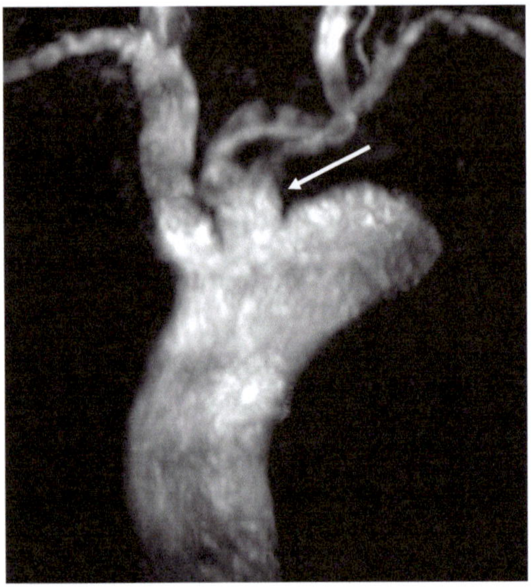

Fig. 1.5 LAO projection of partial MIP MR angiography shows a common origin of the left CCA and left SA, forming bilateral BCTs (*arrow*)

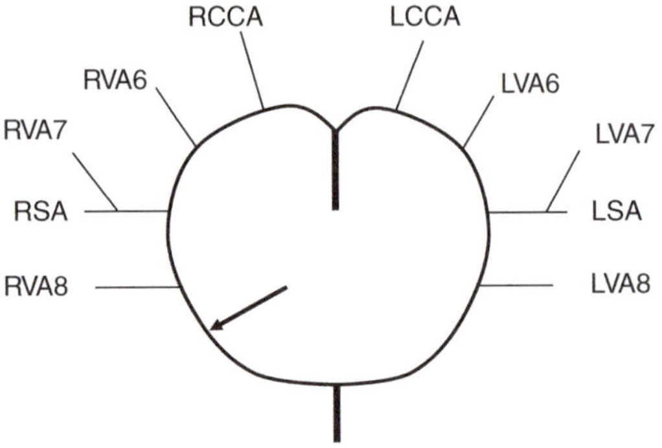

Fig. 1.7 Schematic illustration of the double aortic arch model. (Modified from [6]). Normally, LVA6, LVA8, RVA6, and RVA8 regress, and the right aortic arch regresses at the segment distal to the RSA (*arrow*). *CCA* common carotid artery, *L* left, *R* right, *SA* subclavian artery, *VA* vertebral artery

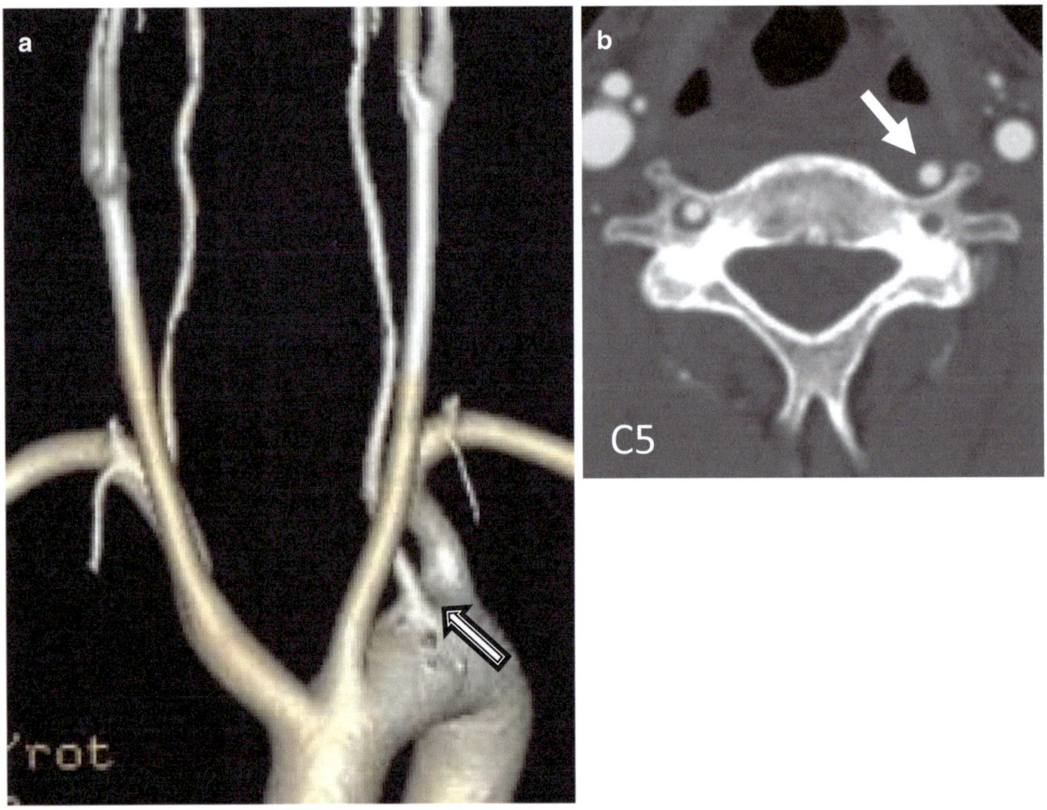

Fig. 1.6 (**a**) A-P projection of CT angiography shows the left VA arising directly from the AA proximal to the left SA (*arrow*). (**b**) CT angiographic source image at the level of the C5, the left VA is not observed in the TF but is located anteriorly (*arrow*)

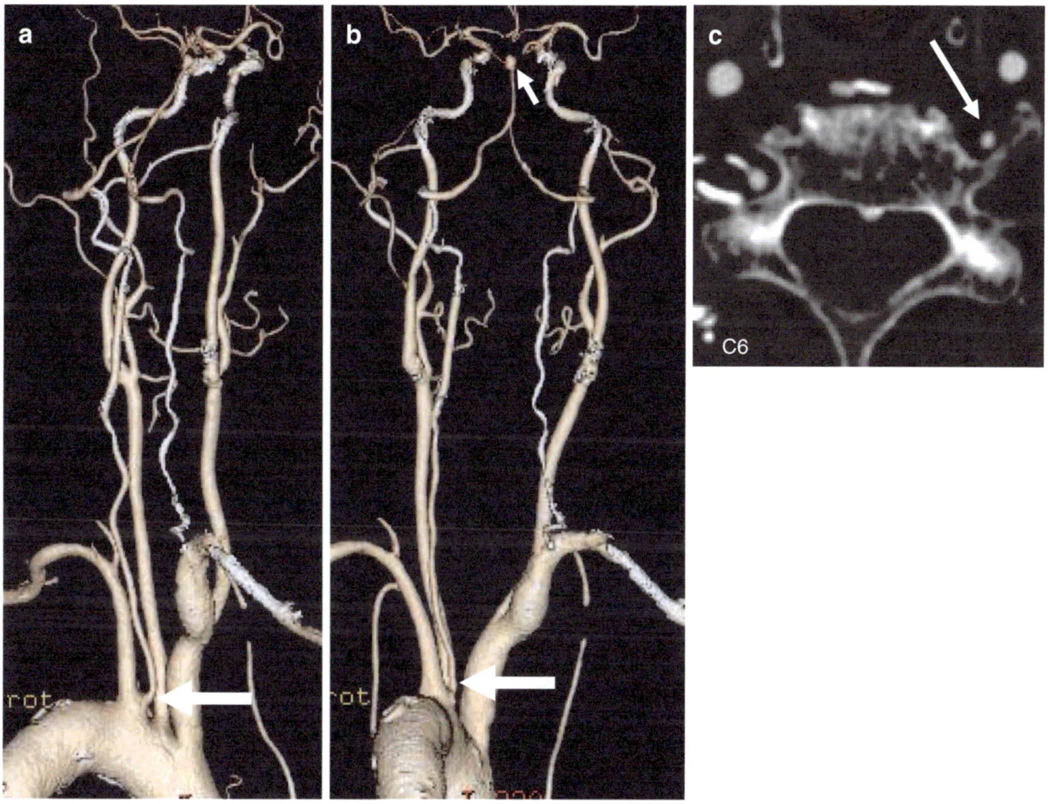

Fig. 1.8 (**a**) RPO and (**b**) P-A projections of CT angiography show the left VA of common origin with the left SA (*long arrows*). An aneurysm is seen at the BA tip (*short arrow*). (**c**) CT angiographic source image at the level of the C6, the left VA is not observed in the TF but is located anteriorly (*arrow*)

formed if both the seventh and sixth segmental arteries (LVA7 and LVA6 in Fig. 1.7) persist. The prevalence of this rare variation is unknown. If one of the two channels is occluded, the remaining channel will provide collateral circulation. Laminar flow may cause this rare variation to be misdiagnosed as dissection by catheter angiography [10].

1.2.3 Direct Origin of the Left VA from the AA Distal to the Left SA

Rarely, the left VA arises from the AA distal to the left SA (Fig. 1.10) [11]. Its prevalence on CT angiography was reported to be 0.2% [6]. This type of VA enters the seventh TF, not the sixth TF. This rare variation is formed when the eighth segmental artery (LVA8 in Fig. 1.7) persists. During total arch replacement, this variation should be kept in mind [12].

1.3 Right VA Origin Variations

1.3.1 Right VA Arising from the Extreme Proximal Right SA

The origin of the right VA from the proximal segment of the right SA, rather than at the usual point of origin (less than half the distance from the origin of the right SA to the usual point), can be regarded as "extreme proximal right SA origin." This right VA variation is the same develop-

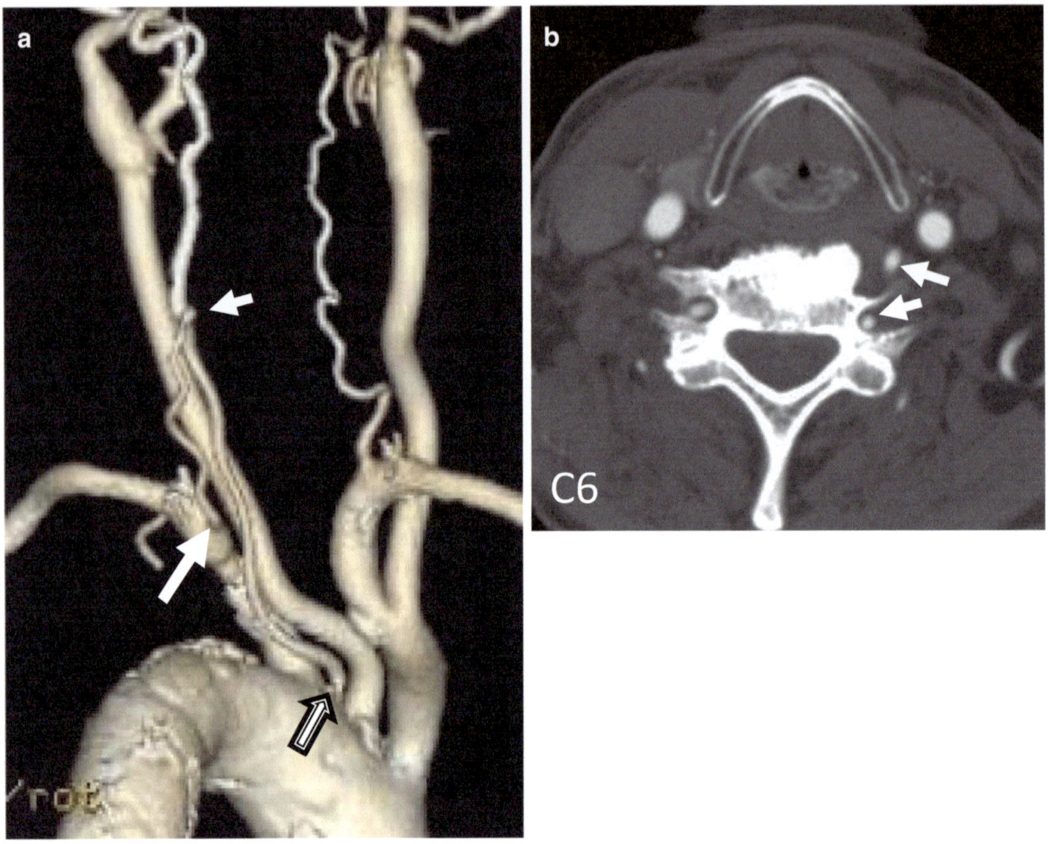

Fig. 1.9 (**a**) RPO projection of CT angiography shows the duplicate origin of the left VA (*long arrows*), with one vessel arising from the AA. The two channels fuse at the C5 level (*short arrow*). (**b**) CT angiographic source image of the level of the C6 shows two channels of the left VA (*short arrows*); the channel originating from the AA is seen anteriorly

mental failure as left VA of direct AA origin, persistence of the right sixth segmental artery (RVA6 in Fig. 1.7). It has not been recognized previously. Its prevalence on CT angiography was reported to be approximately 3% [6]. Just like the left VA of direct AA origin, the majority of the extreme proximal right SA origin right VA enters the fifth, fourth, or third TF, not the sixth TF (Fig. 1.11).

Extremely rarely, the right VA arises from the origin of the right CCA (Fig. 1.12). This is regarded as an extreme type of this variation. In the case of aberrant right SA, the right VA rarely arises from the right CCA (Sect. 1.4.3).

1.3.2 Duplicate Origin of the Right VA

Duplicate origin of the right VA is extremely rare. Most patients have a right VA of both normal origin and of extreme proximal right SA origin (Sect. 1.3.1) that fuse together at the fifth TF (Fig. 1.13) [6]. As mentioned for the left side, persistence of both the seventh and sixth segmental arteries (RVA7 and RVA6 in Fig. 1.7) forms this rare variation.

A patient in whom both channels arose from the extreme proximal segment of the right SA was also reported (Fig. 1.14) [13].

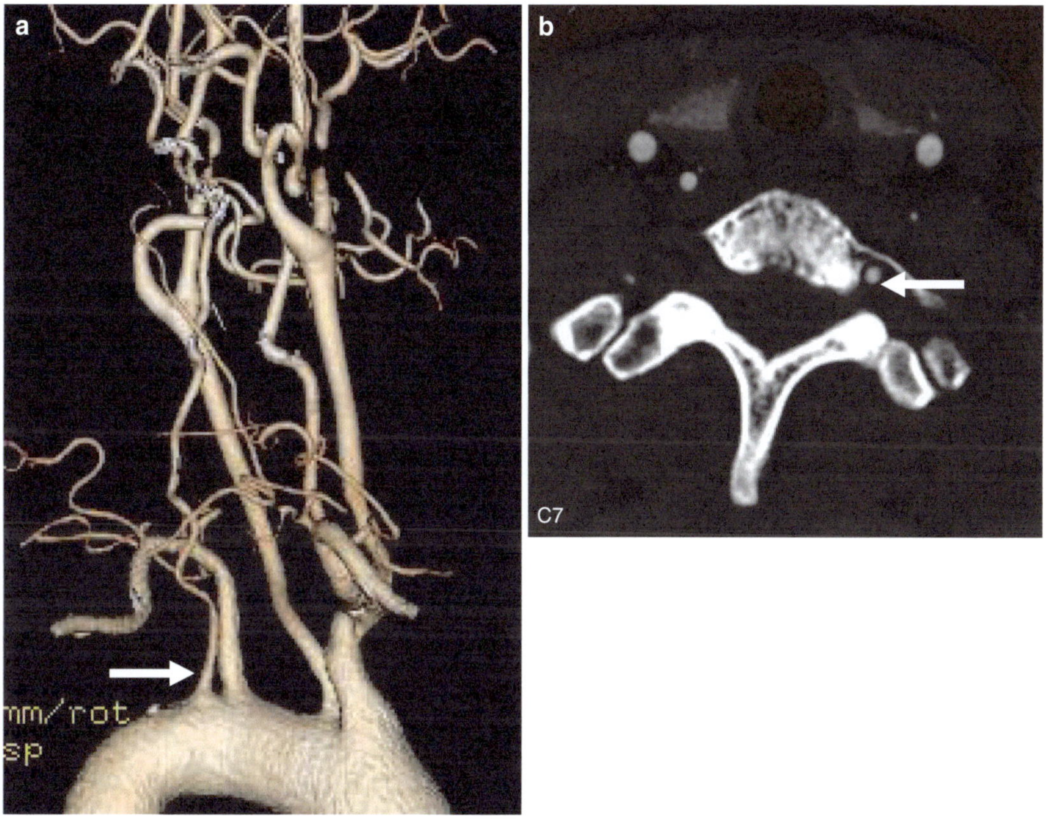

Fig. 1.10 (**a**) RPO projection of CT angiography shows the left VA arising directly from the AA distal to the left SA (*arrow*). (**b**) CT angiographic source image at the level of the C7 shows the left VA in the TF (*arrow*)

1.3.3 Aberrant Right VA (Arising from the AA Distal to the Left SA)

Extremely rarely, the right VA arises from the AA distal to the left SA and crosses the midline via the retroesophageal space, following a similar course to that of an aberrant right SA (Sect. 1.4.1). This type of VA enters the seventh TF, not the sixth TF (Fig. 1.15) [6]. In 2009, Karcaaltincaba et al. [14] initially used the term "aberrant right VA," which seems to suit this variation, which is also termed "vertebral arteria lusoria" [15]. This rare variation is formed when the RVA8 persists and regression of the right AA at the segment between the RSA and RVA8 occurs (Fig. 1.7) [16].

1.4 Right SA Origin Variations and Associated Arterial Variations

1.4.1 Aberrant Right SA (Arising from the AA Distal to the Left SA)

Based on CT angiography [6], it was reported that approximately 0.5% of the general population has a right SA arising from the AA distal to the left SA, called aberrant right SA. Previously reported prevalence of aberrant right SA is 0.4–2% [17]. Regression of the right aortic arch at the segment between the right CCA and right SA in Fig. 1.7 would yield such aberrant right SA. This artery crosses midline via the retroesophageal space

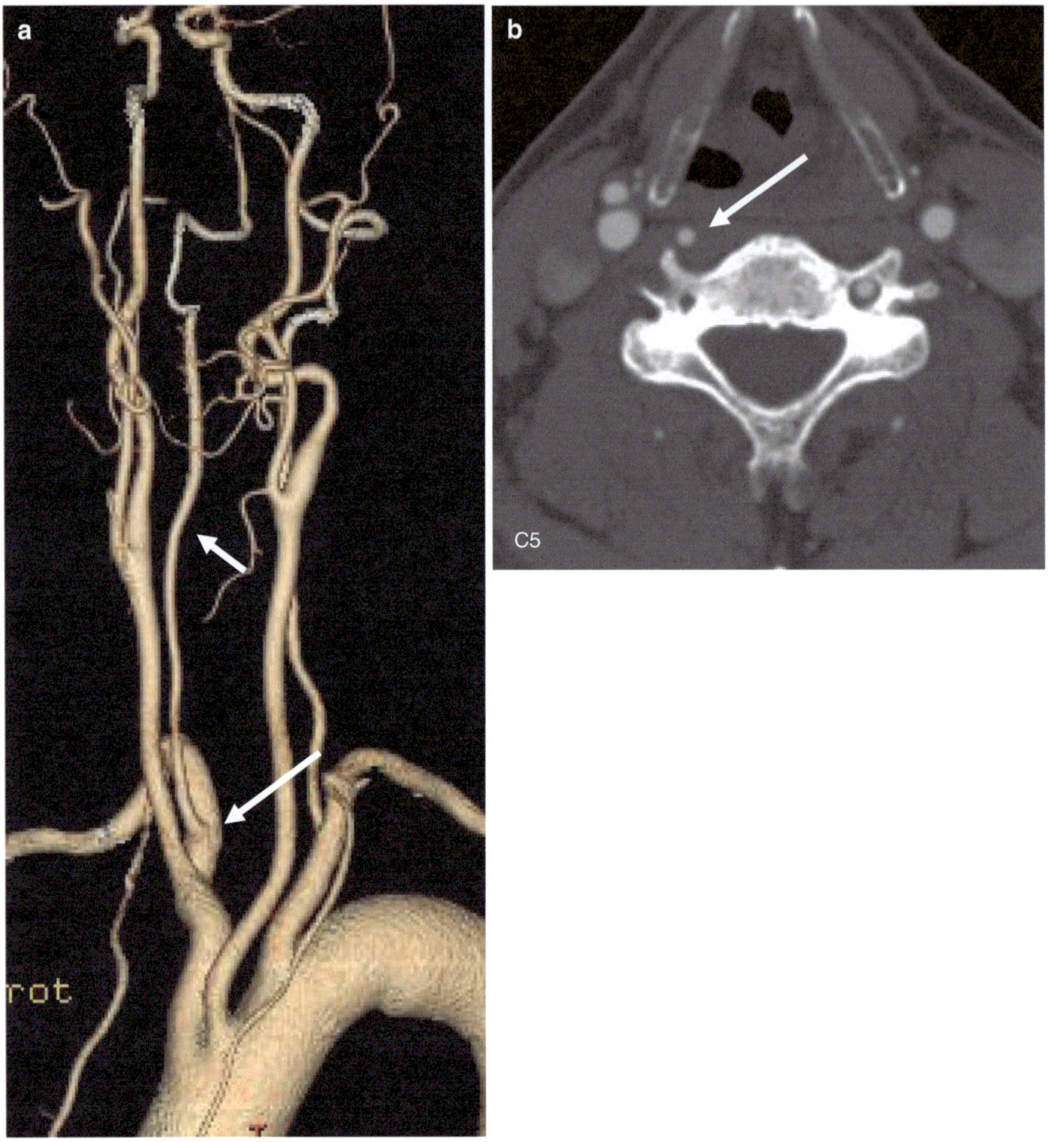

Fig. 1.11 (**a**) LAO projection of CT angiography shows an extreme proximal right SA origin of the right VA (*long arrow*). The right VA enters the fourth TF (*short arrow*). (**b**) CT angiographic source image of the level of the C5 shows the right VA located anteriorly (*arrow*). The right VA enters the fourth TF (not shown)

(Fig. 1.16). Most examples of this variation in the adult population are found incidentally, however, it may cause esophageal disfunction, especially in children, and it is called "dysphagia lusoria" [18]. Because neither a right transradial nor a transbrachial approach can be successfully performed for craniocervical intervention, this common variation should be recognized before the procedure.

1.4.2 Aberrant Right SA with Bicarotid Trunk

In approximately one-third of cases, the right CCA and left CCA of the aberrant right SA have a common origin, forming a bicarotid trunk (Fig. 1.17) [6]. The reason for this highly frequent association is unknown.

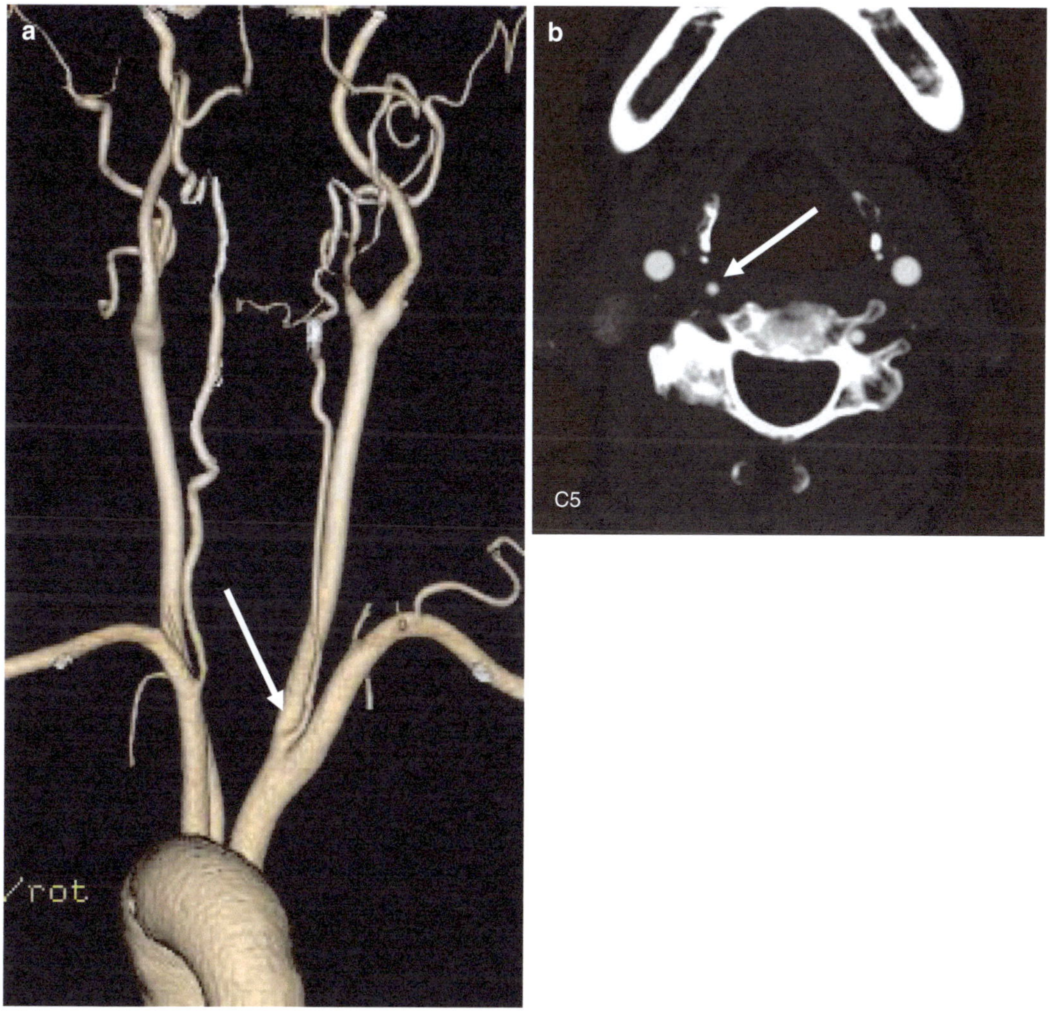

Fig. 1.12 (**a**) P-A projection of CT angiography shows the right VA arising from the origin of the right CCA (*arrow*). (**b**) CT angiographic source image of the level of the C5 shows the right VA located anteriorly (*arrow*). The right VA enters the fourth TF (not shown)

1.4.3 Aberrant Right SA with the Right VA Arising from the Right CCA

Extremely rarely, the right VA arises from the right CCA instead of the aberrant right SA (Fig. 1.18). This type of right VA usually enters the fifth or fourth TF, not the sixth TF [6]. Thus, this VA variation can be regarded as the same as the artery arising from the extreme proximal right SA (Sect. 1.3.1). In Fig. 1.7, when the RVA6 persists and right AA regression occurs between RVA6 and RSA, this extremely rare variation is formed.

1.5 Aortic Arch (AA) Anomaly and Related Variations

1.5.1 Aberrant Left SA Arising from a Right-Sided AA (Type 2)

The majority of right-sided AA is associated with an aberrant left SA, called type 2 right-sided AA. The left CCA arises as the first branch, followed by a right CCA, right SA, and finally, aberrant left SA. The origin of the left SA is usually dilated, and this characteristic configuration is named Kommerell's diverticulum (Fig. 1.19) [19].

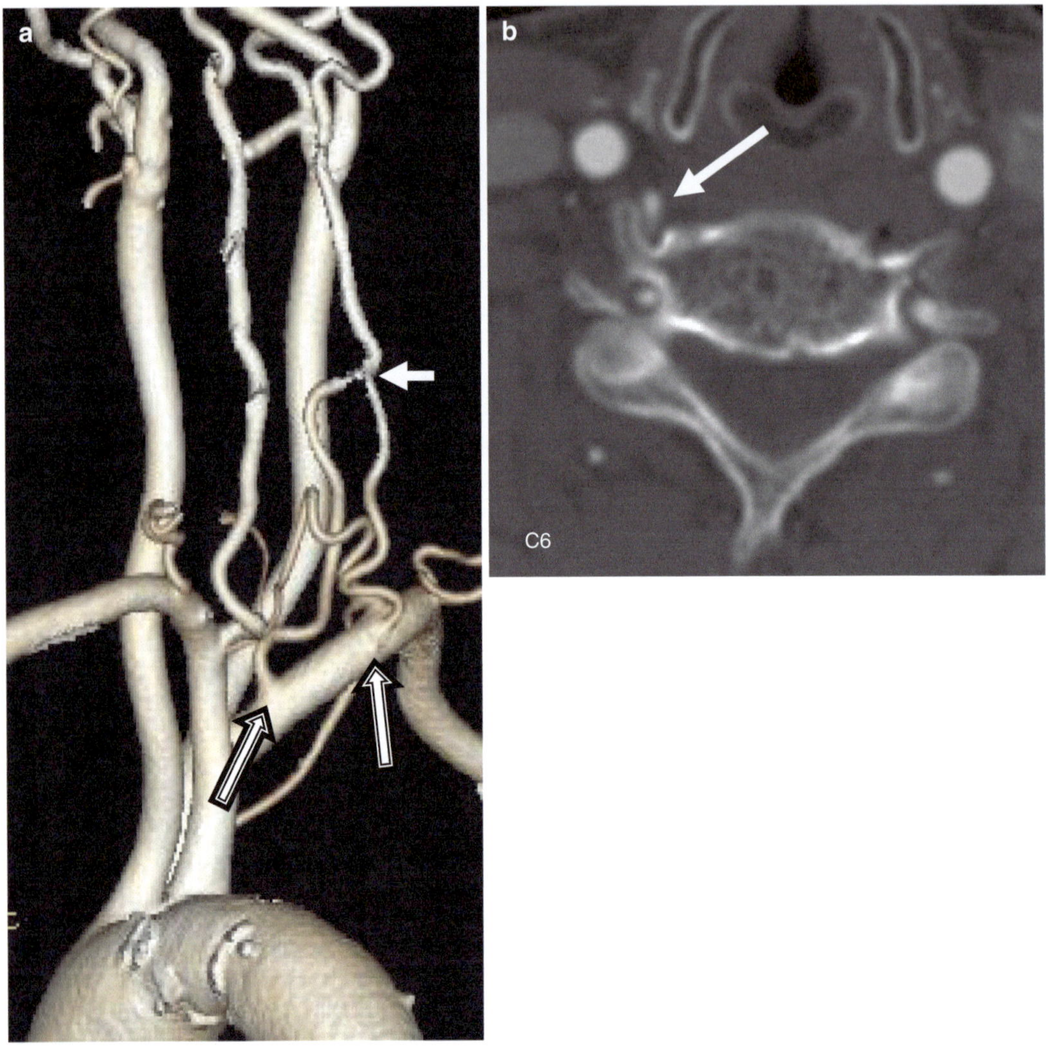

Fig. 1.13 (**a**) RPO projection of CT angiography shows the duplicate origin of the right VA (*long arrows*), one of the two branches arises from an extreme proximal right SA. The two branches fuse at the level of the C5 (*short arrow*). (**b**) CT angiographic source image of the level of the C6 shows one of the two branches of the right VA is located anteriorly (*arrow*)

1.5.2 Right-Sided AA with Mirror-Image Branching (Type 1)

Mirror-image right AA is called type 1 and is extremely rare (Fig. 1.20). Its prevalence in the adult population was reported to be 0.012–0.018% [20]. Associated congenital cardiovascular diseases are frequently observed.

1.5.3 Double AA

Double AA is extremely rare, especially in the adult population. The prevalence of the aortic ring in the pediatric population was reported to be 0.021% [21]. Two AAs are asymmetric, and the right AA is usually located higher than the left AA (Fig. 1.21). Double AA is frequently

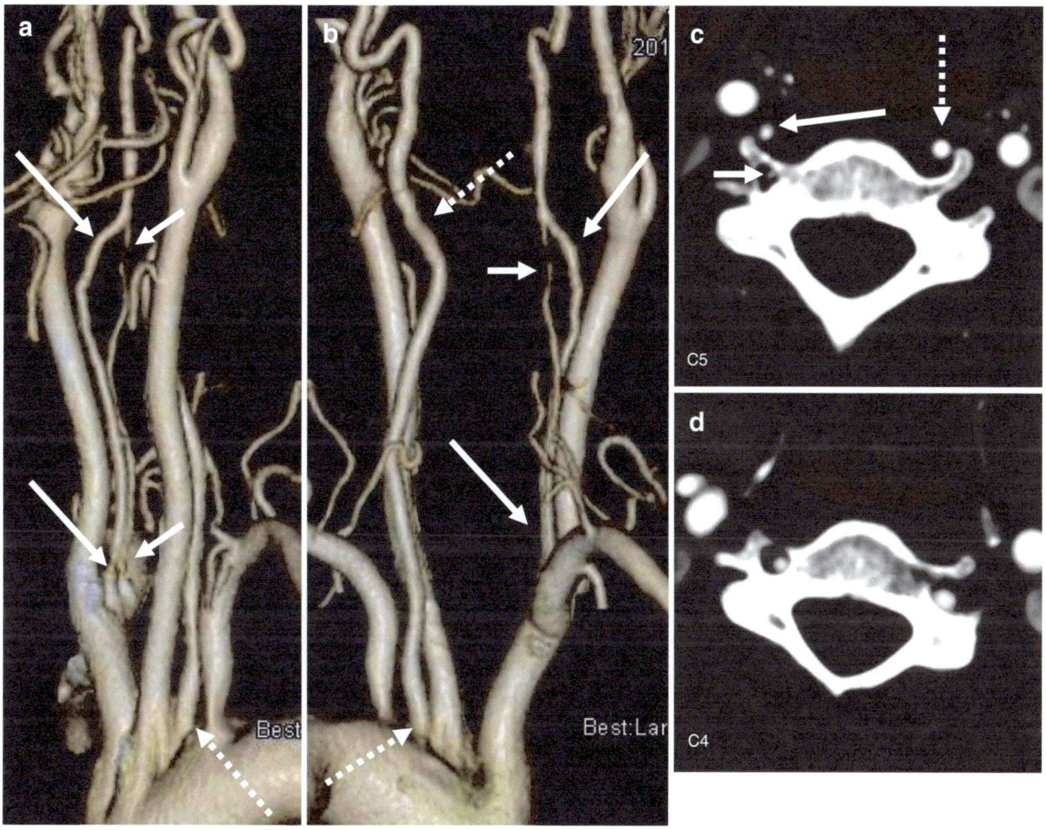

Fig. 1.14 (**a**) LAO and (**b**) RPO projections of CT angiography show duplicate origin of the right VA in which both channels arise from the extreme proximal right SA and fuse at the level of the C4 (*long and short arrows*). The left VA arises directly from the AA (*dotted arrows*). (**c**) CT angiographic source image of the level of the C5 shows the smaller channel of the right VA is located in the TF (*short arrow*), but both the larger channel of the right VA and the left VA are located anteriorly (*long and dotted arrows*). (**d**) At the level of C4, bilateral VAs are seen in the TFs

associated with congenital cardiovascular diseases. It also frequently causes respiratory disturbance due to compression by the aortic ring. Therefore, in the majority of cases, this anomaly can be detected before or immediately after birth.

1.5.4 Cervical AA

Cervical AA, located at an abnormally high position and extending into the neck, is extremely rare. It is usually asymptomatic but may cause symptoms of compression of the trachea and esophagus. Embryologically, abnormal regression of the fourth brachial arch with persistence of the third brachial arch forms a cervical AA. According to Zhong et al. [22], among 35 patients with a surgically repaired cervical AA, 30 (85.7%) had a left-sided AA and 5 (14.3%) had a right-sided AA. Co-existing abnormality of the AA, such as aneurysmal dilatation and coarctation of the aorta can be seen (Fig. 1.22) [23].

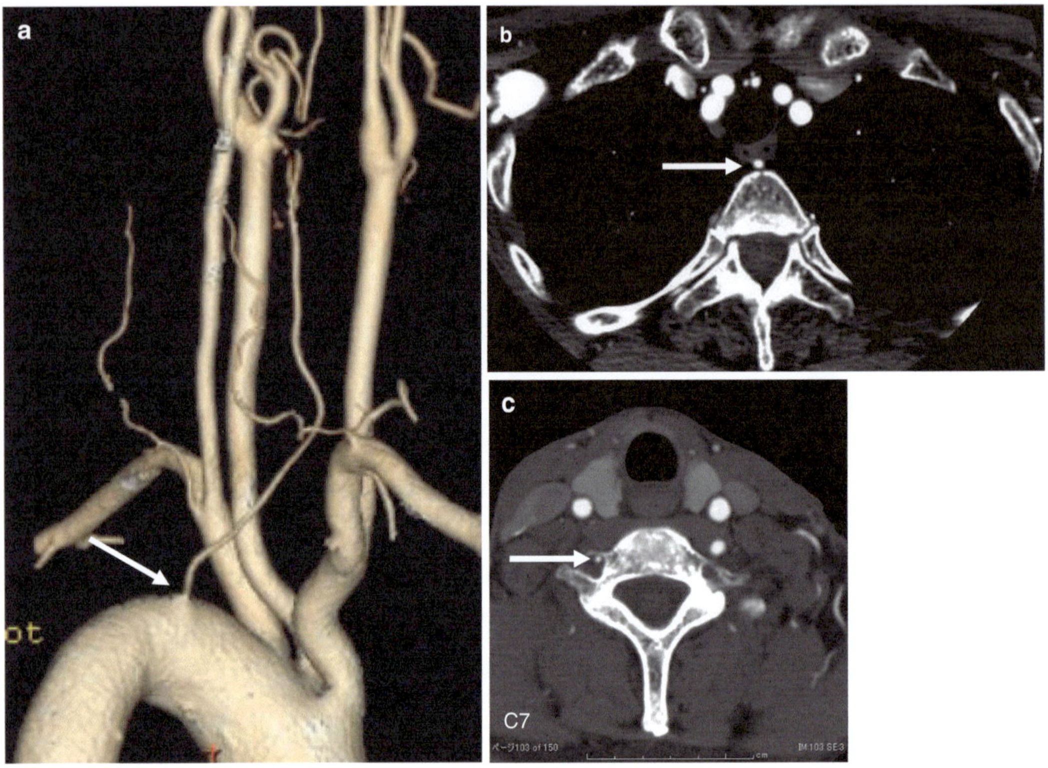

Fig. 1.15 (**a**) RPO projection of CT angiography shows the right VA arising directly from the AA distal to the left SA, indicative of an aberrant right VA (*arrow*). (**b**) CT angiographic source image at the upper thoracic level shows the right VA running in the retroesophageal space (*arrow*). (**c**) CT angiographic source image at the level of the C7 shows the right VA in the TF (*arrow*)

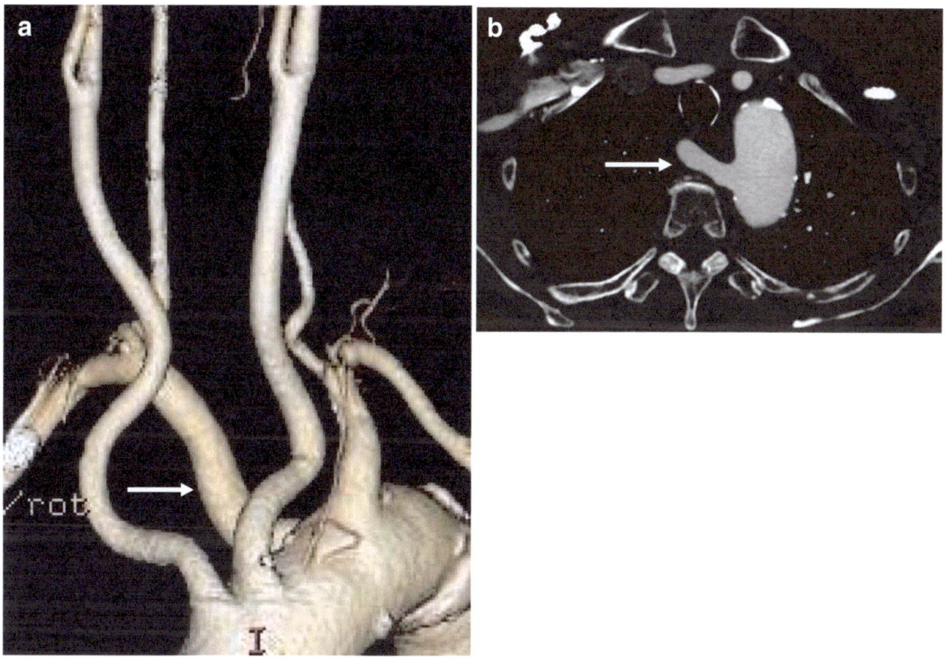

Fig. 1.16 (**a**) Slightly LAO projection of CT angiography shows the right SA arising from the AA distal to the left SA, indicative of an aberrant right SA (*arrow*). (**b**) CT angiographic source image at the upper thoracic level shows the right SA running in the retroesophageal space (*arrow*)

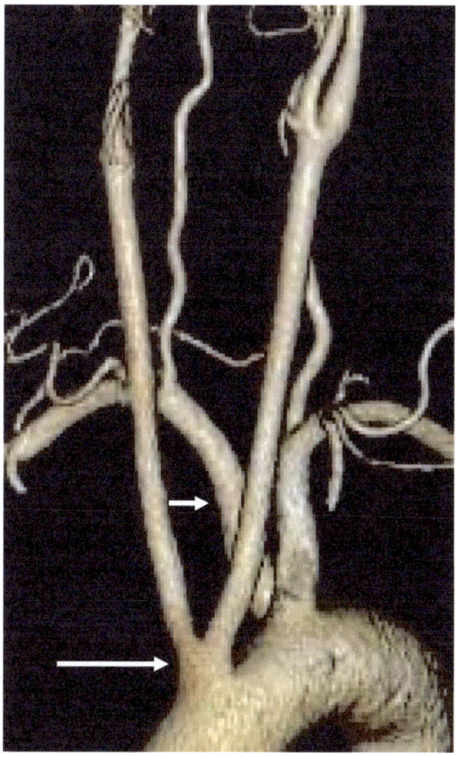

Fig. 1.17 Slightly LAO projection of CT angiography shows an aberrant right SA (*short arrow*). *Long arrow* indicates the bicarotid trunk

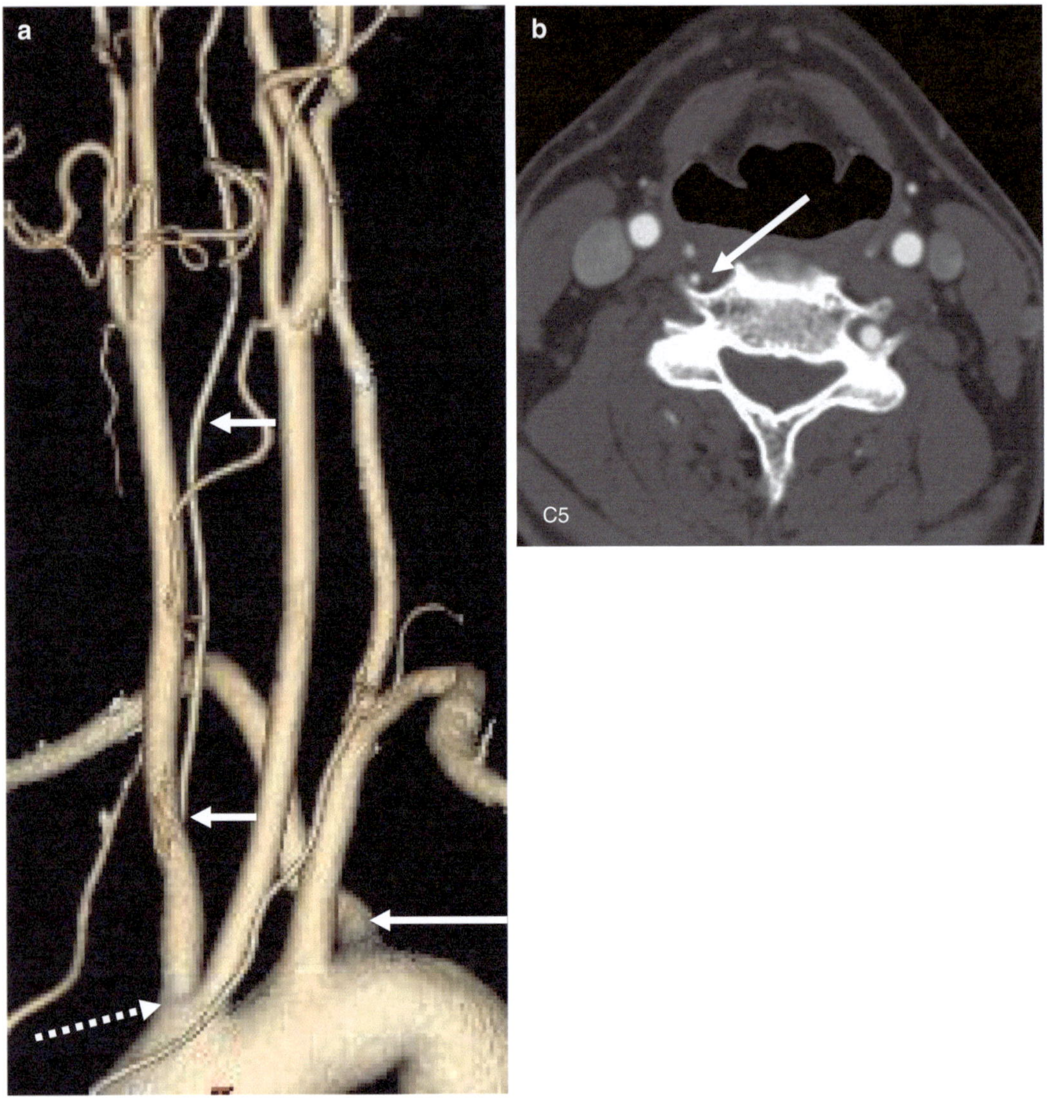

Fig. 1.18 (**a**) LAO projection of CT angiography shows an aberrant right SA (*long arrow*). The right VA arises from the right CCA (*short arrow*). There is also bicarotid trunk (*dotted arrow*). (**b**) CT angiographic source image at the C5 level shows an anteriorly located right VA, not in the TF (*arrow*)

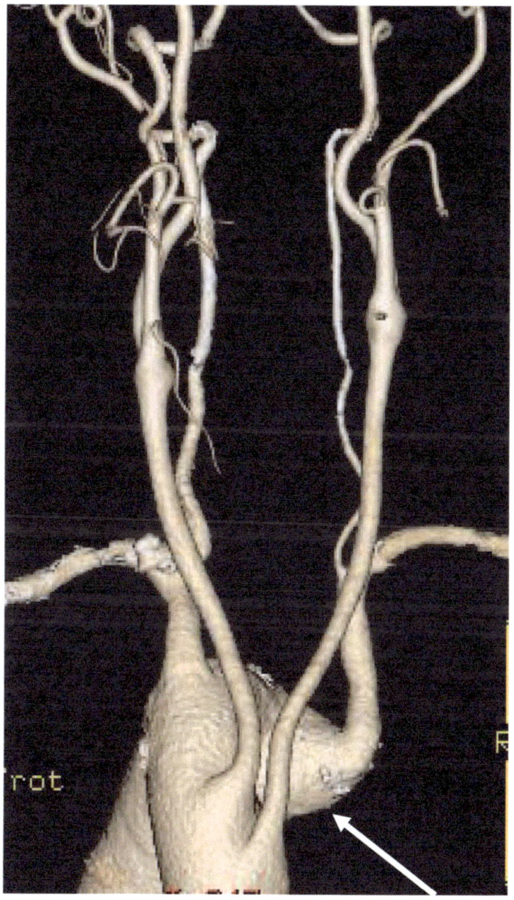

Fig. 1.19 A-P projection of CT angiography shows a right-sided AA. The left SA arises from the AA most distally, indicative of an aberrant left SA, and its origin is markedly dilated, so called Kommerell's diverticulum (*arrow*)

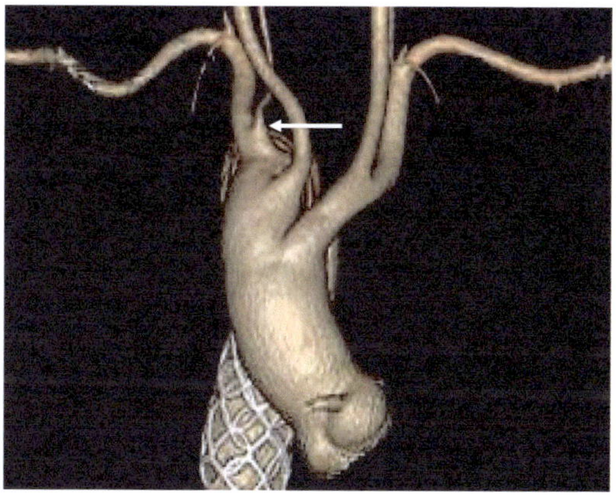

Fig. 1.20 A-P projection of CT angiography shows a right-sided AA with mirror-image branching. The right VA arises from the proximal right SA (*arrow*), otherwise, the branching pattern is normal. A stent-graft was placed in the descending thoracic aorta

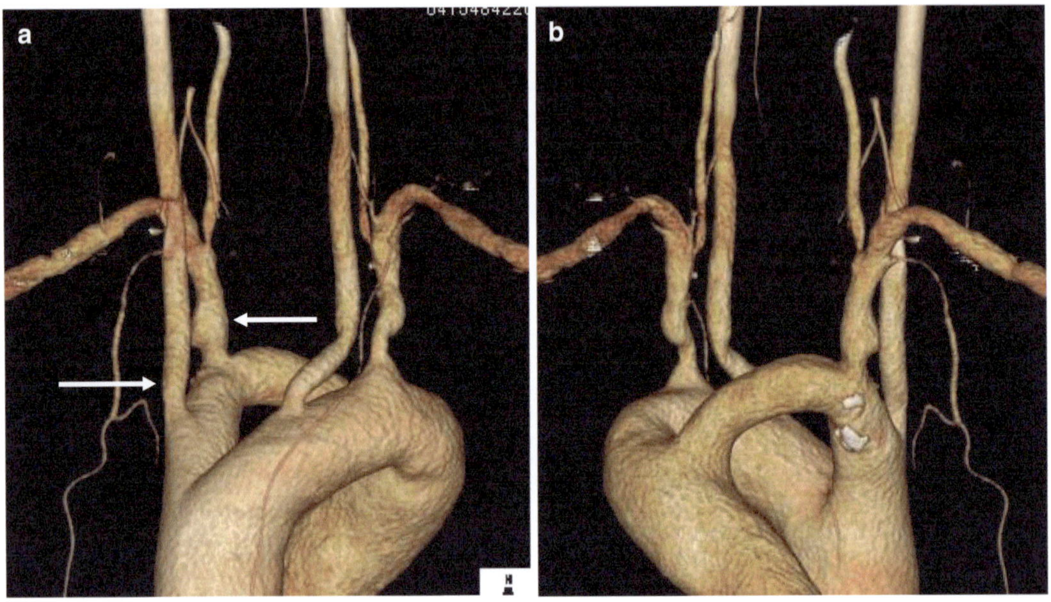

Fig. 1.21 (**a**) Slightly LAO and (**b**) slightly RPO projections of CT angiography show a double AA. The right arch is slightly hypoplastic and located slightly higher than the left arch, but both the right CCA and right SA arise normally (*arrows*)

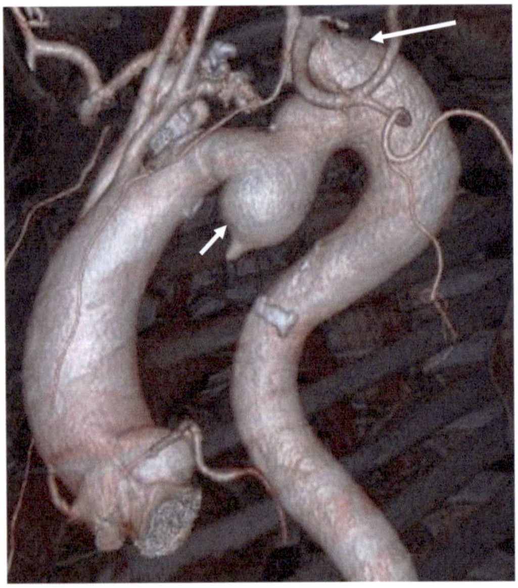

Fig. 1.22 LAO projection of CT angiography shows a left cervical AA with aneurysmal dilatation (*long arrow*). There is also an aneurysm of ductus arteriosus (*short arrow*). (Courtesy of Dr. Tomoki Kaneko)

References

1. Berko NS, Jain VR, Godelman A, Stein EG, Ghosh S, Haramati LB. Variants and anomalies of thoracic vasculature on computed tomographic angiography in adults. J Comput Assist Tomogr. 2009;33:523–8.
2. Uchino A, Saito N, Okada Y, Kozawa E, Nishi N, Mizukoshi W, Nakajima R, Takahashi M, Watanabe Y. Variation of the origin of the left common carotid artery diagnosed by CT angiography. Surg Radiol Anat. 2013;35:339–42.
3. Layton KF, Kallmes DF, Cloft HJ, Lindell EP, Cox VS. Bovine aortic arch variant in humans: clarification of a common misnomer. AJNR Am J Neuroradiol. 2006;27:1541–2.
4. Reinshagen L, Vodiskar J, Mühler E, Hövels-Gürich HH, Vazquez-Jimenez JF. Bicarotid trunk: how much is "not uncommon"? Ann Thorac Surg. 2014;97:945–9.
5. Uchino A. Bilateral brachiocephalic trunks. Surg Radiol Anat. 2018;40:1441–2.
6. Uchino A, Saito N, Takahashi M, Okada Y, Kozawa E, Nishi N, Mizukoshi W, Nakajima R, Watanabe Y. Variations in the origin of the vertebral artery and its level of entry into the transverse foramen

diagnosed by CT angiography. Neuroradiology. 2013;55:585–94.
7. Jakanani GC, Adair W. Frequency of variations in aortic arch anatomy depicted on multidetector CT. Clin Radiol. 2010;65:481–7.
8. Müller M, Schmitz BL, Pauls S, Schick M, Röhrer S, Kapapa T, Schlötzer W. Variations of the aortic arch – a study on the most common branching patterns. Acta Radiol. 2011;52:738–42.
9. Satti SR, Cerniglia CA, Koenigsberg RA. Cervical vertebral artery variations: an anatomic study. AJNR Am J Neuroradiol. 2007;28:976–80.
10. Nogueira TE, Chambers AA, Brueggemeyer MT, Miller TJ. Dual origin of the vertebral artery mimicking dissection. AJNR Am J Neuroradiol. 1997;18:382–4.
11. Goray VB, Joshi AR, Garg A, Merchant S, Yadav B, Maheshwari P. Aortic arch variation: a unique case with anomalous origin of both vertebral arteries as additional branches of the aortic arch distal to left subclavian artery. AJNR Am J Neuroradiol. 2005;26:93–5.
12. Yamashiro S, Kuniyoshi Y, Arakaki K, Inafuku H, Morishima Y, Kise Y. Total arch replacement with associated anomaly of the left vertebral artery. Ann Thorac Cardiovasc Surg. 2010;16:216–9.
13. Uchino A, Kurita H. Duplicate origin of the right vertebral artery in which both channels arose from the extreme proximal right subclavian artery: a case report. Surg Radiol Anat. 2017;39:811–4.
14. Karcaaltincaba M, Haliloglu M, Ozkan E, Kocak M, Akinci D, Ariyurek M. Non-invasive imaging of aberrant right subclavian artery pathologies and aberrant right vertebral artery. Br J Radiol. 2009;82:73–8.
15. Lacout A, Khalil A, Figl A, Liloku R, Marcy PY. Vertebral arteria lusoria: a life-threatening condition for oesophageal surgery. Surg Radiol Anat. 2012;34:381–3.
16. Lemke AJ, Benndorf G, Liebig T, Felix R. Anomalous origin of the right vertebral artery: review of the literature and case report of right vertebral artery origin distal to the left subclavian artery. AJNR Am J Neuroradiol. 1999;20:1318–21.
17. Freed K, Low VH. The aberrant subclavian artery. AJR Am J Roentgenol. 1997;168:481–4.
18. Janssen M, Baggen MG, Veen HF, Smout AJ, Bekkers JA, Jonkman JG, Ouwendijk RJ. Dysphagia lusoria: clinical aspects, manometric findings, diagnosis, and therapy. Am J Gastroenterol. 2000;95:1411–6.
19. Cina CS, Althani H, Pasenau J, Abouzahr L. Kommerell's diverticulum and right-sided aortic arch: a cohort study and review of the literature. J Vasc Surg. 2004;39:131–9.
20. Hayashi T, Ichikawa T, Yamamuro H, Ono S, Kobayashi M, Nomura T, Hashida K, Yashiro H, Okochi T, Koizumi J, Shimura S, Hasebe T, Imai Y. Right aortic arch with mirror-image branching in adults: evaluation using CT. Tokai J Exp Clin Med. 2018;43:30–7.
21. Kaldararova M, Simkova I, Varga I, Tittel P, Kardos M, Ondriska M, Vrsanska V, Masura J. Double aortic arch anomalies in children: a systematic 20-year single center study. Clin Anat. 2017;30:929–39.
22. Zhong Y-L, Ma W-G, Zhu J-M, Qiao Z-Y, Zheng J, Liu Y-M, Sun L-Z. Surgical repair of cervical aortic arch: an alternative classification scheme based on experience in 35 patients. J Thorac Cardiovasc Surg. 2020;159:2202–13.
23. Gomibuchi T, Seto T, Yamamoto T, Nakahara K, Ohashi N, Ohtsu Y, Wada Y, Fukui D, Okada K. Surgical repair of cervical aortic arch with brain circulation anomalu through clamshell incision. Ann Thorac Surg. 2017;104:e235–7.

2 Variations of the Common Carotid Artery (CCA) and Carotid Bifurcation

Abstract

This chapter includes (1) Absent left common carotid artery (Separate origin of the left internal and external carotid arteries from the aortic arch), (2) Absent right common carotid artery (Separate origin of the right internal and external carotid arteries from the brachiocephalic trunk), (3) Low carotid bifurcation, (4) High carotid bifurcation, (5) Non-bifurcating cervical carotid artery, and (6) External carotid-internal carotid artery anastomosis at the mid-cervical segment. There are 9 figures and 3 illustrations.

Because these variations are dangerous during anterior neck surgery, it is important to make a correct diagnosis before surgery.

Keywords

Carotid bifurcation · Common carotid artery · External carotid artery · Internal carotid artery

2.1 Absent Left CCA (Separate Origin of the Left Internal and External Carotid Arteries from the AA)

Extremely rarely, the left ICA and ECA arise separately from the AA, resulting in absent left CCA [1]. Usually, the left ECA arises first, and the ICA follows (Fig. 2.1).

The fourth brachial arch forms the AA (left) and BCT (right). The third brachial arch forms the carotid sinus and proximal portion of the ICA. The ductus caroticus is the part of the dorsal aorta between the third and fourth brachial arches. The ventral pharyngeal artery is a primitive ECA that arises directly from the aortic sac. Normally, the ductus caroticus regresses. When the third brachial arch regresses instead of the ductus caroticus, absent CCA is formed (Fig. 2.2) [2].

2.2 Absent Right CCA (Separate Origin of the Right Internal and External Carotid Arteries from the BCT)

Extremely rarely, the right ICA and ECA arise separately from the BCT, resulting in absent right CCA [3]. The same as on the left side, the right ECA arises first, and right ICA follows (Fig. 2.3). Reported arch variations associated with this variation include right (Sect. 1.5.1), double (Sect. 1.5.3), and cervical (Sect. 1.5.4) AA [2]. Aberrant right SA (Sect. 1.4.1) can also be associated with this variation [2].

2.3 Low Carotid Bifurcation

The CCA usually bifurcates at the level of the C4 vertebral body. However, there is a wide range in

A. Uchino, *Atlas of the Supraaortic Craniocervical Arterial Variations*, https://doi.org/10.1007/978-981-16-6803-6_2

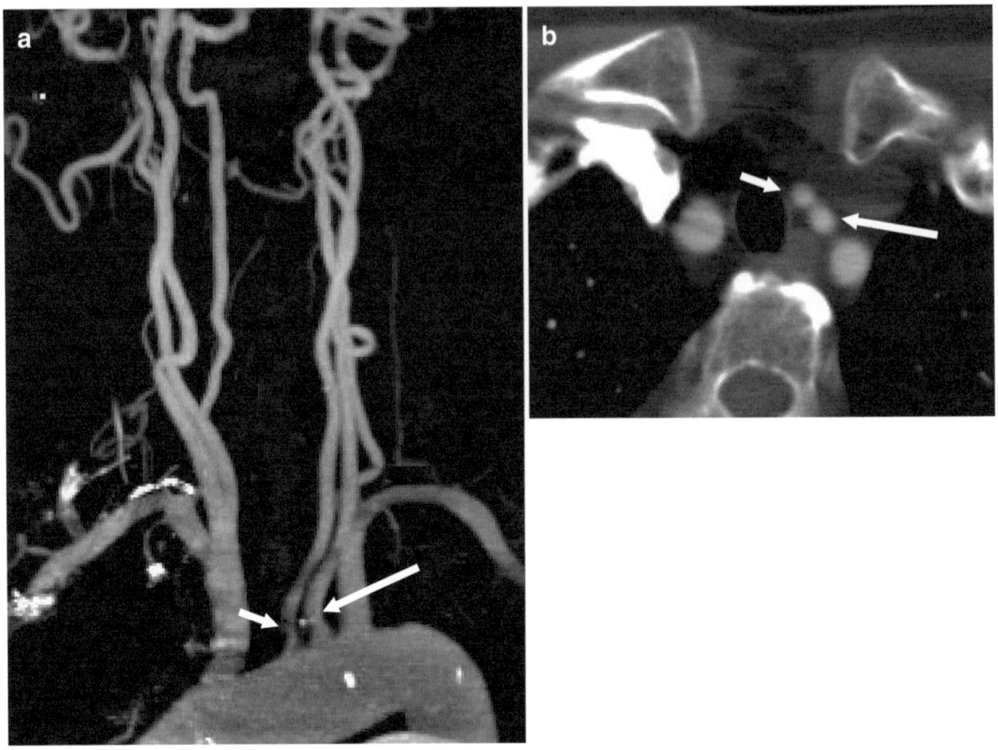

Fig. 2.1 (**a**) LAO projection MIP image of CT angiography shows the separate origin of the left ICA (*long arrow*) and left ECA (*short arrow*), indicative of an absent left CCA. Low right carotid bifurcation (2.3) is also observed. (**b**) CT angiographic source image just above the level of the AA shows two arteries. The smaller and anteriorly located artery is the ECA (*short arrow*) and the other is the ICA (*long arrow*). (Courtesy of Dr. Kiyotaka Liu)

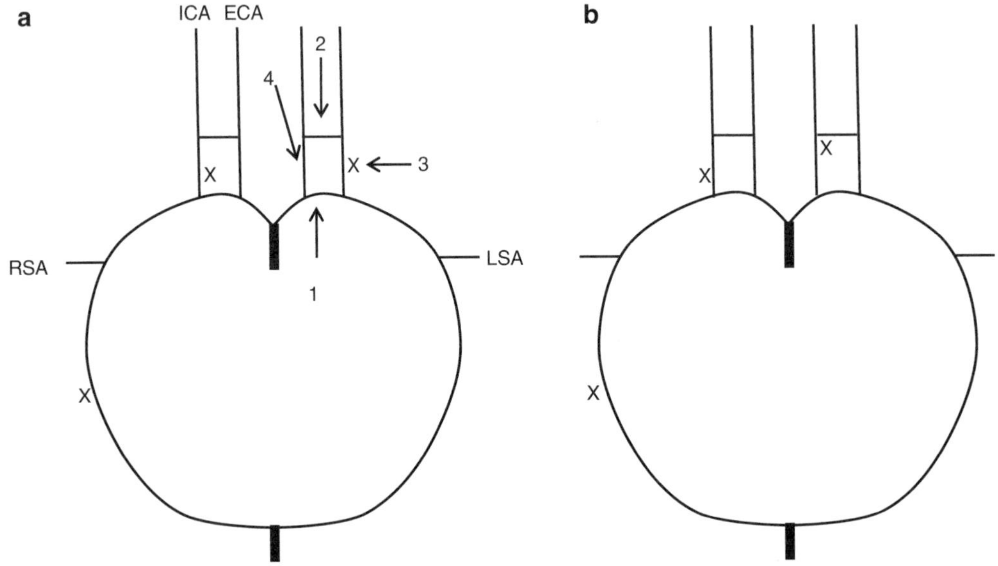

Fig. 2.2 Schematic illustration of the double aortic arch model. (Modified from [2]). 1: Fourth brachial arch, 2: Third brachial arch, 3: Ductus caroticus, 4: Ventral pharyngeal artery. ECA: external carotid artery, ICA: internal carotid artery, RSA: right subclavian artery, LSA: left subclavian artery. X is a primitive artery, which regresses. Normally, 3 regresses (**a**). When 2 regresses instead of 3, absent CCA is formed (**b**)

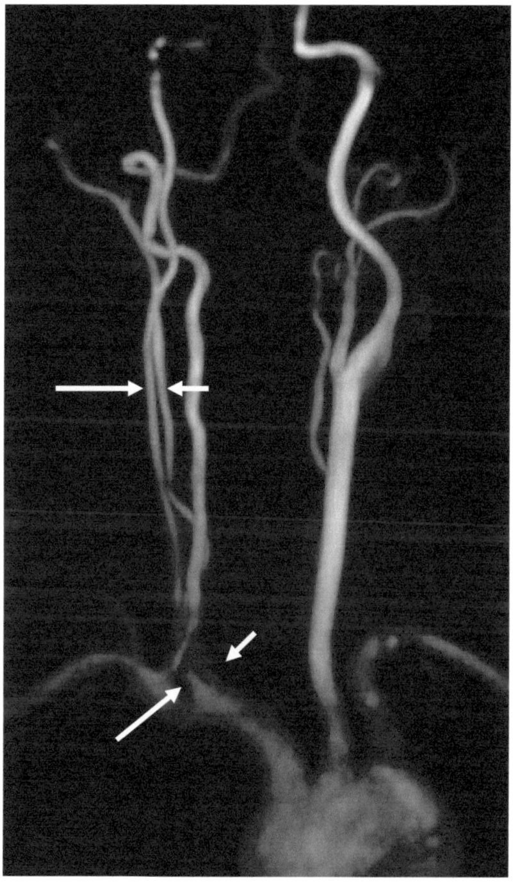

Fig. 2.3 A-P projection of MR angiography shows the separate origin of the right ICA (*long arrows*) and ECA (*short arrows*), indicative of an absent right CCA. (Courtesy of Dr. Takashi Yamamoto)

the level of bifurcation. In the case of the low carotid bifurcation, the ECA has a long main trunk (Fig. 2.4). In the case of anterior neck surgery, this variation should be recognized before the procedure [4].

2.4 High Carotid Bifurcation

As mentioned above (Sect. 2.3), the CCA usually bifurcates at the level of the C4 vertebral body. However, there is a wide range in the bifurcation level. In the case of high carotid bifurcation, the ECA has a short main trunk (Fig. 2.5). For the treatment of stenosis of ICA origin, carotid endarterectomy is usually difficult and dangerous for patients with high carotid bifurcation [5]. This variation should not be confused with a non-bifurcating cervical carotid artery, which is described in the next section (Sect. 2.5).

2.5 Non-bifurcating Cervical Carotid Artery

Rarely, the major branches of the proximal ECA, such as the lingual artery, facial artery, or their common trunk, the distal trunk of the ECA, and the occipital artery, arise separately from the terminal segment of the CCA, resulting in the ECA having no proximal main trunk (Fig. 2.6) [6]. This variation is called a non-bifurcating cervical carotid artery and may be caused by segmental agenesis of the most proximal ICA, not the ECA (Fig. 2.7). Because the affected artery does not show physiological dilatation or mild curvature of the origin of the ICA. Its prevalence on MR angiography was reported to be 0.21% [7]. The non-bifurcating cervical carotid artery shows no significant lateral predominance, and it can be seen bilaterally (Fig. 2.8). This rare variation should not be confused with high carotid bifurcation, which is described above (Sect. 2.4). A correct diagnosis is necessary to avoid complications, such as embolic cerebral infarctions, during interventional radiologic procedures [8, 9], or head and neck surgeries.

2.6 External Carotid-Internal Carotid Artery Anastomosis at the Mid-cervical Segment

Extremely rarely, a hypoplastic proximal ICA and hyperplastic proximal main trunk of the ECA anastomose at the mid-cervical segment of the ICA and form a large arterial ring (Figs. 2.9 and 2.10). This is not exactly fenestration, because the two channels are two different arteries; thus, this variation is congenital EC-ICA anastomosis [10]. It seems to be a variant of the non-bifurcating cervical carotid artery (Sect. 2.5) [7]. A case in which these two variations were combined was reported (Fig. 2.11) [11]. The arterial ring repre-

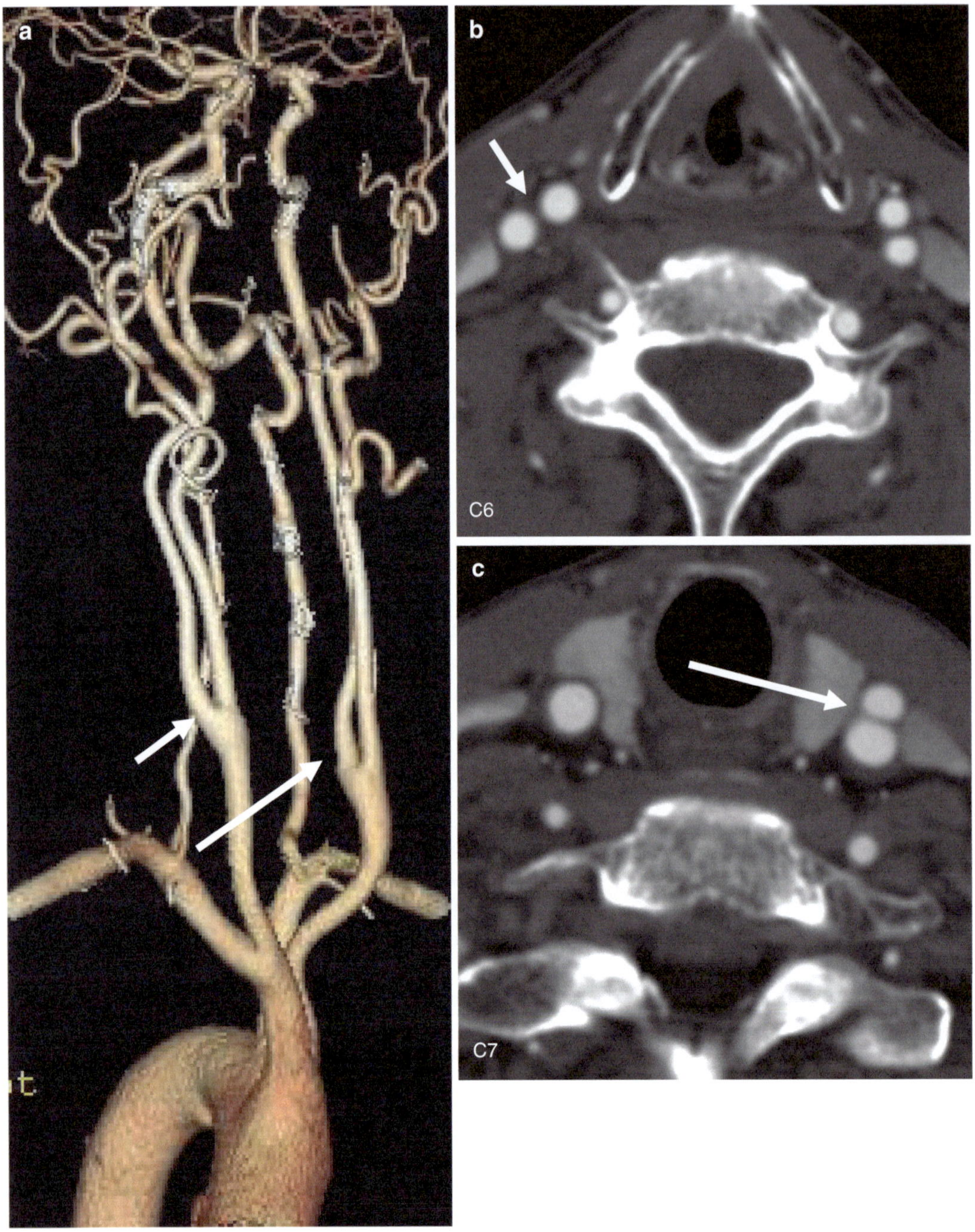

Fig. 2.4 (**a**) RAO projection of CT angiography shows low carotid bifurcation, bilaterally. The left carotid bifurcation (*long arrow*) is lower than the right (*short arrow*). (**b**) CT angiographic source image at the level of the C7 shows that the left CCA has already bifurcated (*arrow*). (**c**) CT angiographic source image at the level of the C6 shows that the right CCA has also bifurcated (*arrow*)

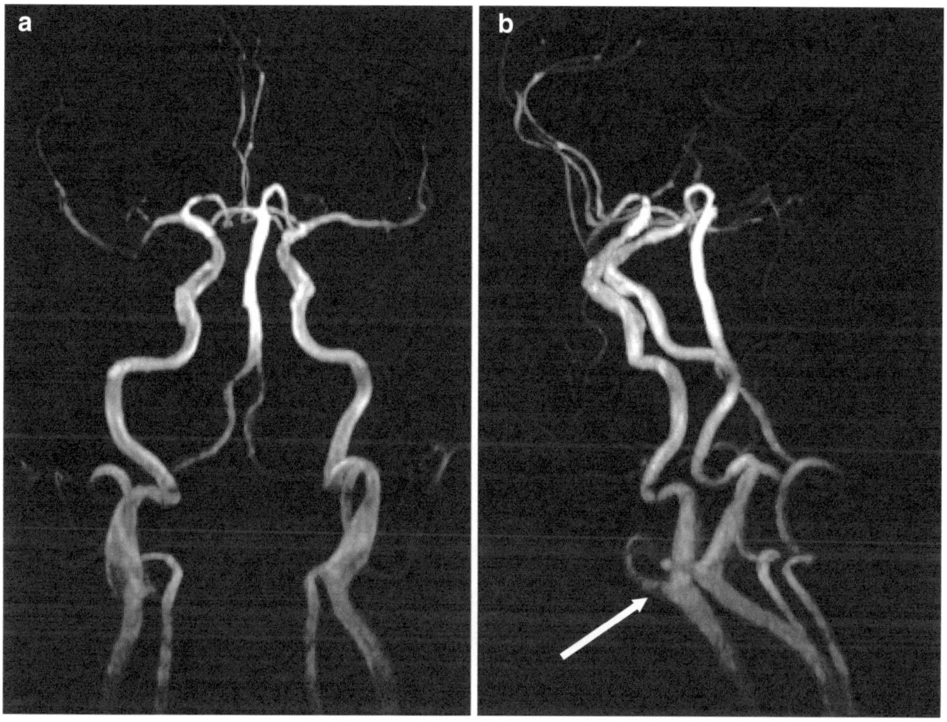

Fig. 2.5 (**a**) A-P and (**b**) lateral projections of MR angiography show bilateral high carotid bifurcations, located at the level of the C2/3 intervertebral space. The main trunks of the ECAs are short (*arrow*)

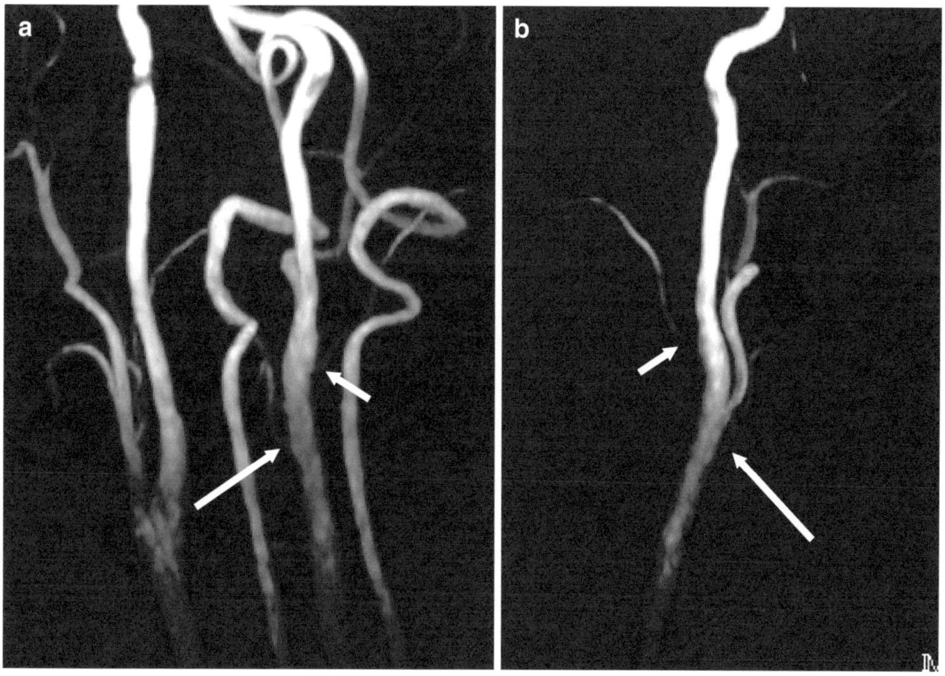

Fig. 2.6 (**a**) LAO projection of MR angiography and (**b**) partial MIP right lateral image show a left non-bifurcating cervical carotid artery. The branching order is lingual artery (*long arrows*), facial artery, distal trunk of the ECA, and finally occipital artery (*short arrows*)

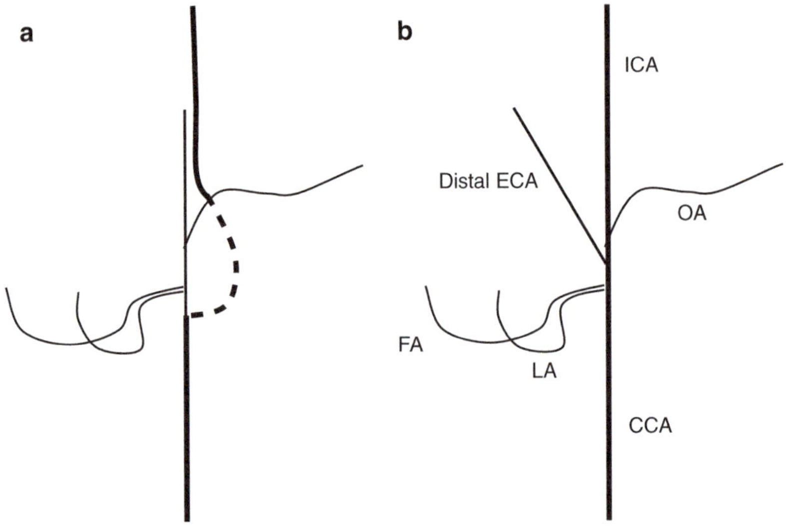

Fig. 2.7 Schematic illustration of a non-bifurcating cervical carotid artery in lateral projection. (Modified from [7]). (**a**) Agenesis of the most proximal ICA. (**b**) Final configuration of this variation. *CCA* common carotid artery, *ECA* external carotid artery, *FA* facial artery, *ICA* internal carotid artery, *LA* lingual artery, *OA* occipital artery

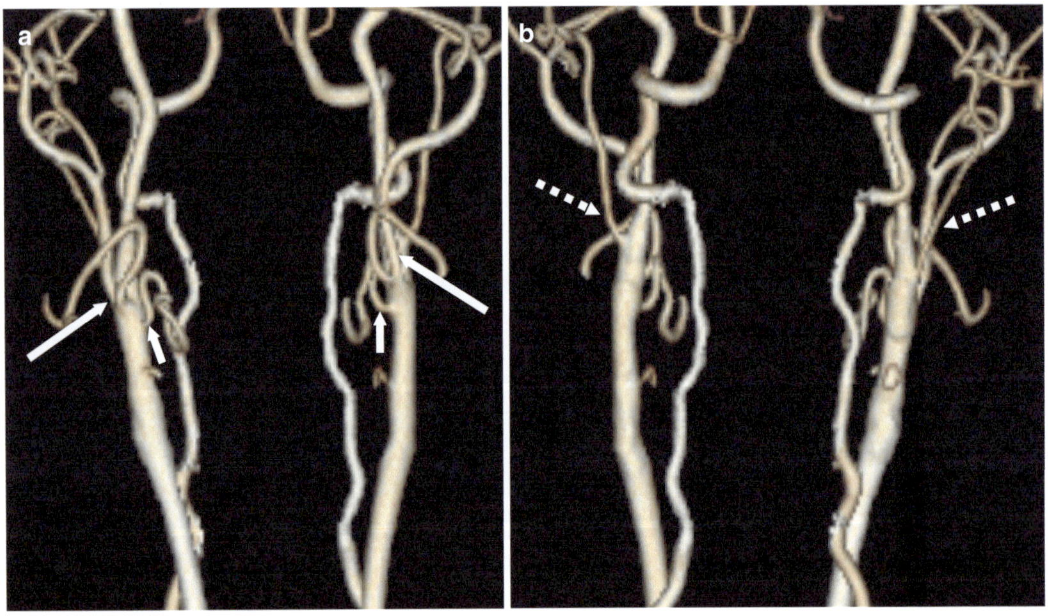

Fig. 2.8 (**a**) A-P and (**b**) P-A projections of CT angiography show bilateral non-bifurcating cervical carotid arteries. The lingual artery (*short arrows*), common origin of the facial artery-distal ECA trunk (*long arrows*), and occipital artery (*dotted arrows*) arise separately. Neither physiological dilatation nor mild curvature is observed at the origins of the ICAs

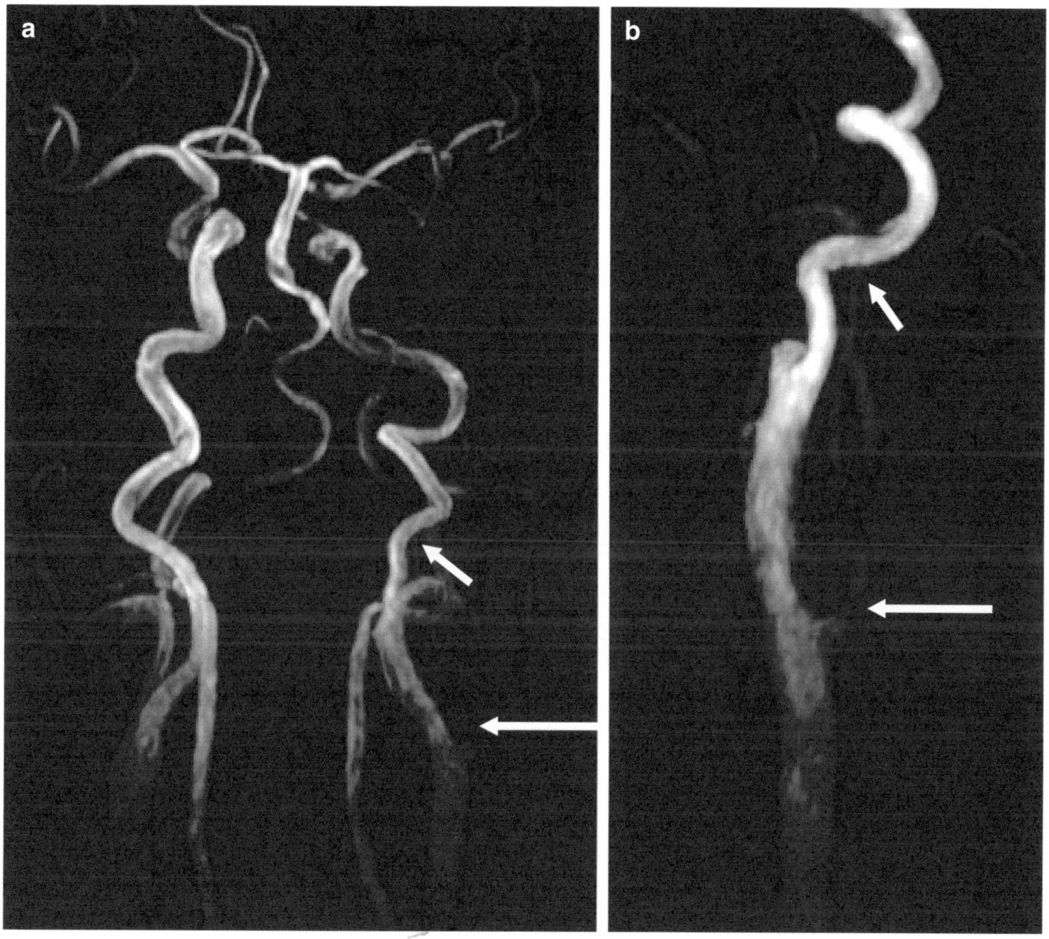

Fig. 2.9 (**a**) Slightly LAO projection of MR angiography and (**b**) right lateral projection of a partial MIP image show a hypoplastic proximal left ICA (*long arrows*) and hyperplastic left ECA. They fuse at the mid-cervical segment of the ICA (*short arrows*), indicative of an EC-ICA anastomosis

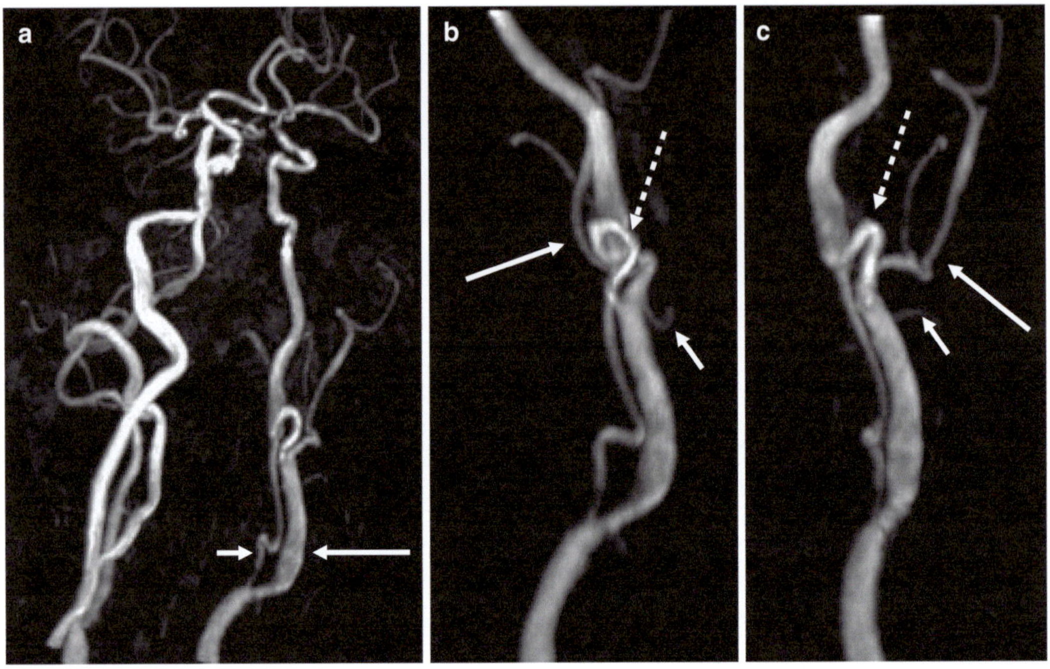

Fig. 2.10 (**a**) RAO projection of MR angiography shows a hyperplastic left ECA (*long arrow*) and a hypoplastic left ICA (*short arrow*). (**b**, **c**) Partial MIP RAO and A-P projections show a large arterial ring at the proximal cervical segment of the ICA, indicative of an EC-ICA anastomosis. *Long arrows* indicate the distal segment of the ECA, *short arrows* indicate the lingual artery, and *dotted arrows* indicate the anastomotic vessel

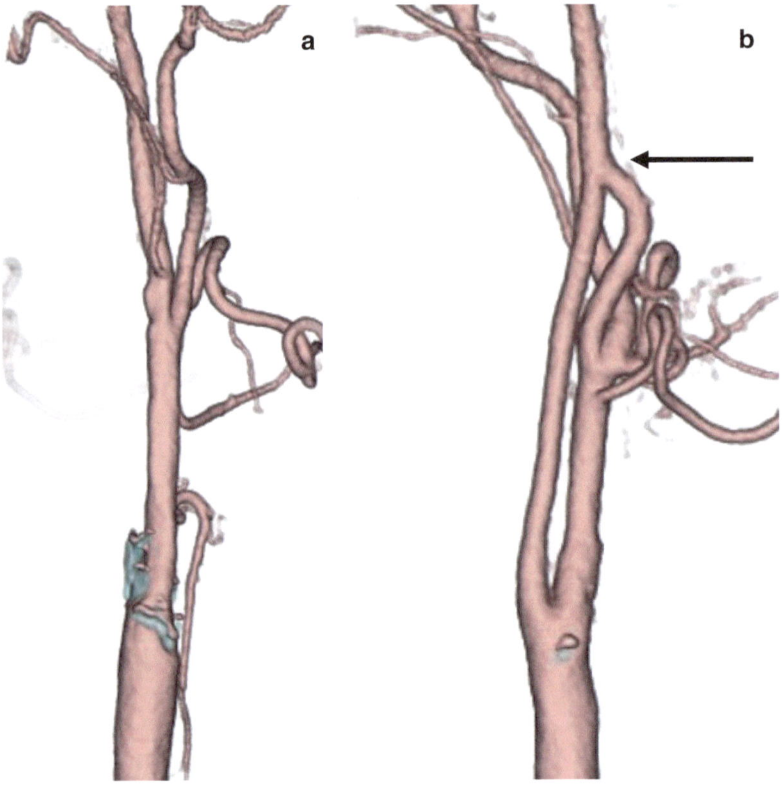

Fig. 2.11 (**a**) RAO projection of CT angiography of the right carotid system shows a non-bifurcating cervical carotid artery. (**b**) Right lateral projection of CT angiography of the left carotid system shows an EC-ICA anastomosis (*arrow*)

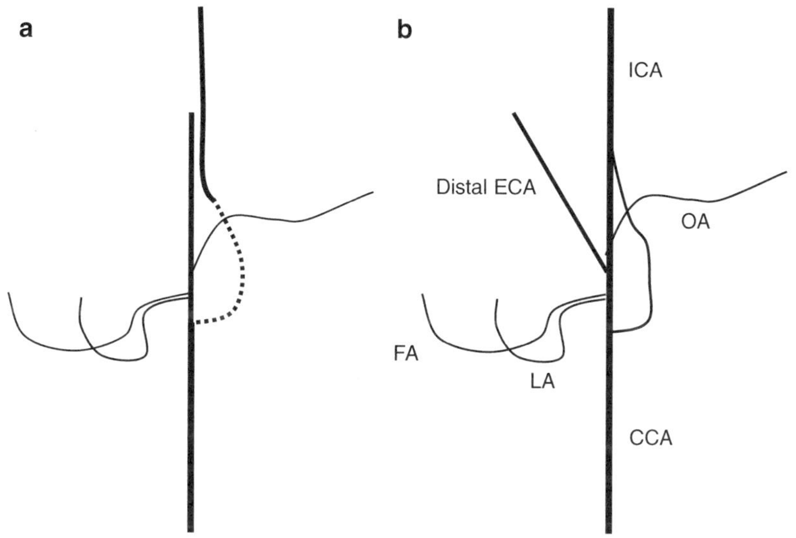

Fig. 2.12 Schematic illustration of EC-ICA anastomosis in lateral projection. (Modified from [10]), (**a**) Hypoplasia of the most proximal ICA; (**b**) Final configuration of this variation. If the hypoplastic proximal ICA is occluded, the variation transforms to the non-bifurcating cervical carotid artery (Fig. 2.8b). *CCA* common carotid artery, *ECA* external carotid artery, *FA* facial artery, *ICA* internal carotid artery, *LA* lingual artery, *OA* occipital artery

sents an incomplete form or preceding stage of a variant, non-bifurcating cervical carotid artery, before the small rudimentary channel of the primary ICA regresses. If the hypoplastic proximal ICA is occluded before or after birth, it forms a non-bifurcating cervical carotid artery (Fig. 2.12).

References

1. Cakirer S, Karaarslan E, Kayabali M, Rozanes I. Separate origins of the left internal and external carotid arteries from the aortic arch: MR angiographic findings. AJNR Am J Neuroradiol. 2002;23:1600–2.
2. Uchino A, Uwabe K, Osawa I. Absent right common carotid artery associated with aberrant right subclavian artery. Neuroradiol J. 2018;31:305–8.
3. Berczi V, Bottomley JR, Gopalan D, Griffiths PD, Gaines PA, Cleveland TJ. Absent right common carotid artery with stenting of symptomatic internal carotid artery stenosis. J Vasc Surg. 2014;59:1418–21.
4. Gulsen S, Caner H, Altinors N. An anatomical variant: low-lying bifurcation of the common carotid artery, and its surgical implications in anterior cervical discectomy. J Korean Neurosurg Soc. 2009;45:32–4.
5. Farhat-Sabet A, Aicher BO, Tolaymat B, Coca-Soliz V, Nagarsheth KH, Ucuzian AA, Lubek JE, Toursavadkohi S. An alternative approach to carotid endarterectomy in the high catotid bifurcation. Ann Vasc Surg. 2020;65:240–6.
6. Morimoto T, Nitta K, Kazekawa K, Hashizume K. The anomaly of a non-bifurcating cervical carotid artery. Case report. J Neurosurg. 1990;72:130–2.
7. Uchino A, Saito N, Watadani T, Mizukoshi W, Nakajima R. Nonbifurcating cervical carotid artery diagnosed by MR angiography. AJNR Am J Neuroradiol. 2011;32:1119–22.
8. Murono S, Nakanishi Y, Minami T, Matsui O, Furukawa M, Yoshizaki T. Case report. Intra-arterial chemotherapy for laryngeal cancer via a non-bifurcating carotid artery. Br J Radiol. 2009;82:e197–9.
9. Kiyosue H, Mori H, Tanoue S, Sagara Y, Hori Y, Miyamoto S, Abe T, Komiyama M. Non-bifurcating carotid artery coexisting with transverse sinus dural arteriovenous fistula. Neuroradiology. 2009;51:697–8.
10. Uchino A, Saito N, Watadani T. Congenital external carotid-internal carotid artery anastomosis diagnosed by MR angiography. J Neuroimaging. 2013;23:96–7.
11. Nakai K, Kaji T, Uchino A, Kawauchi T, Tamura C, Otani N, Nawashiro H. Congenital external carotid-internal carotid artery anastomosis associated with contralateral non-bifurcating cervical carotid artery. Neuroradiology. 2012;54:521–3.

3 Variations of the Internal Carotid Artery (ICA)

Abstract

This chapter includes (1) The retropharyngeal course of the ICA, Kissing carotid, (2) Coiling (Tonsillar loop) of the cervical ICA, (3) Aberrant course of the petrous segment of the ICA (4) Duplication of the ICA, (5) Six types of agenesis and hypoplasia of the ICA, (6) ICA fenestration, and (7) Dolichoectasia of the distal ICA. There are 26 figures and 1 illustration.

Recognition of these arterial variations before surgery of the retropharyngeal space, middle ear, the pituitary gland is important for the prevention of bleeding complications during surgery.

Keywords

Aberrant course · Agenesis · Fenestration · Internal carotid artery · Retropharyngeal course

3.1 Retropharyngeal Course of the ICA, Kissing Carotids

The origin of the ICA has a physiological dilatation and mild curve. The proximal ICA is usually directed dorsolaterally. However, the ICA arises medially in approximately 10% of patients. Some ICAs with a medial course reach the midline retropharyngeal space. In the case of the bilateral type of this variation, the arteries touch each other, and this condition is called kissing carotids (Fig. 3.1). Because this variation mimics a retropharyngeal submucosal tumor, a needle biopsy is contraindicated [1]. Atherosclerotic elongation of the cervical ICA may partly contribute to this variation.

Kissing carotids are also found in the sellar region [2]. Bilateral cavernous segments of the ICAs deviate medially and touch each other (Fig. 3.2). This variation is important because it may cause pituitary disease and is also dangerous during trans-sphenoidal pituitary surgery. Atherosclerotic elongation of the cavernous ICA may partly contribute to this variation.

3.2 Coiling (Tonsillar Loop) of the Cervical ICA

The extremely tortuous cervical ICA is referred to as coiling [3] or tonsillar loop [4] (Fig. 3.3). This redundancy is a significant risk factor for ICA dissection [5]. This variation is believed to result from anomalous embryological development of the third aortic arch and the dorsal aorta. In addition, atherosclerotic elongation of the cervical ICA may partly contribute to this variation.

A. Uchino, *Atlas of the Supraaortic Craniocervical Arterial Variations*,
https://doi.org/10.1007/978-981-16-6803-6_3

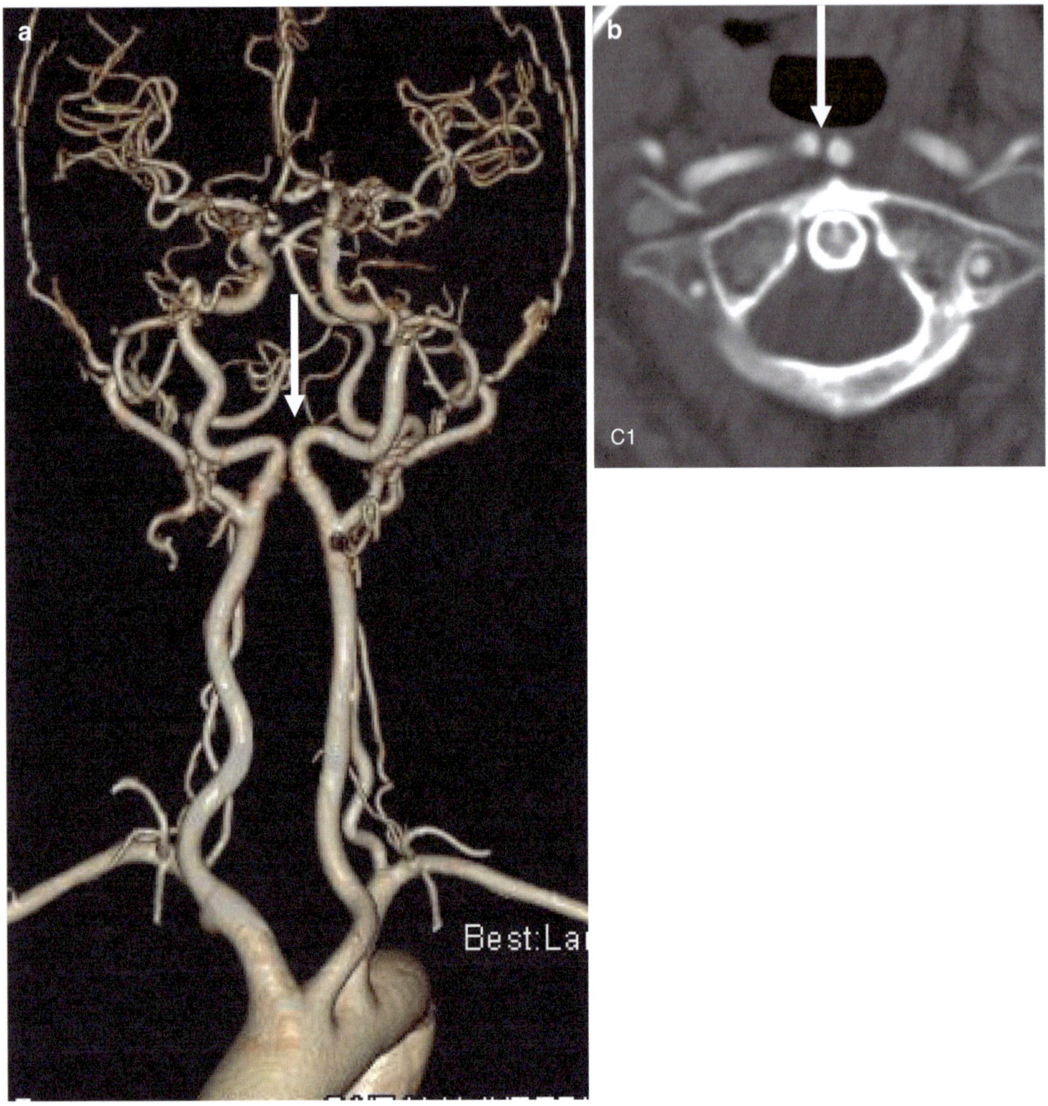

Fig. 3.1 (**a**) A-P projection of CT angiography shows the bilateral retropharyngeal course of the ICAs (*arrow*). This patient also has a common origin of the left CCA with BCT (Sect. 1.1.2) and bilateral high carotid bifurcations (Sect. 2.4). (**b**) CT angiographic source image obtained at the level of C1 shows the kissing point at the retropharyngeal space, indicative of kissing carotids (*arrow*)

3.3 Aberrant Course of the Petrous Segment of the ICA

The petrous segment of the ICA rarely takes an abnormally lateral course and makes a hairpin turn. The most lateral portion is in the middle ear cavity (Fig. 3.4). Thus, this variation is dangerous during middle ear surgery. In this variation, there is right-side and female predominance [6]. It is caused by segmental agenesis of the petrous ICA and collateral circulation via the inferior tympanic artery and caroticotympanic artery [7]. Thus, the absence of the vertical segment of the petrous ICA is seen. This variation may be associated with a persistent stapedial artery, which is described in the next chapter (Sect. 4.3) [8, 9].

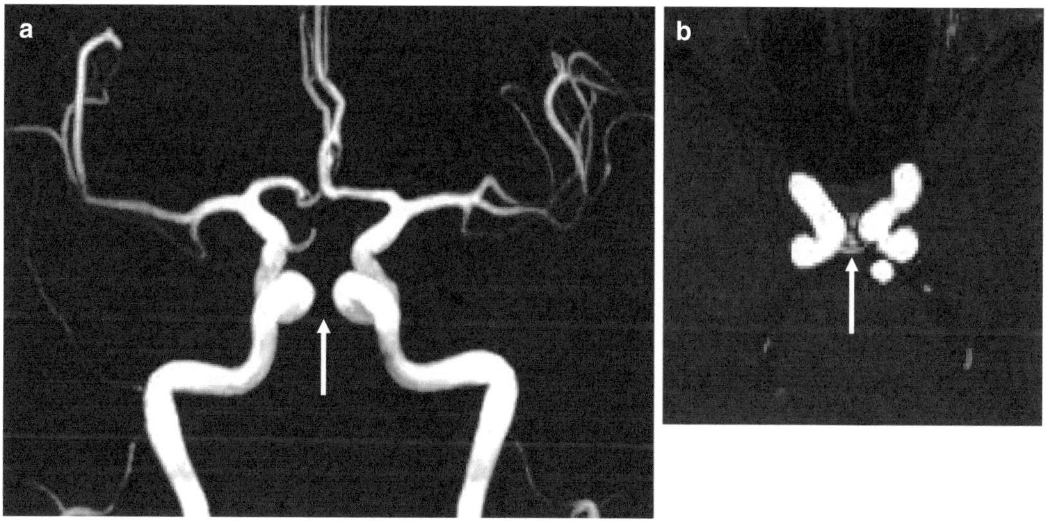

Fig. 3.2 (**a**) A-P projection of partial MIP MR angiography (the vertebrobasilar system was deleted) shows kissing carotids at the cavernous segments (*arrow*). (**b**) MR angiographic source image at the sellar region shows the compressed pituitary gland (*arrow*)

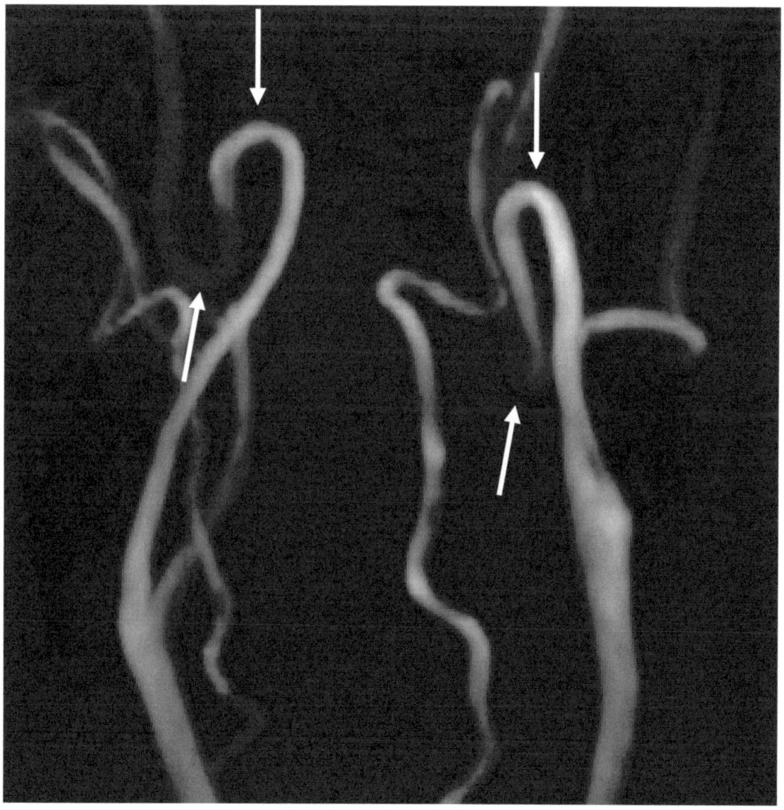

Fig. 3.3 Slightly RAO projection of MR angiography shows extremely tortuous bilateral cervical ICAs (*arrows*). This variation is referred to as coiling or tonsillar loop of the cervical ICA

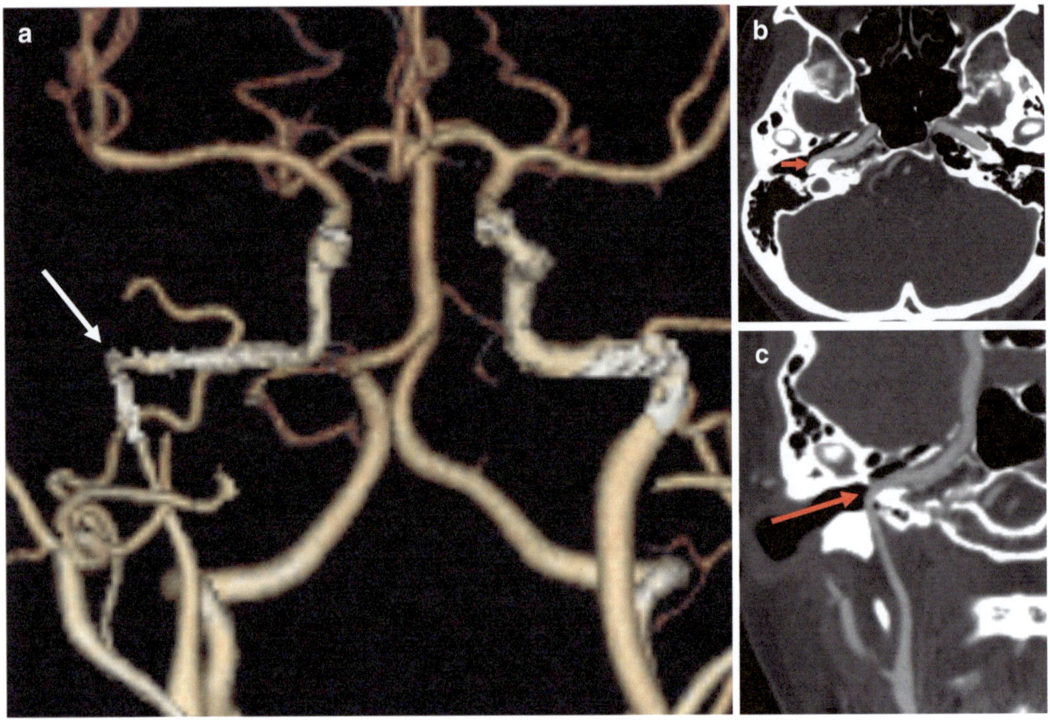

Fig. 3.4 (**a**) A-P projection of CT angiography shows a slightly hypoplastic and abnormally lateral course of the cervical and petrous segments of the right ICA. There is a hairpin turn (*arrow*). (**b**) CT angiographic source image and (**c**) curved reformatted image show the artery passing in the middle ear cavity (*arrow*), indicative of an aberrant course of the petrous segment of the ICA

3.4 Duplication of the ICA

Extremely rarely, the aberrant course of the petrous ICA (Sect. 3.3) can be seen to be associated with the normal course of the ICA, forming a large arterial ring from the cervical segment to the vertical petrous segment of the ICA (Fig. 3.5). This variation is called duplication of the ICA [10], and it can be seen bilaterally [11].

3.5 Agenesis and Hypoplasia of the ICA

3.5.1 ICA Agenesis with Collateral Blood Supply Via the Posterior Communicating Artery (PCoA) (Lie's Type A)

Agenesis of the ICA occurs due to abnormal regression of the first and third aortic arch; the exact etiology is unclear [12]. Lie [13] classified congenital agenesis and hypoplasia of the ICA into 6 types (Fig. 3.6). Type A is the most common but is rare. The MCA is mainly supplied by the PCoA (Fig. 3.7). Its prevalence was considered to be approximately 0.01% in the general population [14]. The prevalence of either the absence of the ICA or hypoplasia of the ICA was also reported to be 0.13% [12]; however, the true prevalence is unclear. Usually, patients with ICA agenesis are asymptomatic due to well-developed collateral circulation; however, an aneurysm is frequently found, probably due to hemodynamic stress (Fig. 3.8). Dilatation and elongation of the vertebrobasilar system may cause neurovascular compression syndrome [14]. Associated variations of the contralateral ICA can rarely be seen (Fig. 3.9).

The absence of the carotid canal is an important finding for the diagnosis of ICA agenesis. Thus, skull base CT is useful for differentiation between congenital ICA agenesis and acquired ICA occlusion.

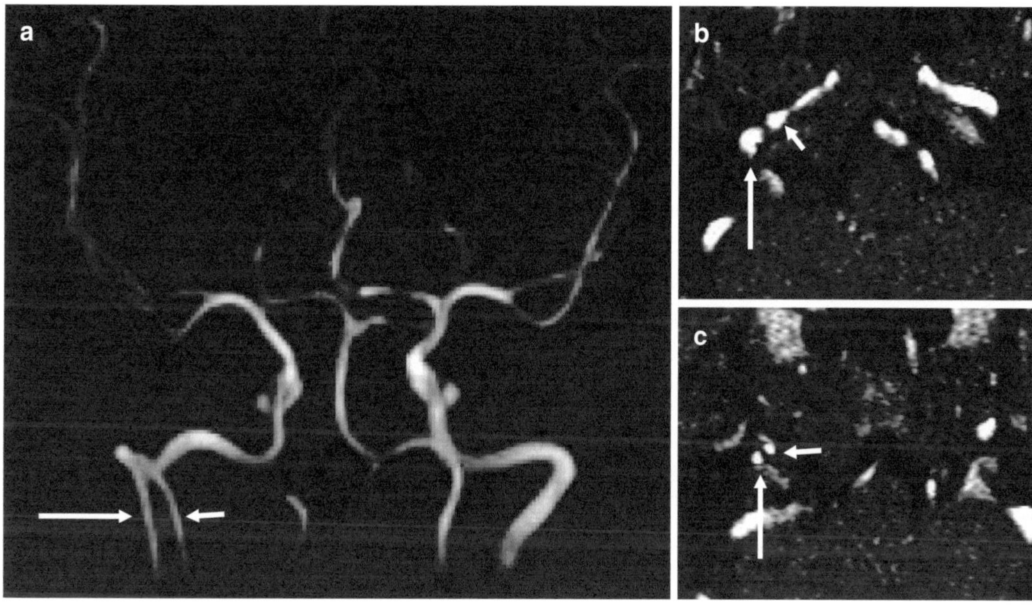

Fig. 3.5 (**a**) A-P projection of MR angiography shows two channels from the cervical segment to the vertical petrous segment of the right ICA, indicative of a duplication of the ICA. The *long arrow* indicates the aberrant course of the ICA and the *short arrow* indicates the normal course of the ICA. (**b**, **c**) MR angiographic source images show that the laterally located artery passes the middle ear cavity (*long arrows*). The *short arrow* indicates the normal course of the ICA. (Courtesy of Drs. Toshiyuki Ohuchida and Yaeko Kanamiya)

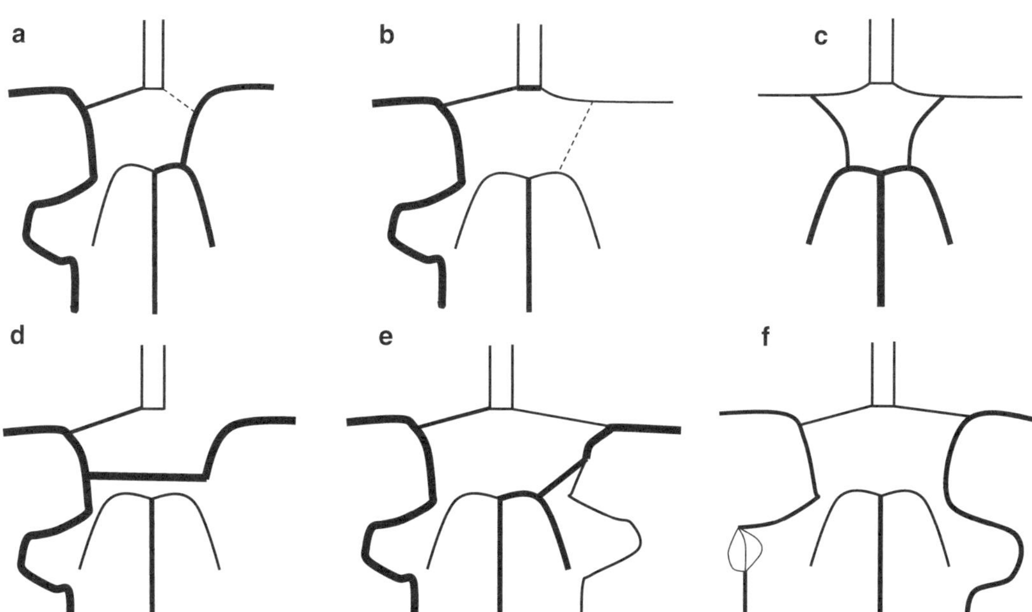

Fig. 3.6 Schematic illustration of Lie's classification of the ICA agenesis. (Modified from [15]). (**a**) Type A: collateral via the PCoA. (**b**) Type B: collateral via the ACoA. (**c**) Type C: bilateral agenesis. (**d**) Type D: intercavernous anastomosis. (**e**) Type E: hypoplasia. (**f**) Type F: rete mirabile (collaterals from ECA with network formation)

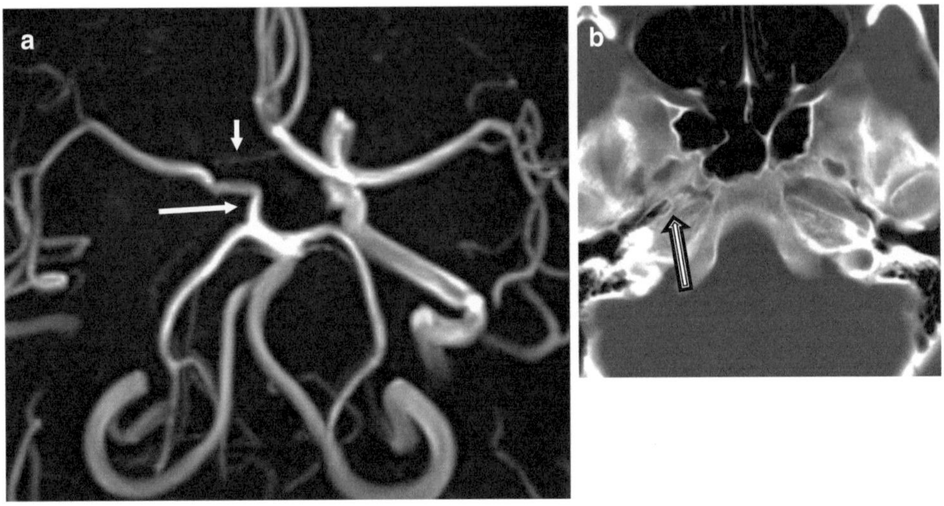

Fig. 3.7 (**a**) I-S projection of MR angiography shows the absence of the right ICA. Large right PCoA supplies the right MCA (*long arrow*), indicative of a Type A ICA agenesis. The tiny A1 segment of the right ACA can be seen (*short arrow*). (**b**) Skull base level CT with bone window shows the absence of the right carotid canal (*arrow*)

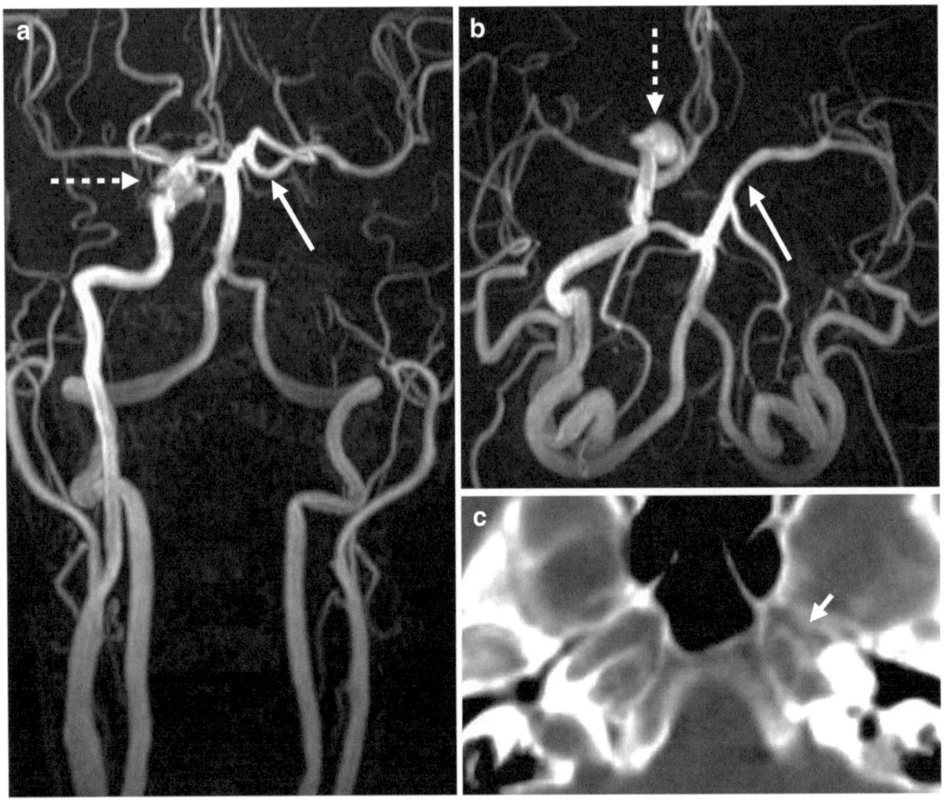

Fig. 3.8 (**a**) A-P and (**b**) I-S projections of MR angiography show the absence of the left ICA. The left MCA is supplied by the left PCoA (*long arrows*), indicative of a Type A ICA agenesis. The A1 segment of the left ACA is absent. There is an aneurysm at the paraclinoid segment of the right ICA (*dotted arrows*). (**c**) Skull base level CT with bone window shows the absence of the left carotid canal (*short arrow*)

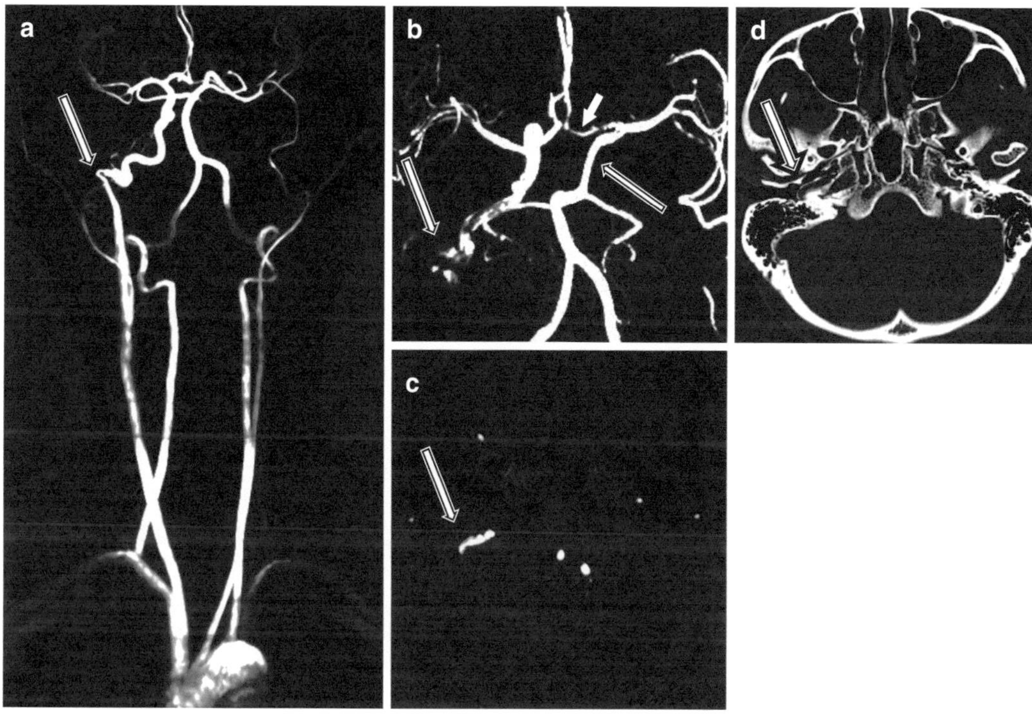

Fig. 3.9 (**a**) A-P and (**b**) I-S projections of MR angiography show the absence of the left ICA. The left MCA is supplied mainly by the PCoA (*long arrow*), indicative of a Type A ICA agenesis. The small left A1 is present (*short arrow*). The right petrous ICA takes an anomalous course, suggesting an aberrant course of the petrous segment of the ICA (Sect. 3.3) (*dotted arrows*). (**c**) MR angiographic source image and (**d**) skull base CT show the absence of both the left carotid canal and right ICA in the middle ear cavity (*dotted arrows*). (Courtesy of Dr. Noriharu Yanagimachi)

3.5.2 ICA Agenesis with Collateral Blood Supply via the Anterior Communicating Artery (ACoA) (Lie's Type B)

Lie's Type B ICA agenesis [13] is extremely rare. The MCA is supplied mainly by the contralateral ACA via the ACoA (Fig. 3.10). As mentioned above (Sect. 3.5.1), the absence of the carotid canal is important for the definite diagnosis of this rare variation.

3.5.3 Bilateral ICAs Agenesis (Lie's Type C)

Bilateral ICA agenesis, Lie's Type C [13], is extremely rare. The bilateral MCAs and ACAs are supplied by the bilateral PCoAs. Thus, the vertebrobasilar system is extremely hyperplastic (Fig. 3.11). According to a review of 60 reported cases, approximately one-quarter of the cases showed no pathological findings [16]. Segmental agenesis of the bilateral ICAs is also seen [17].

3.5.4 ICA Agenesis with Intercavernous Anastomosis (Lie's Type D)

Lie's Type D [13] is rare. Its prevalence is unknown. From the cervical segment to the precavernous segment of the ICA is absent. The distal ICA is supplied by the contralateral cavernous ICA (Fig. 3.12). This type of ICA agenesis is called intercavernous anastomosis [18] or transsellar anastomosis [19]. Because the anastomotic

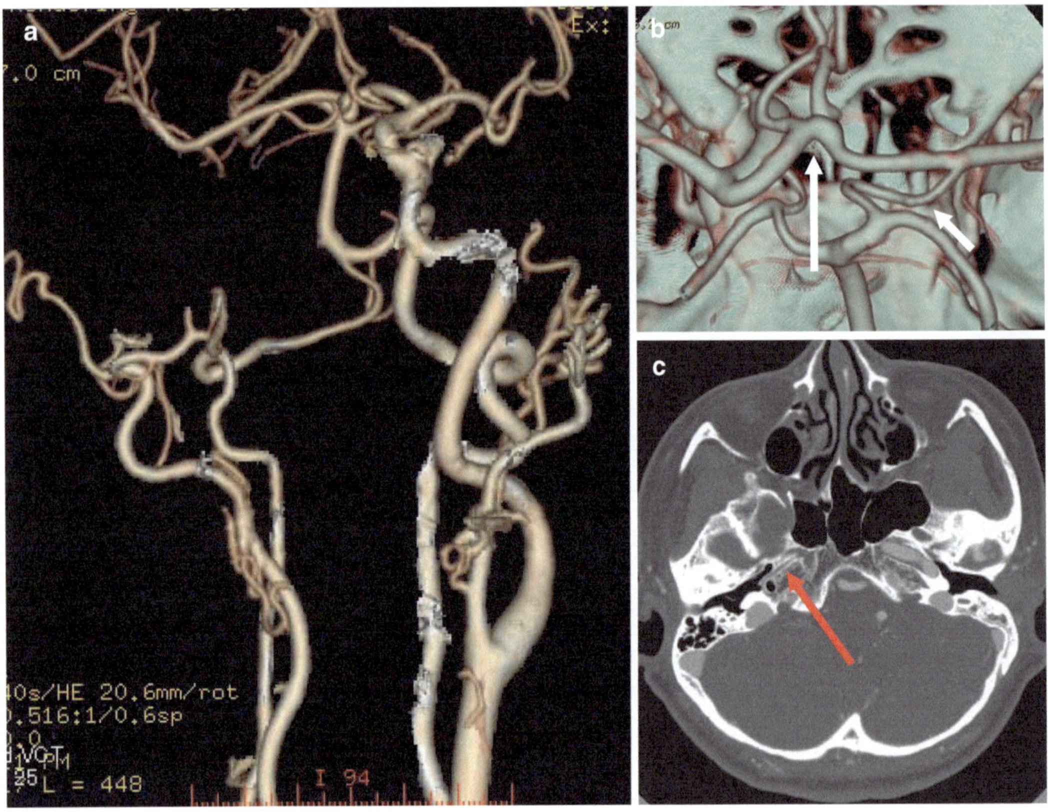

Fig. 3.10 (**a**) A-P projection of CT angiography shows the absence of the right ICA. (**b**) S-I projection of CT angiography shows the markedly dilated ACoA (*long arrow*), suggestive of a Type B ICA agenesis. The right PCoA is patent but small (*short arrow*). (**c**) CT angiographic source image shows a tiny right carotid canal (*arrow*). Therefore, there is a possibility of an occluded hypoplastic ICA, not congenital agenesis

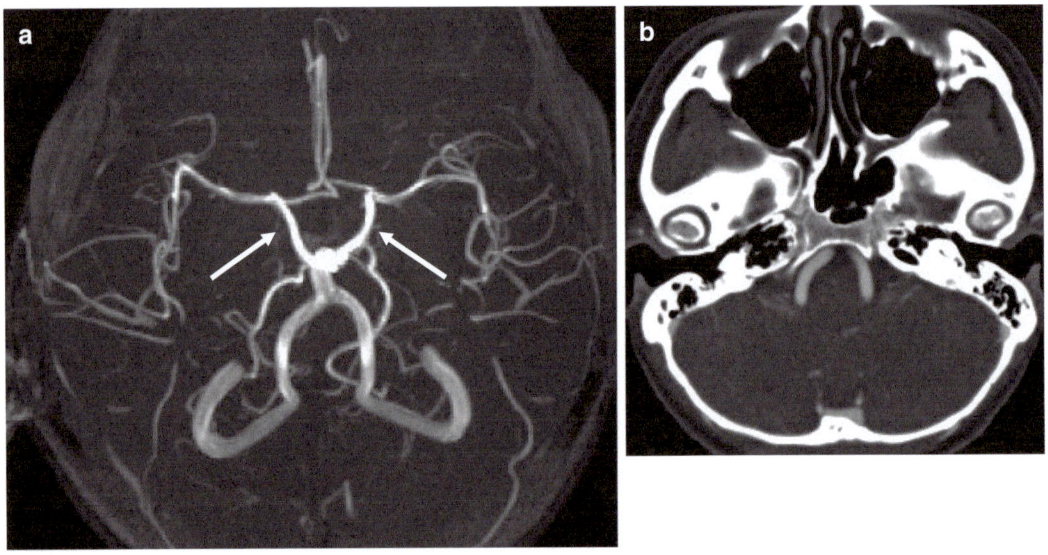

Fig. 3.11 (**a**) I-S projection of MR angiography shows bilateral ICA agenesis (Type C). The bilateral PCoAs are markedly dilated (*arrows*). (**b**) CT angiographic source image shows the absence of the bilateral carotid canals

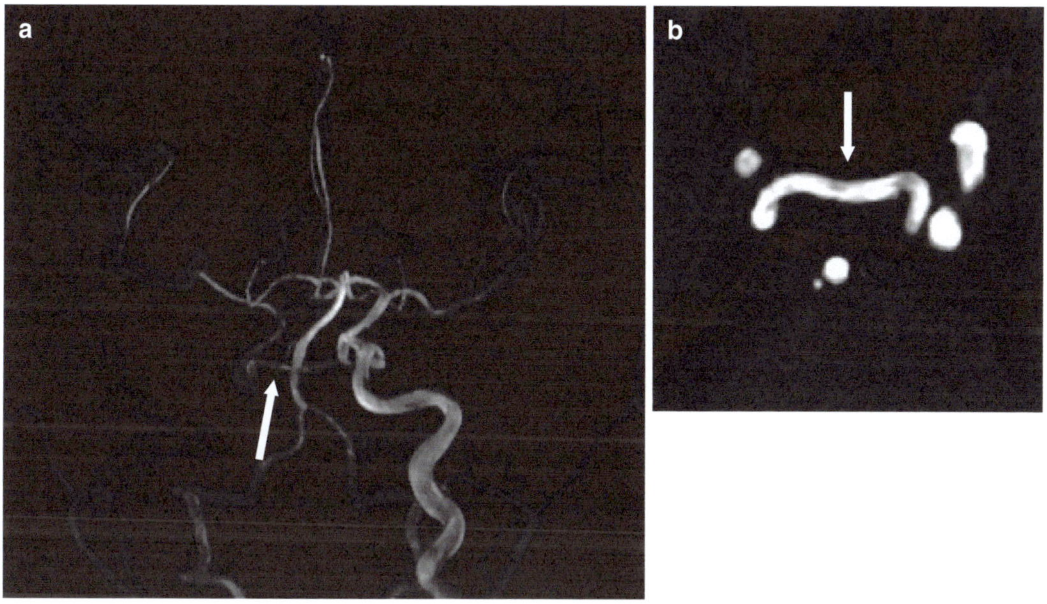

Fig. 3.12 (**a**) A-P projection of MR angiography shows the absence of the right ICA except for the distal segment. The collateral channel is seen between the bilateral cavernous segments (*arrow*), indicative of a Type D ICA agenesis. (**b**) MR angiographic source image shows the anastomotic artery at the sellar floor (*arrow*)

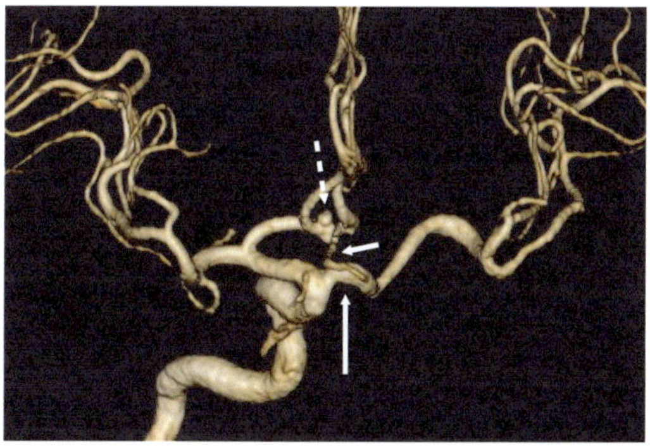

Fig. 3.13 A-P projection of partial VR MR angiography (the vertebrobasilar system was deleted) shows the absence of the left ICA, except for the distal segment. The collateral channel is seen between the bilateral paraclinoid segments (*long arrow*). This patient also has left carotid-ACA anastomosis (Sect. 9.2) (*short arrow*). There is an aneurysm at the right ACA-ACoA junction (*dotted arrow*). (Courtesy of Dr. Koji Yamashita)

channel runs through the sellar region, this variation is dangerous during transsphenoidal pituitary surgery.

ICA agenesis with interparaclinoid anastomosis (Fig. 3.13) and paraclinoid-supraclinoid anastomosis are also seen (Figs. 3.14 and 3.15) [15], but they are extremely rare.

3.5.5 ICA Hypoplasia (Lie's Type E)

Lie's Type E [13], ICA hypoplasia, is relatively common. However, this type should not be confused with acquired stenotic ICA. In the case of the origin of the ICA is severely stenotic with reduced blood flow, the appearance on both MR and CT angiography is similar to the hypoplastic ICA. A hypoplastic carotid canal is a definite criterion for congenital hypoplasia (Fig. 3.16). Associated variations in the vertebrobasilar system have been reported (Fig. 3.17) [20]. In rare cases, ICA hypoplasia can be seen bilaterally (Fig. 3.18). ICA hypoplasia is usually asymptomatic; however, it may cause ischemic brain diseases [21].

3.5.6 Rete Mirabile (ICA Agenesis with Collaterals from the ECA with Network Formation) (Lie's Type F)

Rete mirabile is a normal structure in some lower mammals, such as sheep, cows, and pigs [22]. This arterial network has physiological

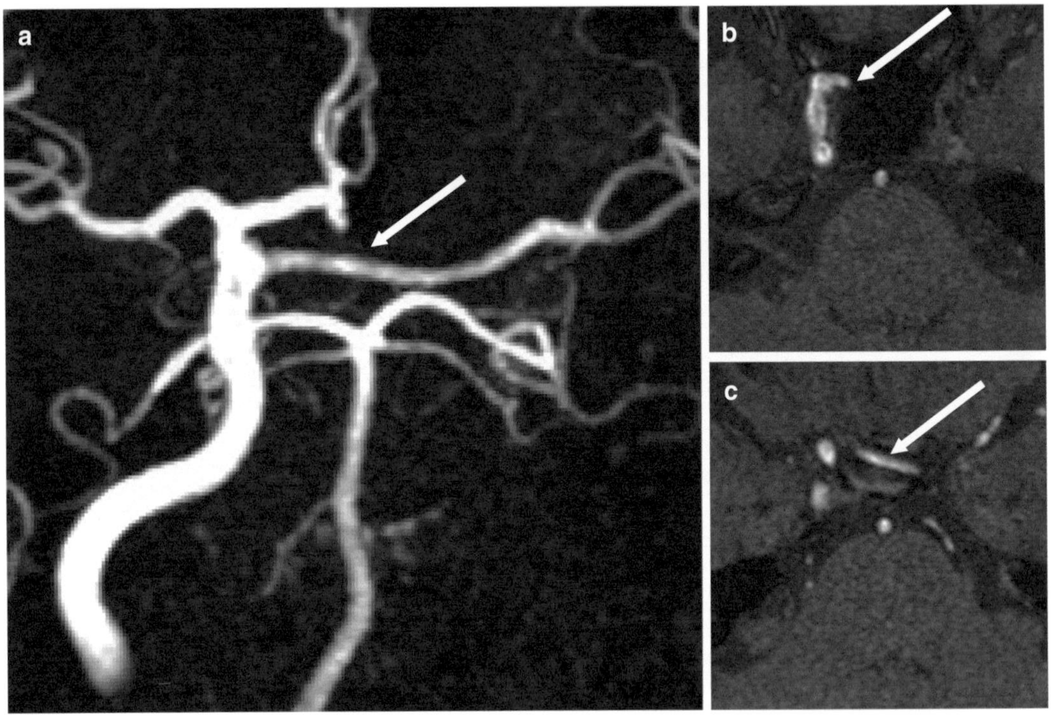

Fig. 3.14 (**a**) AI-PS projection of MR angiography shows the absence of the left ICA, except for the distal segment. The left MCA is supplied by the collateral channel arising from the right ICA (*arrow*). (**b**, **c**) MR angiographic source images show the connecting artery between bilateral ICAs arising from the paraclinoid right ICA and passing through the suprasellar cistern (*arrows*), indicative of a paraclinoid-supraclinoid anastomosis. (Courtesy of Dr. Naomi Fujiwara)

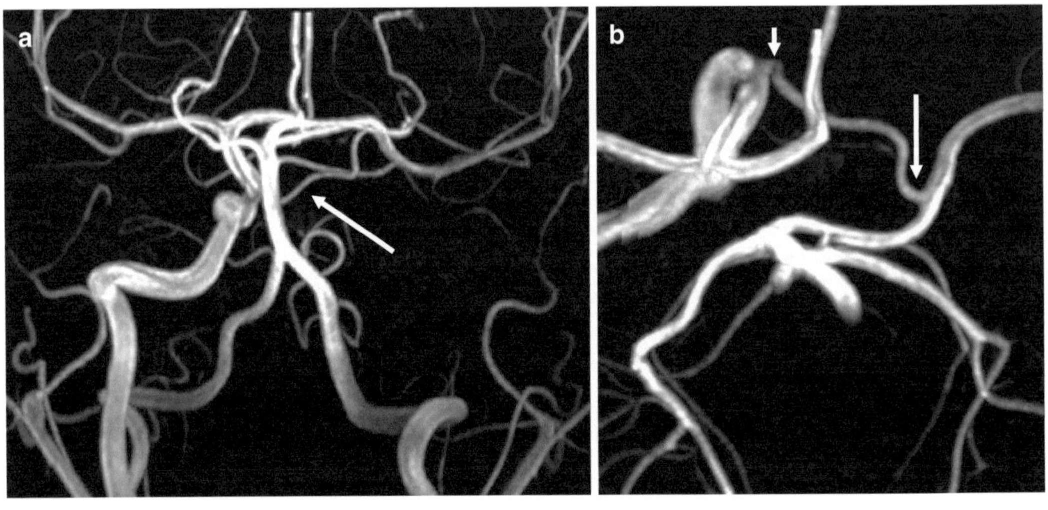

Fig. 3.15 (**a**) A-P projection of MR angiography shows left ICA agenesis. The left MCA is mainly supplied by the left PCoA (Type A). A small artery is crossing the midline (*arrow*). (**b**) I-S projection of partial MIP MR angiography shows a small anastomotic artery arising from the right paraclinoid ICA (*short arrow*) and fusing with the left supraclinoid ICA (*long arrow*), indicative of a paraclinoid-supraclinoid anastomosis

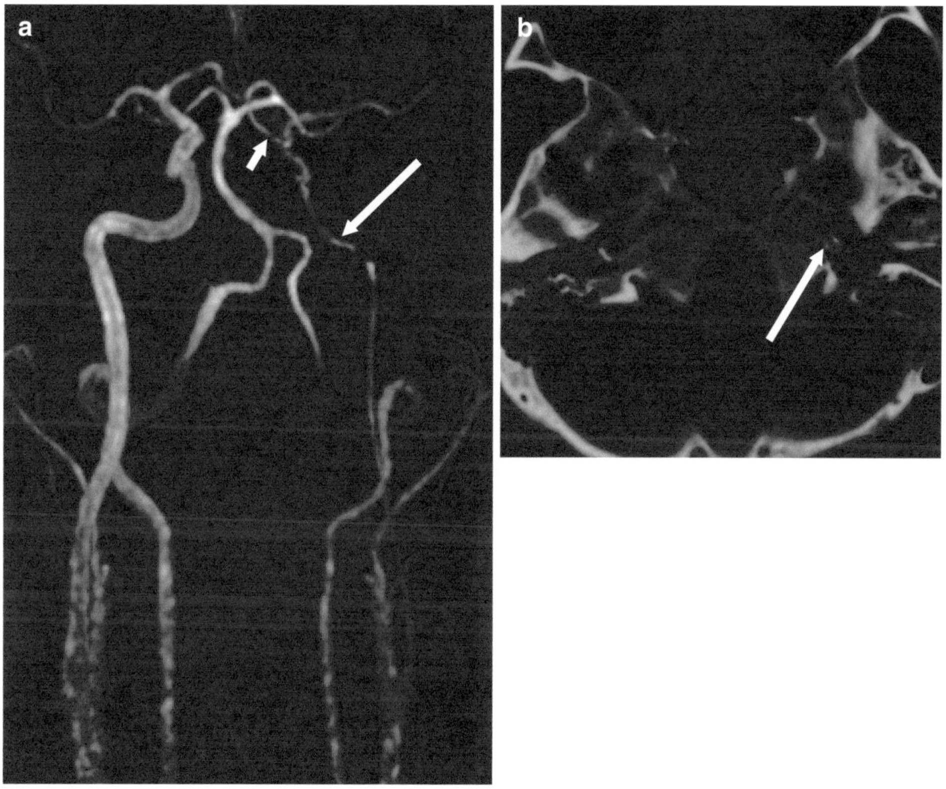

Fig. 3.16 (**a**) A-P projection of MR angiography shows a hypoplastic left ICA (*long arrow*). The left PCoA is dilated (*short arrow*). (**b**) Skull base CT with bone window shows a hypoplastic left carotid canal (*arrow*)

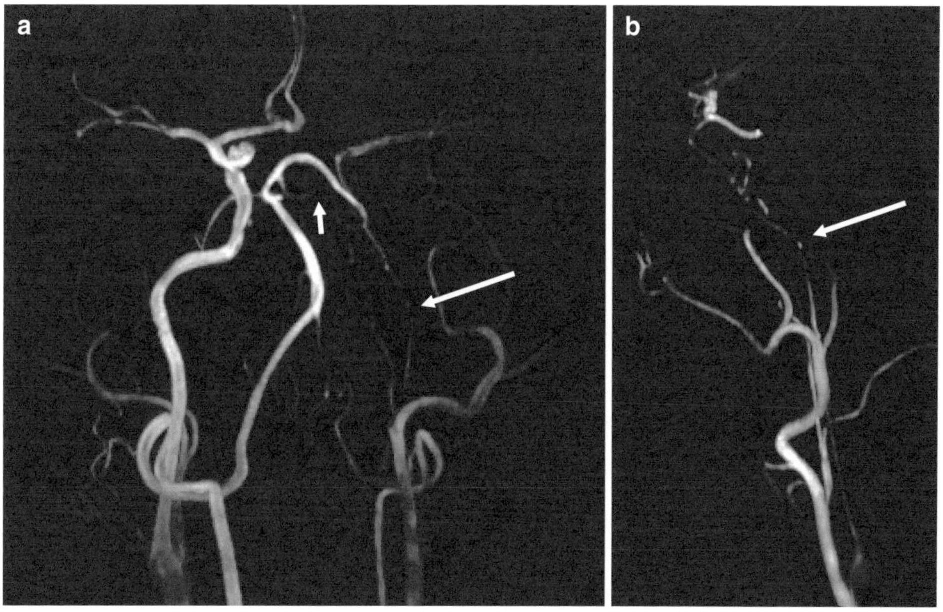

Fig. 3.17 (**a**) A-P projection of MR angiography and (**b**) partial MIP lateral image show a hypoplastic left ICA (*long arrows*). A large fenestration and long P1 segment of the left PCA (*short arrow*) are present (Sect. 7.8)

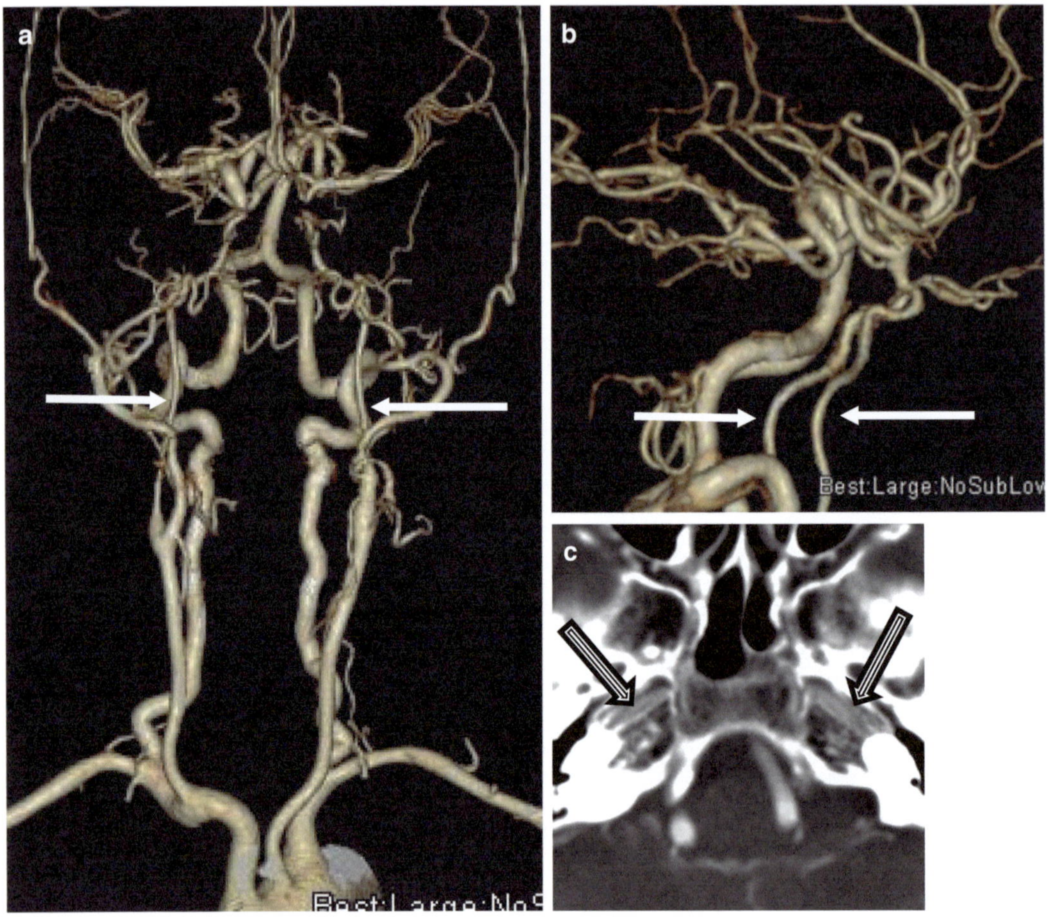

Fig. 3.18 (**a**) A-P and (**b**) lateral projections of CT angiography show bilateral narrow ICAs (*arrows*). (**c**) CT angiographic source image shows bilateral narrow carotid canals (*arrows*), indicative of bilateral hypoplastic ICAs

roles, including functioning as a heat exchanger and pressure absorber for the intracranial blood flow. In humans, rete mirabile is extremely rarely formed for the collateral circulation from extradural to intradural arteries in a patient with congenital dysplastic ICA (Fig. 3.19) [23]. This segmental agenesis of the ICA with a collateral arterial network can be seen bilaterally with involvement of the VA (Figs. 3.20 and 3.21) [22].

3.6 ICA Fenestration

Characteristically, fenestration occurs when a single artery divides into two arterial channels that fuse together, forming an arterial ring. It is most prevalent in the vertebrobasilar system (Sects. 10.3 and 11.1). ICA fenestration is relatively rare. However, it is most frequently observed at the supraclinoid segment (Figs. 3.22 and 3.23), and is frequently associated with an aneurysm at the proximal end of the fenestrated segment (Fig. 3.24) [24]. Extremely rarely, fenestration can be seen at the cavernous segment (Fig. 3.25) [25]. Chronic dissection with a patent pseudolumen of the cervical ICA may be misdiagnosed as a fenestration (Fig. 3.26).

3.7 Dolichoectasia of the Distal ICA

Marked arterial elongation and tortuosity (dolichoectasia) is rarely seen at the distal segment of the ICA, even in pediatric patients (Fig. 3.27)

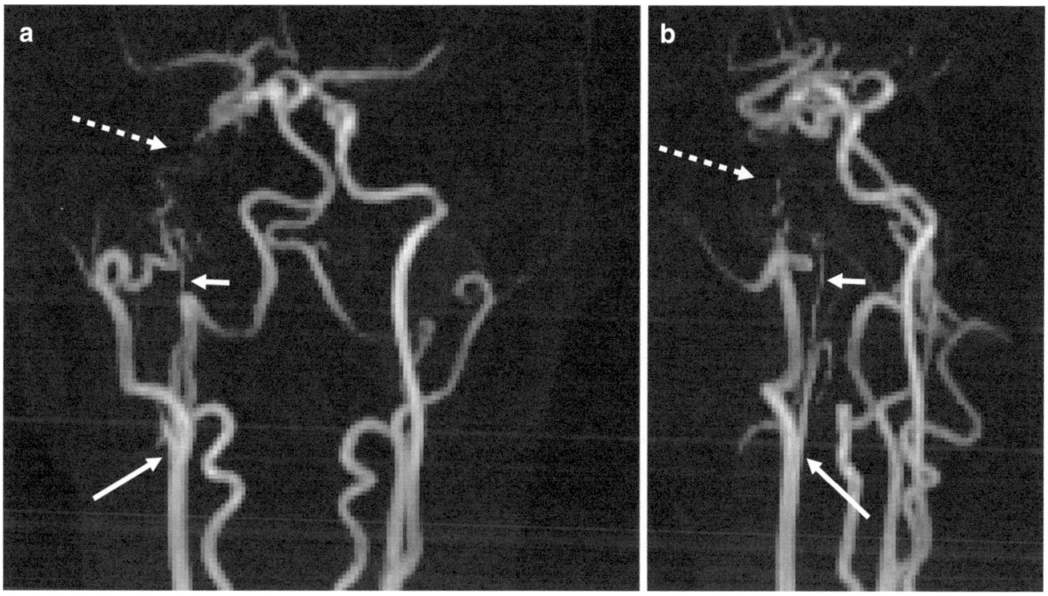

Fig. 3.19 (**a**) A-P and (**b**) LAO projections of MR angiography show right high carotid bifurcation (*long arrows*). The cervical segment of the right ICA is hypoplastic (*short arrows*). A collateral arterial network from the ECA to the cavernous segment of the ICA is formed (*dotted arrows*), indicative of a rete mirabile. (Courtesy of Dr. Hideki Sato)

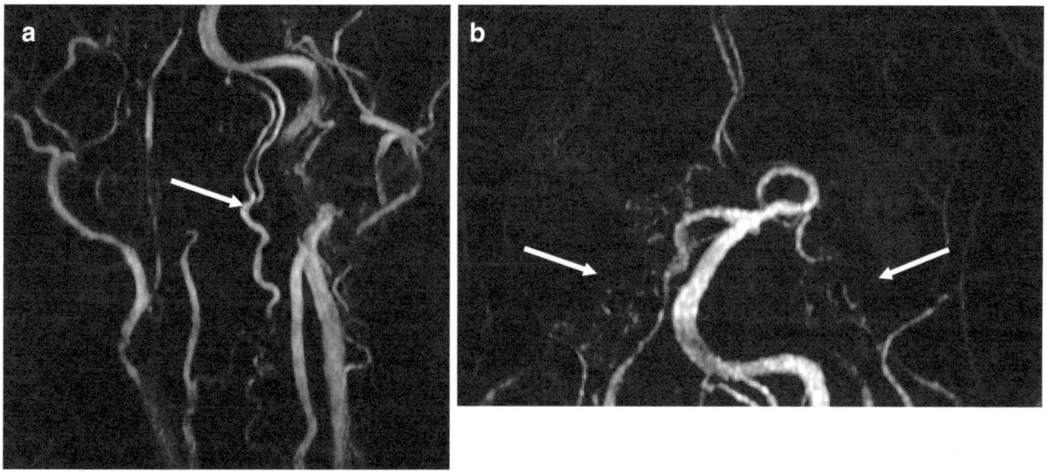

Fig. 3.20 (**a**) A-P projection of MR angiography of the neck region shows no cervical ICA. The bilateral ECAs and anterior spinal artery (*arrow*) are dilated. (**b**) A-P projection of MR angiography of the head region shows a fine arterial network at the skull base region, bilaterally (*arrows*). The anterior circulation is faintly visualized, indicative of a rete mirabile. (Courtesy of Dr. Morio Nagahata)

[26, 27]. This anomalous artery can be seen in patients with or without PHACE (posterior fossa malformations, hemangiomas, arterial anomalies, cardiac defects, and eye abnormalities) syndrome [26]. Dolichoectasia can also be seen in other intracranial arteries, especially in the vertebrobasilar system. However, because the majority of patients with dolichoectatic BA are aged and hypertensive, prolonged hypertension might contribute to its development [27].

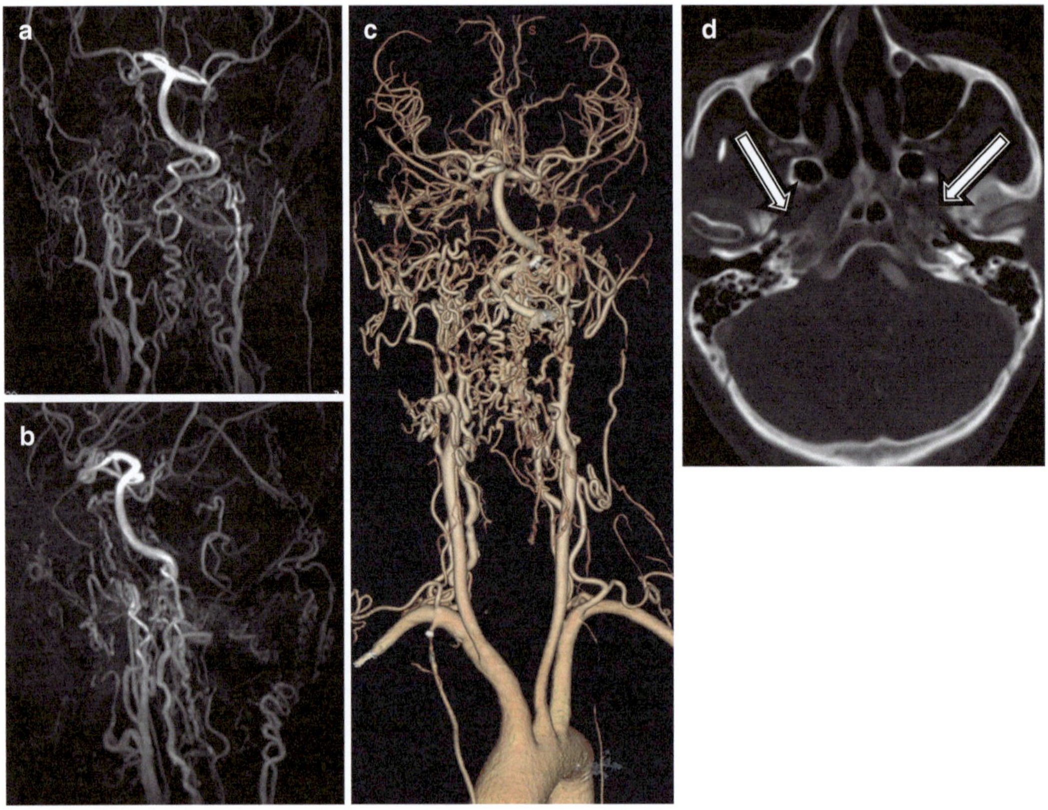

Fig. 3.21 (**a**) A-P and (**b**) LAO projections of MR angiography show agenesis of the bilateral ICAs and VAs with a network of numerous collateral arteries, indicative of a rete mirabile. (**c**) A-P projection of CT angiography from the aortic arch to the intracranial region shows normal arterial development at the lower cervical level. The intracranial arterial systems are well visualized by collateral circulation. (**d**) CT angiographic source image shows the absence of the bilateral carotid canals (*arrows*)

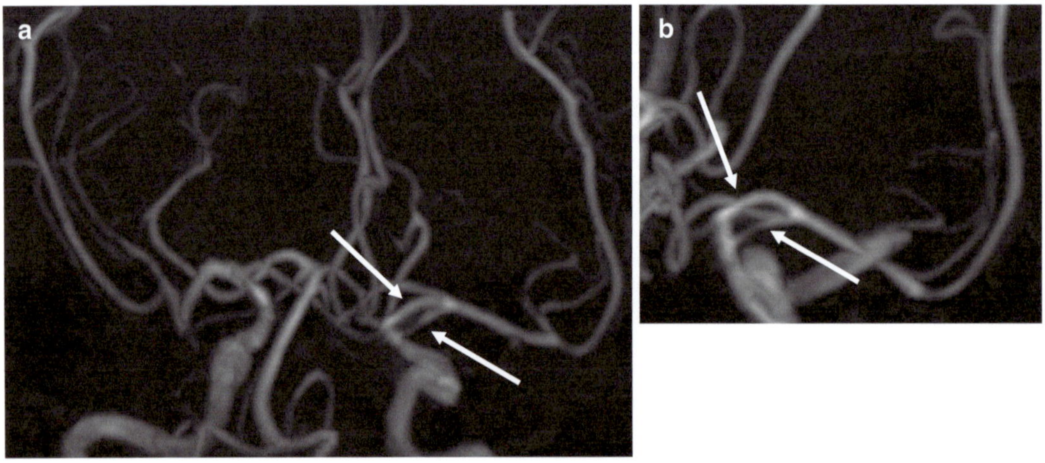

Fig. 3.22 (**a**) Slightly RAO projection of MR angiography shows two arterial channels at the left supraclinoid ICA (*arrows*). (**b**) S-I projection of MR angiography shows the large fenestration more clearly (*arrows*)

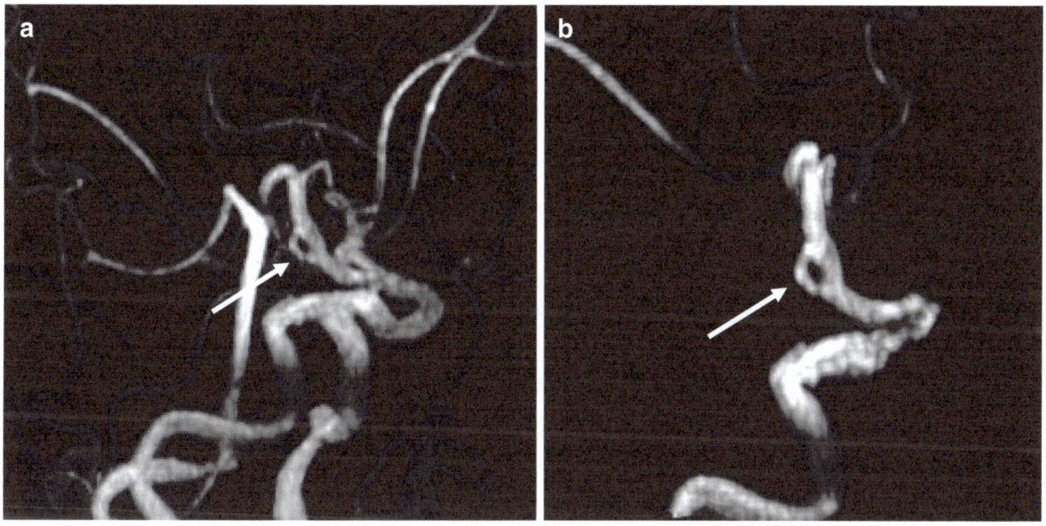

Fig. 3.23 (**a**) Lateral projection of MR angiography and (**b**) partial MIP image show a small fenestration at the supraclinoid segment of the right ICA (*arrows*)

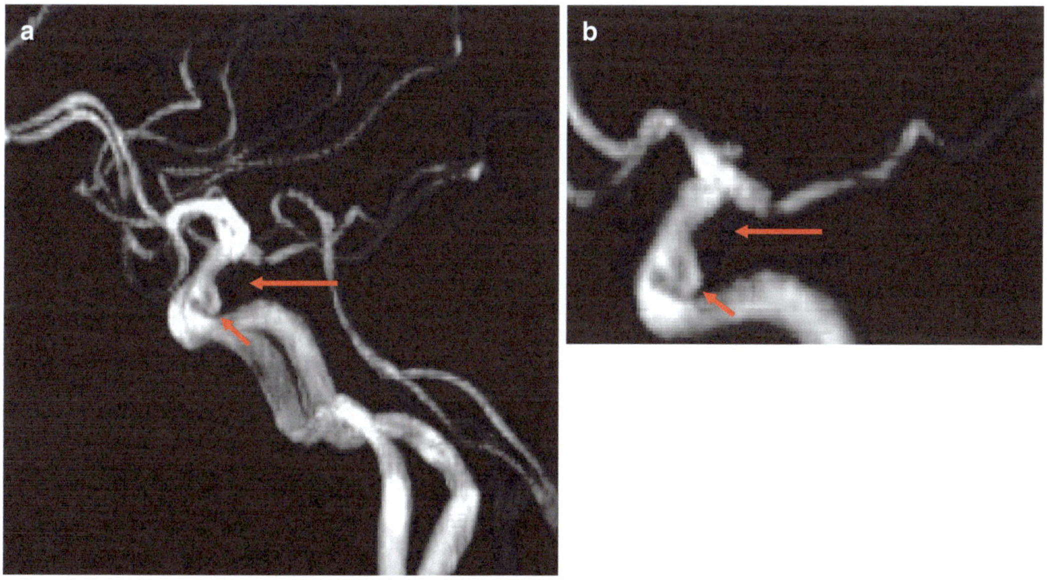

Fig. 3.24 (**a**) Lateral projection of MR angiography shows an aneurysm of the left paraclinoid ICA (*black short arrow*). A tiny artery can be seen posterior to the left supraclinoid ICA (*white long arrow*). (**b**) LAO projection of partial MIP image demonstrates a fenestration (*white long arrow*) and associating aneurysm (*black short arrow*)

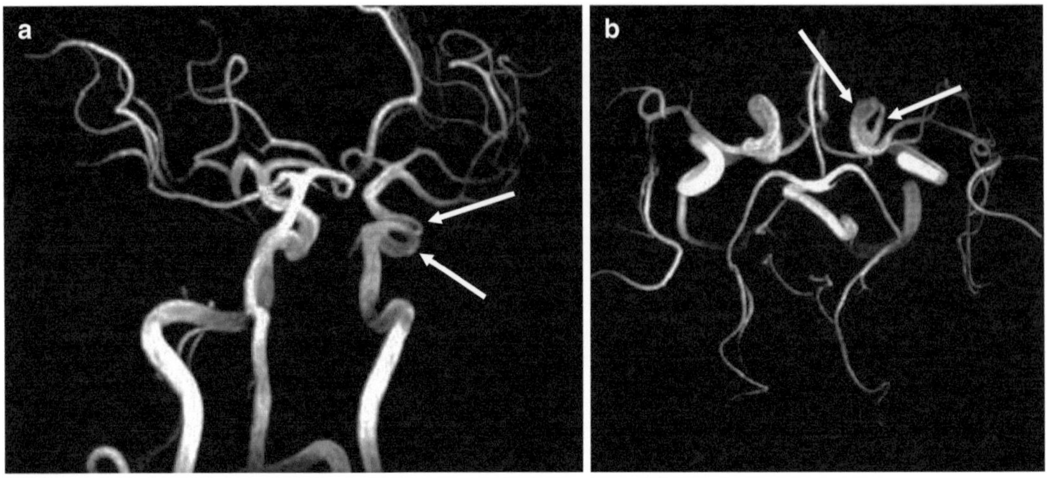

Fig. 3.25 (**a**) RAO and (**b**) I-S projections of MR angiography show a fenestration at the left cavernous ICA (*arrows*). (Courtesy of Dr. Yuji Numaguchi)

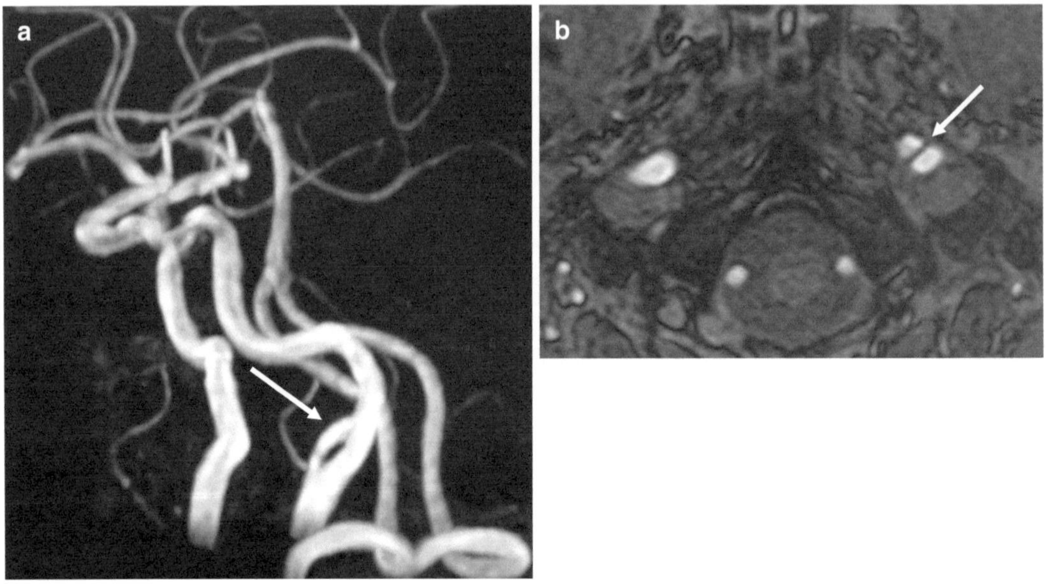

Fig. 3.26 (**a**) Slightly LAO projection of MR angiography shows a segmental double lumen at the cervical ICA (*arrow*). (**b**) MR angiographic source image shows a slit-like septum (*arrow*), indicating the possibility of both true fenestration and chronic dissection with a patent pseudolumen

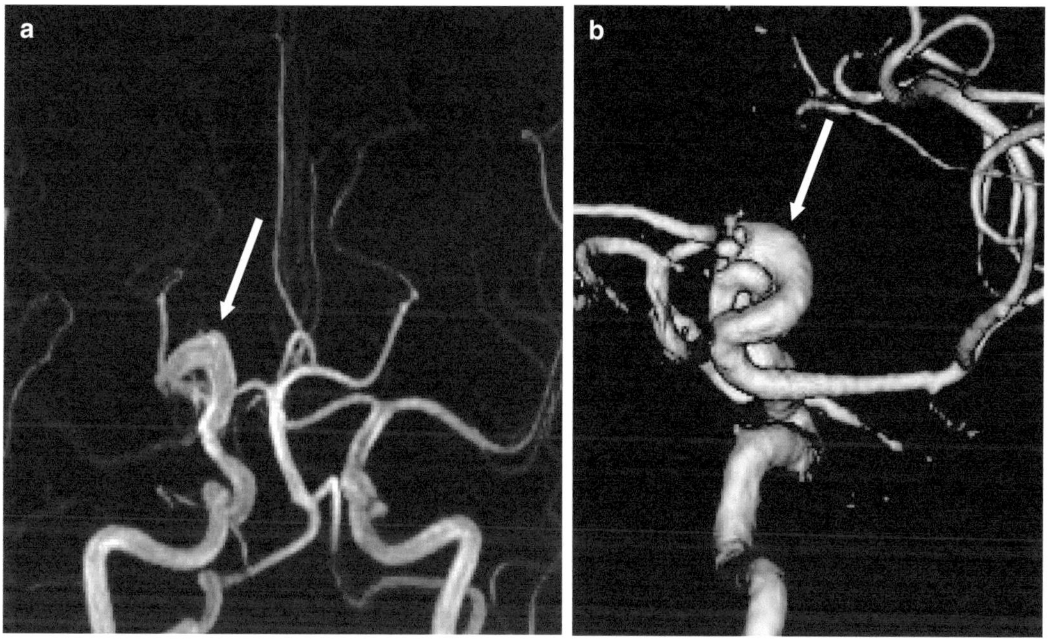

Fig. 3.27 (**a**) AS-PI projection of MR angiography shows dilated and extremely elongated right distal ICA, indicative of a dolichoectasia (*arrow*). (**b**) P-A projection of a partial VR image clearly shows anomalous terminal segment of the right ICA (*arrow*)

References

1. Gowdh NS, Gill FJ, Regan LA, Wilkie SW. Kissing carotid arteries: an unusual cause of prevertebral swelling. BMJ Case Rep. 2014 Oct;01:2014.
2. Pereira Filho Ade A, Gobbato PL, Pereira Filho Gde A, Silva SB, Kraemer JL. Intracranial intrasellar kissing carotid arteries: case report. Arq Neuropsiquiatr. 2007;65:355–7.
3. Weibel J, Fields WS. Tortuosity, coiling, and kinking of the internal carotid artery: etiology and radiographic anatomy. Neurology. 1965;15:7–18.
4. Rahal JP, Gao B, Safain MG, Malek AM. Stent recanalization of carotid tonsillar loop dissection using the Enterprise vascular reconstruction device. J Clin Neurosci. 2014;21:1141–7.
5. Barbour PJ, Castaldo JE, Rae-Grant AD, Gee W, Reed JF III, Jenny D, Longennecker L. Internal carotid artery redundancy is significantly associated with dissection. Stroke. 1994;25:1201–6.
6. Uchino A, Saito N, Okano N, Kakehi Y. Aberrant internal carotid artery associated with occipital artery arising from the internal carotid artery. Surg Radiol Anat. 2015;37:1137–40.
7. Lasjaunias P, Moret J, Manelfe C, Theron J, Hasso T, Seeger J. Arterial anomalies at the base of the skull. Neuroradiology. 1977;13:267–72.
8. Roll JD, Urban MA, Larson TC 3rd, Gailloud P, Jacob P, Harnsberger HR. Bilateral aberrant internal carotid arteries with bilateral persistent stapedial arteries and bilateral duplicated internal carotid arteries. AJNR Am J Neuroradiol. 2003;24:762–5.
9. Hatipoglu HG, Cetin MA, Yuksel E, Dere H. A case of a coexisting aberrant internal carotid artery and persistent stapedial artery: the role of MR angiography in the diagnosis. Ear Nose Throat J. 2011;90:E17–20.
10. Aladwan A, Mack M, Gstöttner W, Vogl TJ. Duplication of internal carotid artery: a rare case of tympanic mass. Eur Radiol. 2005;15:2525–7.
11. Gartrell BC, Kennedy TA, Gubbels SP. Bilateral duplicated internal carotid arteries presenting as middle ear masses: a case report and review of the literature. Ann Otol Rhinol Laryngol. 2012;121:521–4.
12. Li S, Hooda K, Gupta N, Kumar Y. Internal carotid artery agenesis: a case report and review of literature. Neuroradiol J. 2017;30:186–91.
13. Lie TA. Congenital anomalies of the carotid arteries. Excerpta Media, Amsterdam, 1968; pp 16–51.
14. Uchino A, Sawada A, Hirakawa N, Totoki T, Kudo S. Congenital absence of the internal carotid artery diagnosed during investigation of trigeminal neuralgia. Eur Radiol. 2002;12:2339–42.
15. Uchino A, Saito N, Kohyama S. Agenesis of the internal carotid artery with paraclinoid-supraclinoid anastomosis and basilar artery-posterior communicating

artery anastomosis diagnosed by magnetic resonance angiography. Surg Radiol Anat. 2015;37:685–7.
16. Vasović L, Trandafilović M, Vlajković S, Radenković G. Congenital absence of the bilateral internal carotid artery: a review of the associated (ab)normalities from a newborn status to the eighth decade of life. Childs Nerv Syst. 2018;34:35–49.
17. Giragani S, Kumar RK, Kasireddy AR, Alwala S. Bilateral internal carotid artery agenesis and posterior circulation stroke: a rare association. J Stroke Cerebrovasc Dis. 2020;29:105342.
18. Quint DJ, Boulos RS, Spera TD. Congenital absence of the cervical and petrous internal carotid artery with intercavernous anastomosis. AJNR Am J Neuroradiol. 1989;10:435–9.
19. Mellado JM, Merino X, Ramos A, Salvadó E, Sauri A. Agenesis of the internal carotid artery with a transsellar anastomosis: CT and MRI findings in late-onset congenital hypopituitarism. Neuroradiology. 2001;43:237–41.
20. Uchino A, Ehara T, Kurita H. Hypoplasia of the internal carotid artery with associated fenestration and extremely long P1 segment of the ipsilateral posterior cerebral artery diagnosed by MR angiography. Surg Radiol Anat. 2019;41:707–11.
21. Nardone R, Venturi A, Ausserer H, Buffone E, Covi M, Lochner P, Psenner K, Tezzon F. Transient ischemic attacks in two cases of internal carotid artery hypoplasia. Neurol Sci. 2005;26:282–4.
22. Nagahata M, Kondo R, Mouri W, Sato A, Ito M, Sato S, Itagaki H, Yamaki T, Nagahata S, Saito S, Kayama T. Bilateral carotid and vertebral rete mirabile presenting with subarachnoid hemorrhage caused by the rupture of spinal artery aneurysm. Tohoku J Exp Med. 2013;230:205–9.
23. Lin E, Linfante I, Dabus G. Unilateral rete mirabile as a result of segmental agenesis of the ascending petrous segment of the internal carotid artery: embryology, differential diagnosis and clinical implications. Interv Neuroradiol. 2013;19:73–7.
24. Uchino A, Tanaka M. Fenestration of the supraclinoid internal carotid artery arising from the paraclinoid aneurysmal dilatation and fusing with the origin of the posterior communicating artery: a case report. Surg Radiol Anat. 2017;39:581–4.
25. Uchino A, Nomiyama K, Takase Y, Kohata T, Kudo S. Intracavernous fenestration of the internal carotid artery. Eur Radiol. 2006;16:1623–4.
26. Jia ZY, Zhao LB, Lee DH. Localized marked elongation of the distal internal carotid artery with or without PHACE syndrome: segmental dolichoectasia of the distal internal carotid artery. AJNR Am J Neuroradiol. 2018;39:817–23.
27. Uchino A, Ohira M. Dolichoectasia of the right internal carotid artery diagnosed incidentally by MR angiography in a 17-year-old girl. Radiol Case Rep. 2019;14:444–7.

4 External Carotid Artery (ECA) Branches Arising from the Internal Carotid Artery (ICA)

Abstract

This chapter includes (1) Occipital artery arising from the carotid bulb, (2) Occipital artery arising from the cervical internal carotid artery, (3) Ascending pharyngeal artery arising from the internal carotid artery, and (4) Persistent stapedial artery (Middle meningeal artery arising from the petrous internal carotid artery). There are 10 figures.

Before catheterization to these arteries, recognition of their anomalous origin is important to prevent technical failures and complications.

Keywords

Ascending pharyngeal artery · Internal carotid artery · Occipital artery · Persistent stapedial artery

4.1 Occipital Artery Arising from the ICA

4.1.1 Occipital Artery Arising from the Carotid Bulb

The occipital artery rarely arises from the ICA, especially from the carotid bulb. The prevalence on MR angiography was reported to be 0.09% per occipital artery, with right-side predominance [1]. There are two types: anterior wall origin (Figs. 4.1 and 4.2) [2] and posterosuperior wall origin (Fig. 4.3). In the former type, the ECA has a curved main trunk, while in the latter type, the ECA has a normal straight main trunk. The occipital artery is regarded as a remnant of the proatlantal artery [3]; however, these two types may have different embryonic origins. The occipital artery also rarely arises from the carotid bifurcation (Fig. 4.4).

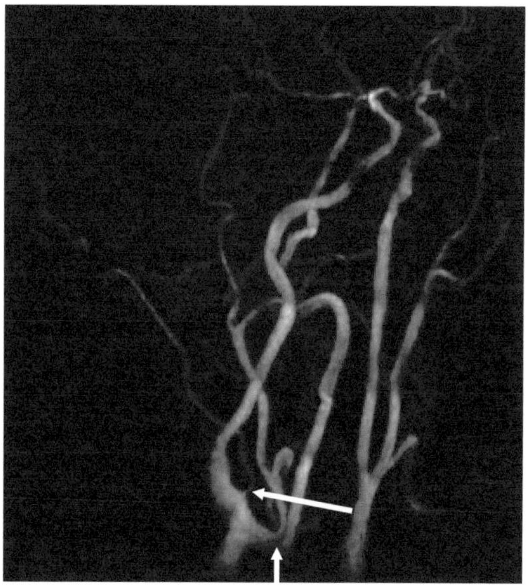

Fig. 4.1 RAO projection of MR angiography shows the right occipital artery arising from the anterior wall of the carotid bulb (*long arrow*). The ECA has a curved main trunk (*short arrow*)

A. Uchino, *Atlas of the Supraaortic Craniocervical Arterial Variations*,
https://doi.org/10.1007/978-981-16-6803-6_4

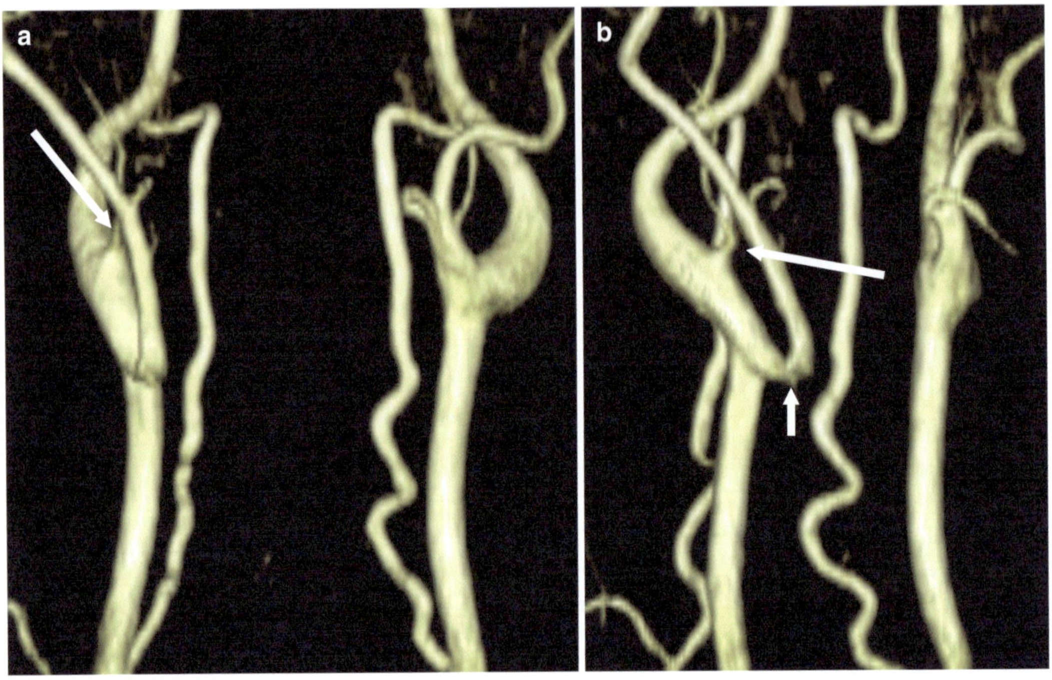

Fig. 4.2 (**a**) A-P and (**b**) RAO projections of VR MR angiography show the right occipital artery arising from the anterior wall of the carotid bulb (*long arrows*). The ECA has a curved main trunk (*short arrow*)

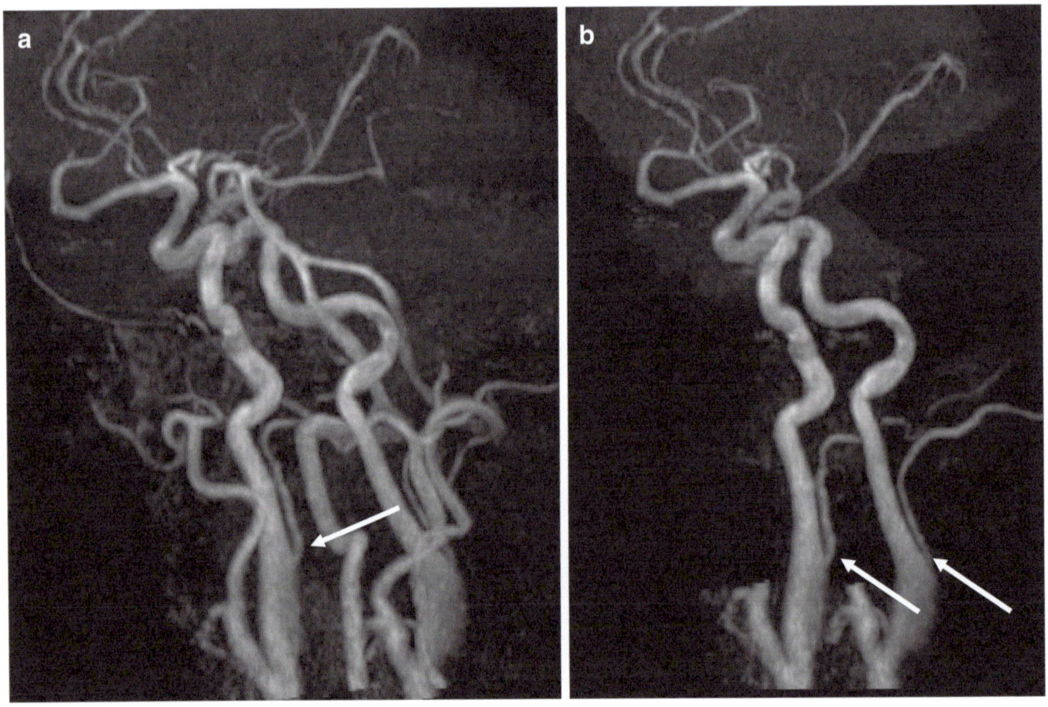

Fig. 4.3 (**a**) LAO projection of MR angiography and (**b**) partial MIP image show bilateral occipital arteries arising from the posterosuperior wall of the carotid bulb (*arrows*). The ECAs have normal straight main trunks, bilaterally

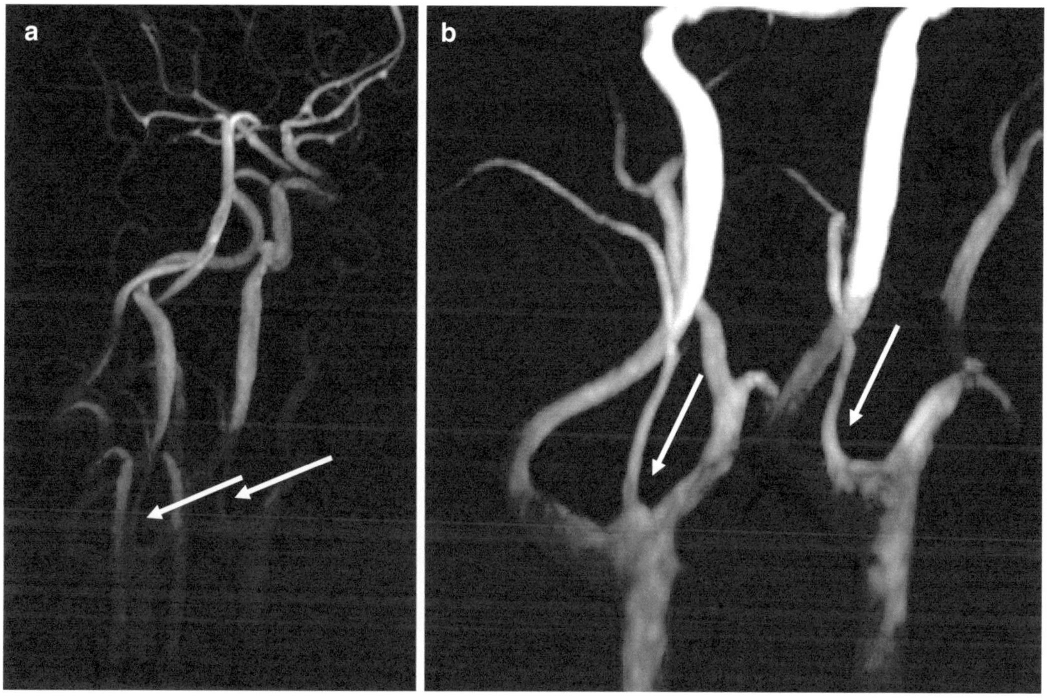

Fig. 4.4 (**a**) RAO projection of MR angiography and (**b**) partial MIP image show bilateral occipital arteries arising from the carotid bifurcations (*arrows*)

4.1.2 Occipital Artery Arising from the Cervical Segment of the ICA

The occipital artery arising from the cervical ICA at the level of the C2 vertebral body is extremely rare (Fig. 4.5) [4]. This variation may be formed when all but the distal part of anastomosis of the primitive proatlantal artery between the ICA and VA persists [3]. It is usually asymptomatic; however, it may cause atherosclerotic stenosis [5]. This variation can be associated with an aberrant course of the petrous segment of the ICA (Sect. 3.3) (Fig. 4.6) [6]. In the case of a non-bifurcating cervical carotid artery (Sect. 2.5), the occipital artery also arises from the cervical ICA, but not as high as the level of the C2 vertebral body.

4.2 Ascending Pharyngeal Artery (APA) Arising from the ICA

The APA is regarded as a remnant of the hypoglossal artery and rarely arises from the ICA. This variation is called an aberrant or ectopic origin of the APA [7]. Because the APA is usually a tiny vessel, it frequently cannot be visualized or is overlooked on MR or CT angiography (Fig. 4.7). Because the presence of APA variation is a significant condition during carotid endarterectomy, it should be detected before surgery [8]. The neuromeningeal trunk of the APA has hypoglossal and jugular branches [9]. If the posterior meningeal artery arises from the APA, it is hyperplastic, and can easily be detected by MR angiography

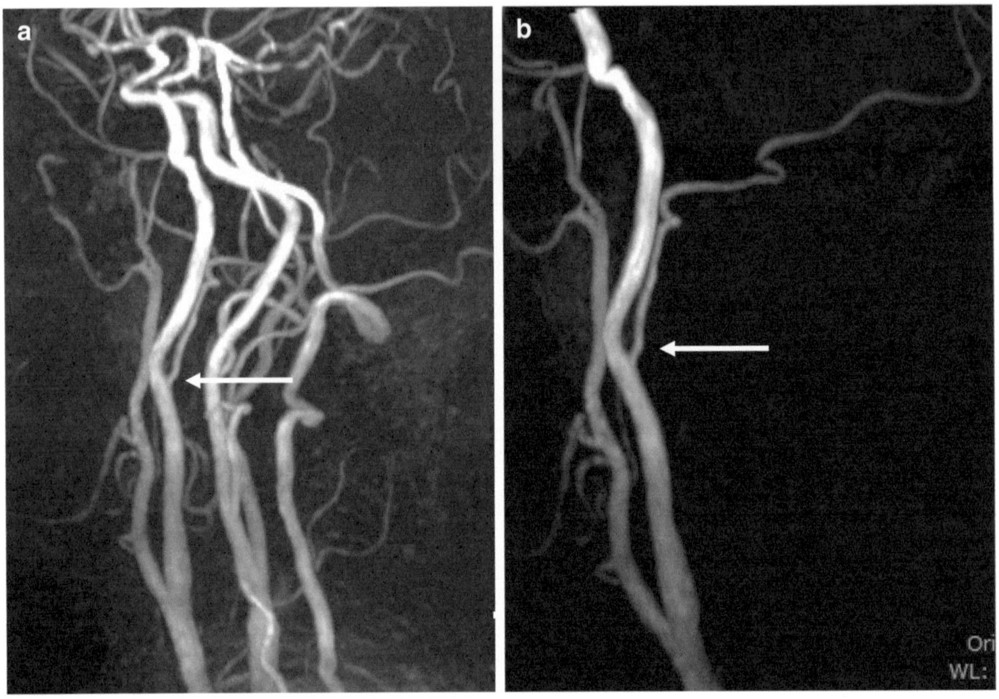

Fig. 4.5 (**a**) Slightly LAO projection of MR angiography and (**b**) partial MIP image show the right occipital artery arising from the cervical ICA at the level of the C2 vertebral body (*arrows*)

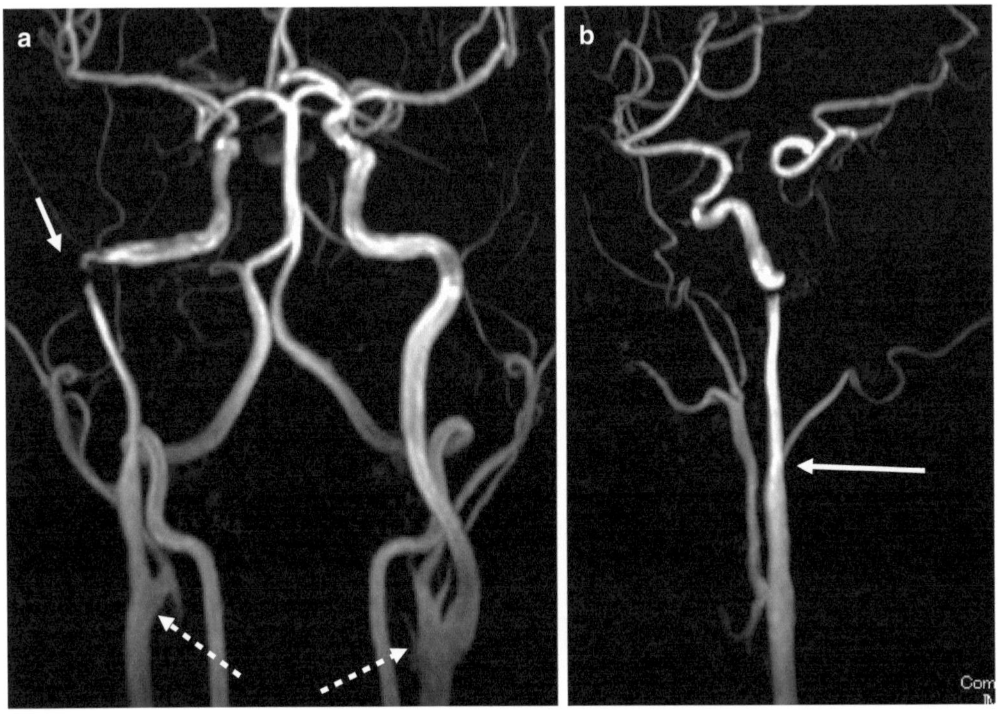

Fig. 4.6 (**a**) A-P projection of MR angiography and (**b**) partial MIP left lateral image show an aberrant course of the petrous segment of the right ICA (*short arrow*) (Sect. 3.3) and right occipital artery arising from the cervical right ICA (*long arrow*). Bilateral carotid bifurcations are high (*dotted arrows*) (Sect. 2.4)

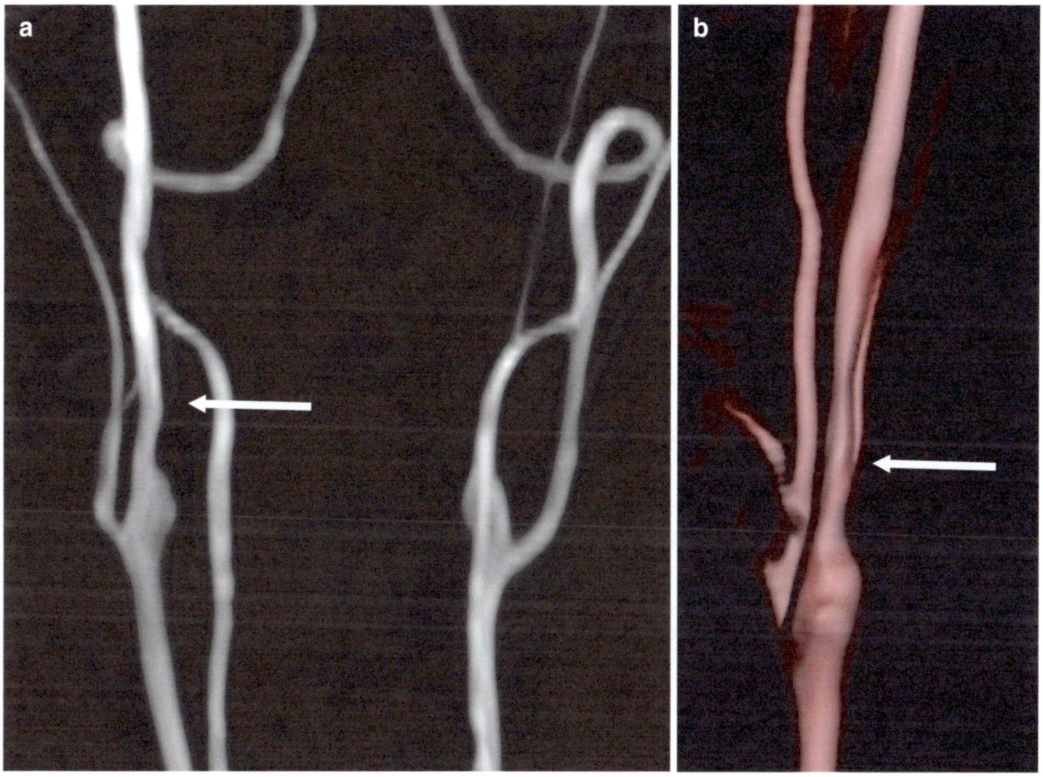

Fig. 4.7 (**a**) A-P projection of MR angiography and (**b**) partial VR left lateral image show a small artery arising from the right proximal ICA and ascending parallel to the cervical ICA, indicative of an aberrant origin of the APA (*arrows*)

(Fig. 4.8). An APA with this ICA origin plays an important role in collateral circulation in the case of cervical ICA occlusion [10].

4.3 Persistent Stapedial Artery (PSA) (Middle Meningeal Artery Arising from the Petrous ICA)

The MMA arising from the petrous ICA is regarded as a PSA and is an extremely rare variation on MR angiography (Fig. 4.9). A PSA can be seen in approximately 0.4% of the population, however, in the majority of cases, the PSA is a tiny artery and cannot be detected by MR angiography. This variation is dangerous during middle ear surgery because it penetrates the stapes. The foramen spinosum (FS), where the usual MMA penetrates the skull base, is absent [11]. Extremely rarely, the PSA arises from an aberrant course of the ICA [12]. The PSA can rarely be seen in patients with moyamoya disease (Fig. 4.10) [13].

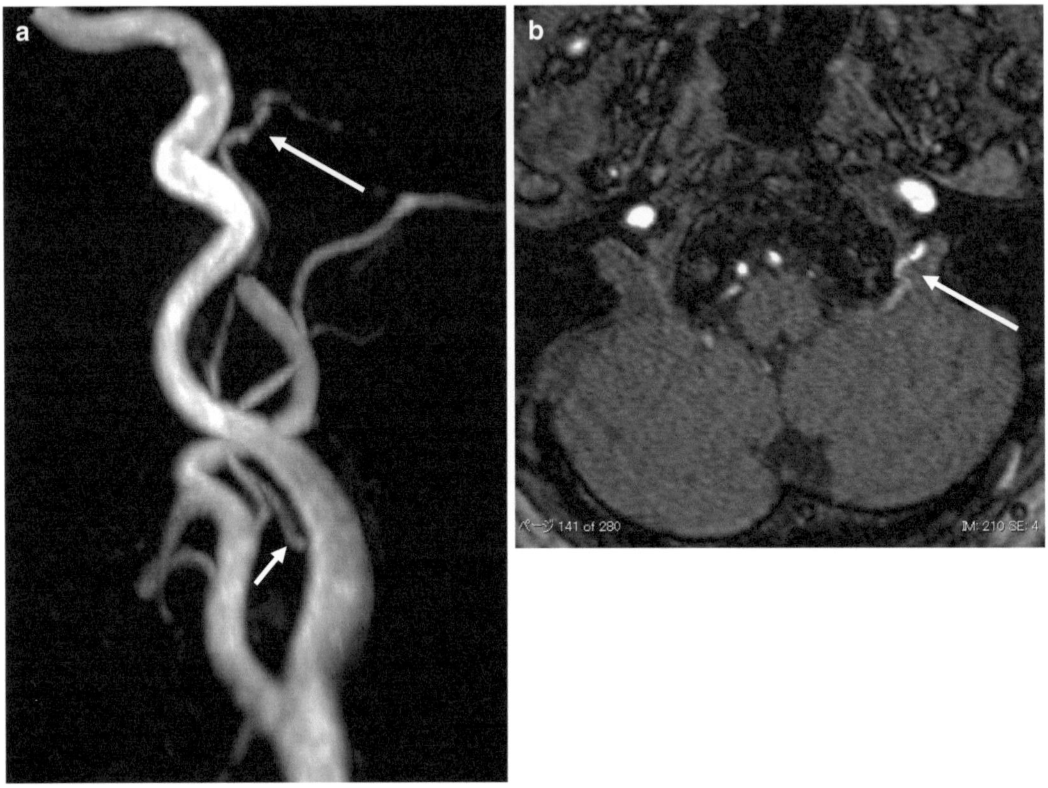

Fig. 4.8 (**a**) Lateral projection of partial MIP MR angiography shows a large left APA arising from the anterior wall of the ICA (*short arrow*). The jugular branch of the APA is hyperplastic (*long arrow*). (**b**) MR angiographic source image shows the posterior meningeal artery passing through the left jugular foramen (*arrow*)

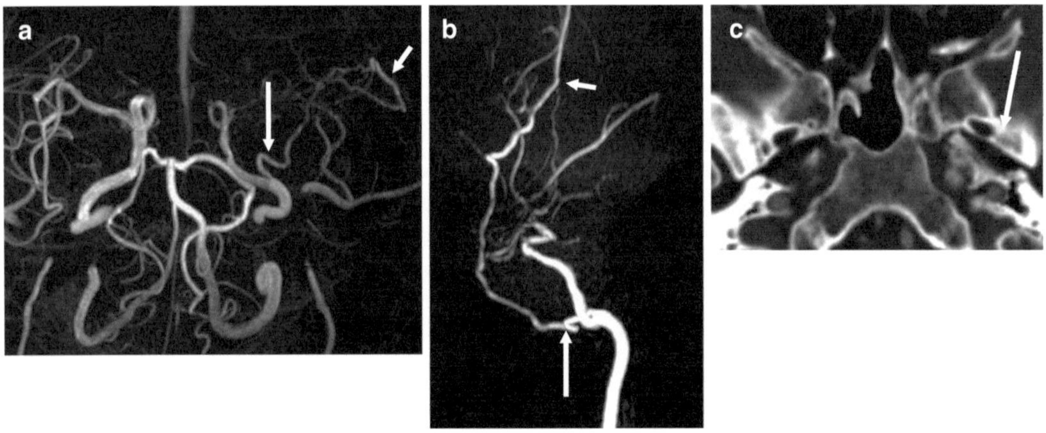

Fig. 4.9 (**a**) I-S projection of MR angiography and (**b**) left lateral projection of a partial MIP image show an anomalous artery arising from the left petrous ICA (*long arrows*) and continuing to the MMA (*short arrows*), indicative of a PSA. This patient has left unilateral moyamoya disease, and the MMA is dilated as a collateral blood supply to the left cerebral hemisphere. (**c**) CT of the skull base with bone window shows the absence of the left FS (*arrow*)

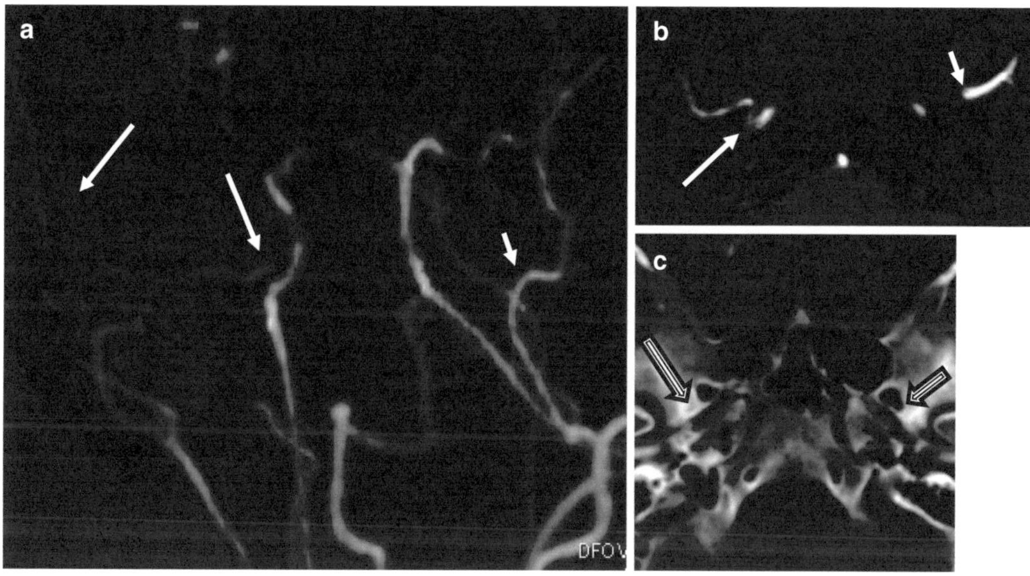

Fig. 4.10 (**a**) Slightly LAO projection of MR angiography shows the typical appearance of moyamoya disease. The right MMA arises from the petrous ICA (*long arrows*). The left MMA is dilated due to transdural collateral circulation (*short arrow*). (**b**) Reformatted MR angiographic source image shows the anomalous origin of the right MMA (*long arrow*). The enlarged left MMA is penetrating the FS (*short arrow*). (**c**) CT of the skull base with bone window shows the absence of the right FS (*long arrow*). The left FS is enlarged and fused with the foramen ovale (*short arrow*)

References

1. Uchino A, Saito N, Mizukoshi W, Okada Y. Anomalous origin of the occipital artery diagnosed by magnetic resonance angiography. Neuroradiology. 2011;53:853–7.
2. Özgür Ö, Sindel M, Hizay A, Öztürk S, Aytaç G, Sindel T. Occipital artery arising from the internal carotid artery: a case report. Surg Radiol Anat. 2017;39:219–22.
3. Lasjaunias P, Théron J, Moret J. The occipital artery. Anatomy—normal arteriographic aspects—embryological significance. Neuroradiology. 1978;15:31–7.
4. Uchino A, Saito N. Occipital artery arising from the cervical internal carotid artery at the level of the C2 vertebral body: three cases detected utilizing magnetic resonance angiography. Surg Radiol Anat. 2020;42:831–4.
5. Yoshikawa G, Kawashima M, Tsutsumi K. Carotid endarterectomy for treatment of tandem carotid stenosis in the presence of the anomalous origin of the occipital artery arising from the cervical internal carotid artery: a case report. J Med Case Rep. 2013;7:254.
6. Uchino A, Saito N, Okano N, Kakehi Y. Aberrant internal carotid artery associated with occipital artery arising from the internal carotid artery. Surg Radiol Anat. 2015;37:1137–40.
7. De Freitas S, Malas MB. Ectopic origin of the ascending pharyngeal artery: implications for carotid surgery. Surg Radiol Anat. 2018;40:1181–3.
8. Maki Y, Kurosaki Y, Ishibashi R, Morita T, Chin M, Yamagata S. The use of the carotid sheath as a rotation anchor to detect an anomalous ascending pharyngeal artery in carotid endarterectomy. Ann Vasc Surg. 2018;53:273.e1–5.
9. Hacein-Bey L, Daniels DL, Ulmer JL, Mark LP, Smith MM, Strottmann JM, Brown D, Meyer GA, Wackym PA. The ascending pharyngeal artery: branches, anastomoses, and clinical significance. AJNR Am J Neuroradiol. 2002;23:1246–56.
10. Uchino A. Collateral circulation via the ascending pharyngeal artery arising from the internal carotid artery (Letter). AJNR Am J Neuroradiol. 2006;27:246.
11. LoVerde ZJ, Shlapak DP, Benson JC, Carlson ML, Lane JI. The many faces of persistent stapedial artery: CT findings and embryologic explanations. AJNR Am J Neuroradiol. 2021;42:160–6.
12. Yilmaz T, Bilgen C, Savas R, Alper H. Persistent stapedial artery: MR angiographic and CT findings. AJNR Am J Neuroradiol. 2003;24:1133–5.
13. Uchino A, Saito N, Takahashi M, Kurita H, Ishihara S. Cerebral arterial variations associated with moyamoya disease diagnosed by MR angiography. Neuroradiol J. 2014;27:697–701.

Carotid-Vertebrobasilar Anastomoses

5

Abstract

This chapter includes (1) Persistent trigeminal artery and its variants, (2) Persistent hypoglossal artery and its variants, (3) Ascending pharyngeal artery-posterior inferior cerebellar artery anastomosis, (4) Ascending pharyngeal artery-vertebral artery anastomosis via the jugular foramen (Transjugular artery), (5) Type 1 proatlantal artery (Persistent proatlantal artery), (6) Type 2 proatlantal artery (Persistent first intersegmental artery), and (7) Persistent second intersegmental artery (True persistent otic artery may not exist). There are 27 figures and 4 illustrations.

The above entities are rare and usually found incidentally, but they can have clinical significance. Their variance can represent aneurysm formation at the origin of the anomalous artery, cerebral ischemia due to unique blood flow, or other complications. Thus, the recognition and correct diagnosis of these anomalous vessels are important when interpreting MR and CT angiography findings.

Keywords

Ascending pharyngeal artery · Carotid-vertebrobasilar anastomoses · Persistent hypoglossal artery · Persistent trigeminal artery · Proatlantal artery

5.1 Persistent Trigeminal Artery (PTA) and Its Variants

5.1.1 Lateral Type (Usual Type) PTA

There are several types of carotid-vertebrobasilar anastomoses (Fig. 5.1) [1]. The PTA is the most cephalically located and frequently occurring anastomosis between the carotid and vertebrobasilar arterial systems. The traditional Salzman's classification [2] of the PTAs is based on the absence of the ipsilateral PCoA (Type 1) or the P1 segment of the ipsilateral PCA (Type 2). This traditional classification and its modified version cited by Weon et al. [3] may be useful for hemodynamic evaluations. However, these classifications seem meaningless, as the PCA is supratentorial, and the PTA is infratentorial, and no developmental relationship exists between the two arteries [4]. Salas et al. [5] classified the PTA into two types according to the relationship to the abducens nerve, lateral and medial types. These two types of PTA may have different embryonic origins. Including PTA variants, there are four types of PTA (Fig. 5.2). Extremely rarely, bilateral PTAs have been reported [6].

According to the large MR angiographic series [4], the prevalence of the PTA is 0.29%, and approximately 90% of PTAs are the lateral type. When PTAs are large, the proximal BA is

A. Uchino, *Atlas of the Supraaortic Craniocervical Arterial Variations*,
https://doi.org/10.1007/978-981-16-6803-6_5

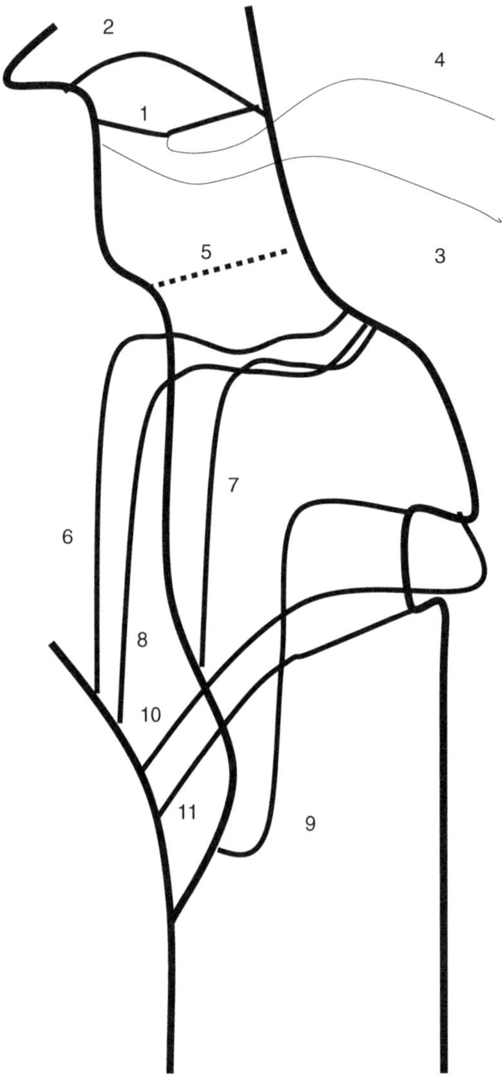

Fig. 5.1 Schematic illustration of carotid-vertebrobasilar anastomoses in the lateral projection. (Modified from [1]). 1: Lateral type persistent trigeminal artery (PTA), 2: Medial type PTA, 3: PTA variants (cerebellar arteries arising from the ICA), 4: Cerebellar artery arising from the lateral type PTA (another rare PTA variant), 5: Persistent otic artery may not exist. 6: Transjugular artery, 7: Persistent hypoglossal artery (PHA), 8: ECA origin PHA, 9: Type 1 proatlantal artery (Persistent proatlantal artery), 10: Type 2 proatlantal artery (Persistent first intersegmental artery), 11: Persistent second intersegmental artery

hypoplastic (Fig. 5.3). An aneurysm can rarely be seen at the origin of the PTA (Fig. 5.4). When the aneurysm ruptures, a carotid-cavernous fistula develops.

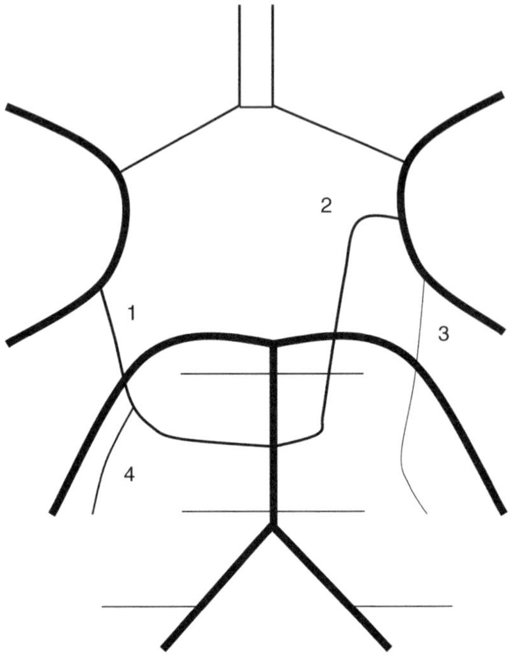

Fig. 5.2 Schematic illustration of persistent trigeminal artery (PTA) and its variants in the I-S projection. (Modified from [1]). 1: Lateral type (usual type) PTA, 2: Medial type (intrasellar type) PTA, 3: PTA variants (cerebellar arteries arising from ICA), 4: Cerebellar artery arising from lateral type PTA (another rare PTA variant)

The lateral type PTA has a tendency to arise more proximally than the medial type (Fig. 5.2). Rarely, lateral type PTA arises from the proximal precavernous segment (Fig. 5.5). This low-lying PTA should not be confused with a persistent otic artery (POA). All previously reported cases of POA diagnosed by catheter angiography seem to have been PTA [7]. Because true POA runs in the internal auditory canal, it can be diagnosed using source images of MR or CT angiography. Lateral type PTA arising from the arterial ring of the cavernous ICA has also been reported (Fig. 5.6) [8].

5.1.2 Medial Type (Intrasellar Type) PTA

As mentioned above, Salas et al. [5] classified the PTA into two types according to the relationship to the abducens nerve. Medial type PTA runs superior to the abducens nerve and takes a medial

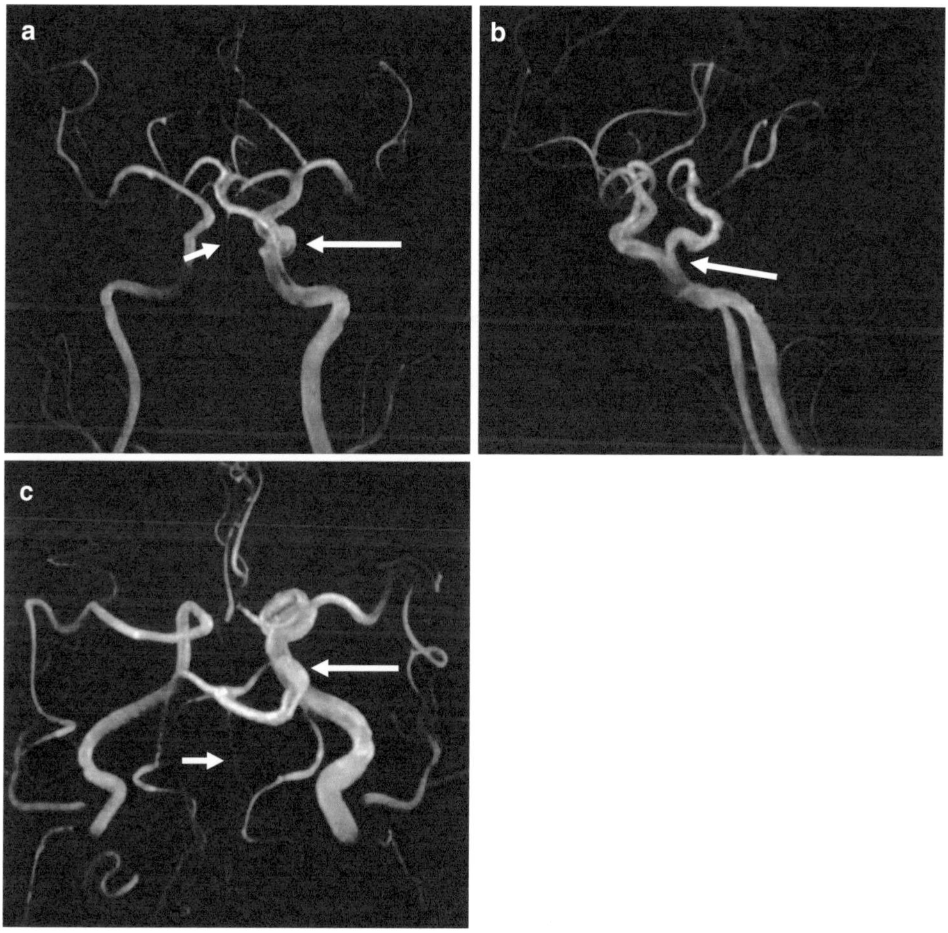

Fig. 5.3 (**a**) A-P, (**b**) lateral and (**c**) I-S projections of MR angiography show large left lateral type PTA arising from the cavernous ICA (*long arrows*). The proximal BA is extremely hypoplastic (*short arrows*). "Tau sign" is seen in the lateral projection (*arrow, b*)

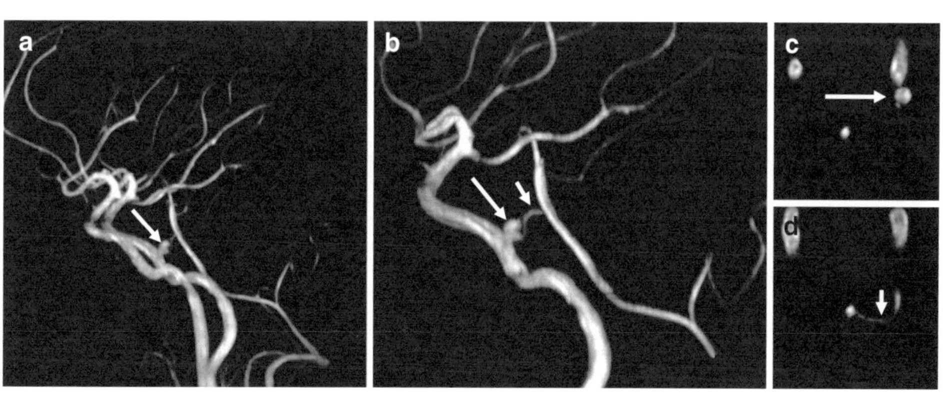

Fig. 5.4 (**a**) Lateral projection of MR angiography, (**b**) partial MIP image and (**c**, **d**) source images show an aneurysm at the cavernous ICA (*long arrow*). A small artery (*short arrow*) arises from the neck of the aneurysm and fuses to the BA, indicating small left lateral type PTA. The proximal BA is normal sized

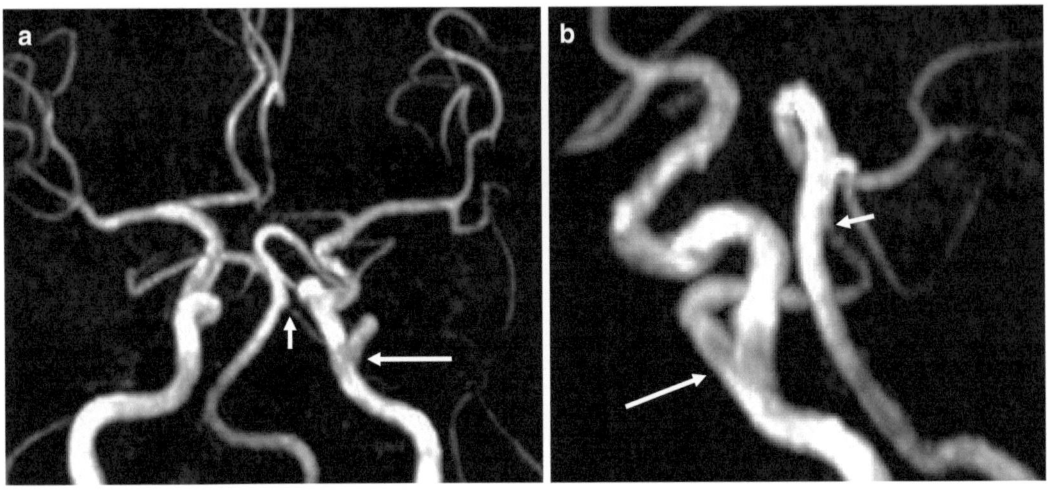

Fig. 5.5 (**a**) A-P and (**b**) lateral partial MIP image show left lateral type PTA arising from the proximal precavernous segment of the ICA (*long arrows*). This low-origin PTA anastomoses to the distal BA (*short arrows*). This type of PTA should not be misinterpreted as a persistent otic artery

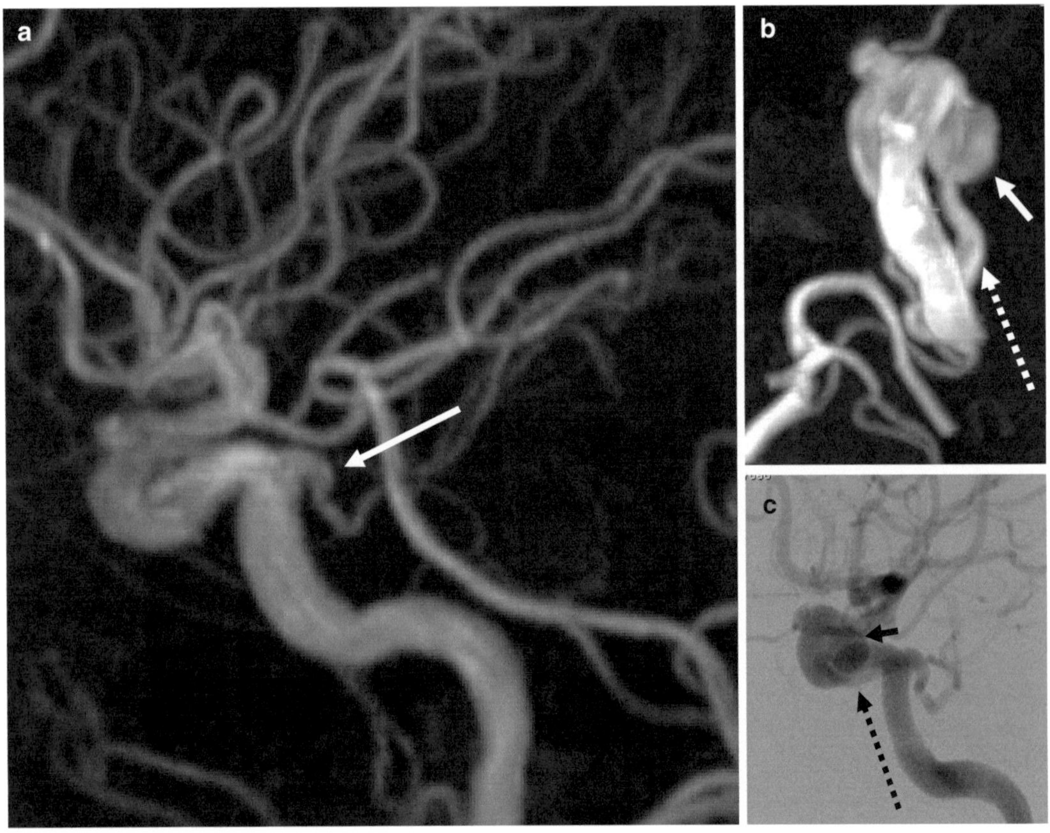

Fig. 5.6 (**a**) Lateral projection of MR angiography shows left PTA (*long arrow*). (**b**) Partial MIP I-S projection of MR angiography and (**c**) lateral projection of left internal carotid angiography show a laterally located connecting artery between the PTA and carotid siphon, forming a large arterial ring (*dotted arrows*). There is a paraclinoid aneurysm (*short arrows*)

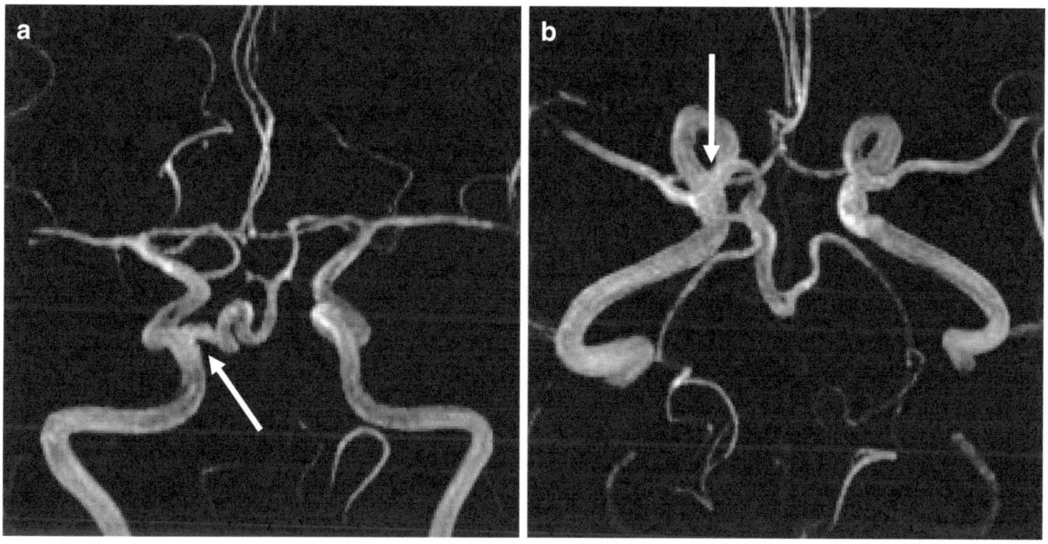

Fig. 5.7 (**a**) A-P and (**b**) I-S projections of MR angiography show a large right PTA. It arises from the cavernous ICA (*arrows*) and takes a medial course, subsequently turning posteriorly, which is indicative of a medial type PTA. The proximal BA is aplastic

course to the pituitary fossa, ultimately penetrating the dorsum sellae and fusing with the anterior wall of the BA (Fig. 5.7). Only approximately 10% of PTAs are classified as the medial type [4, 9]. This is also called intrasellar PTA, and transsphenoidal pituitary surgery is particularly dangerous. The point of origin of the medial type from the ICA is usually more distal than that of the lateral type. It can arise from the carotid siphon (Fig. 5.8), and extremely rarely, an aneurysm can be seen at the trunk of the medial type PTA (Fig. 5.9) [10].

5.1.3 PTA Variants (Cerebellar Arteries Arising from the ICA)

Cerebellar arteries rarely arise directly from the cavernous or precavernous ICA without connection to the BA. These arteries are regarded as PTA variants and had a reported MR angiographic prevalence of 0.34% in a large series using 1.5-Tesla scanners [4]. However, because PTA variants are usually small in caliber, some of the tiny arteries may not be detected on MR angiography. The majority of PTA variants are AICA type (Fig. 5.10) [11]; the SCA type is rare (Fig. 5.11), and the PICA type cannot be diagnosed by MR angiography using a multislab time-of-flight (TOF) technique due to the craniocaudal direction of the blood flow in the PICA (Fig. 5.12). Extremely rarely, bilateral PTA variants can be seen (Fig. 5.13) [12, 13].

5.1.4 Cerebellar Artery Arising from the Lateral Type PTA (Another Rare PTA Variant)

Cerebellar arteries extremely rarely arise from the lateral type PTA [14]. This type of PTA can be regarded as another PTA variant [4]. The SCA arises most commonly (Fig. 5.14), followed by the AICA. Because the distal segment of the PTA is small in caliber and the blood flow in the distal segment may be slow, the distal segment sometimes may not be visualized on MR angiography, resulting in its misinterpretation as a PTA variant.

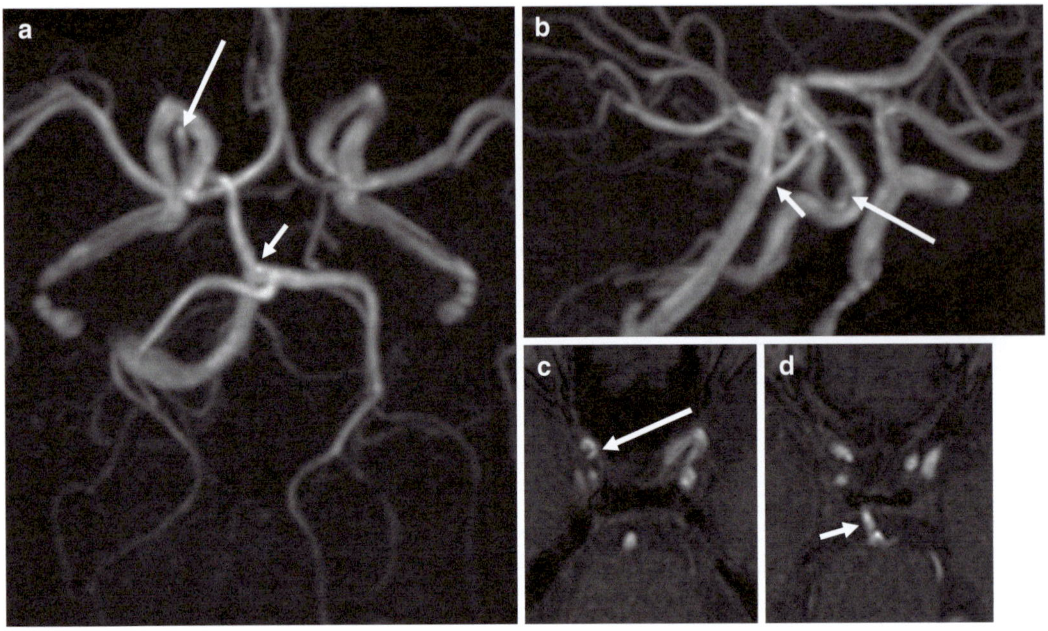

Fig. 5.8 (**a**) I-S and (**b**) RAO projections of MR angiography show a large right PTA arising from the carotid siphon, an extremely distal portion (*long arrows*). It takes a medial course and fuses with the anterior wall of the BA (*short arrows*). (**c**, **d**) MR angiographic source images show the point of origin (*c, long arrow*) and the fusing point (*d, short arrow*). (Courtesy of Dr. Harushi Mori)

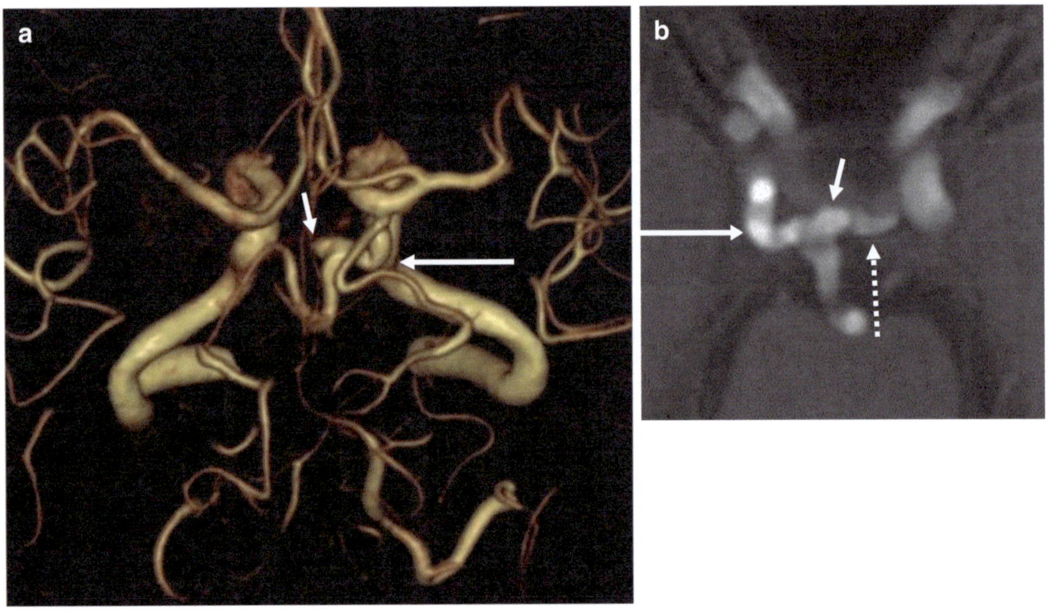

Fig. 5.9 (**a**) S-I projection of VR image of MR angiography and (**b**) reformatted source image at 5-mm thickness show a large anomalous artery arising from the cavernous segment of the right ICA (*long arrows*). The artery takes a medial course and turns posteriorly, finally anastomosing with the BA, which is indicative of a medial type PTA. At the turning point of the PTA trunk, a saccular aneurysm can be seen (*short arrows*). The *dotted arrow* indicates the posterior lobe of the pituitary gland

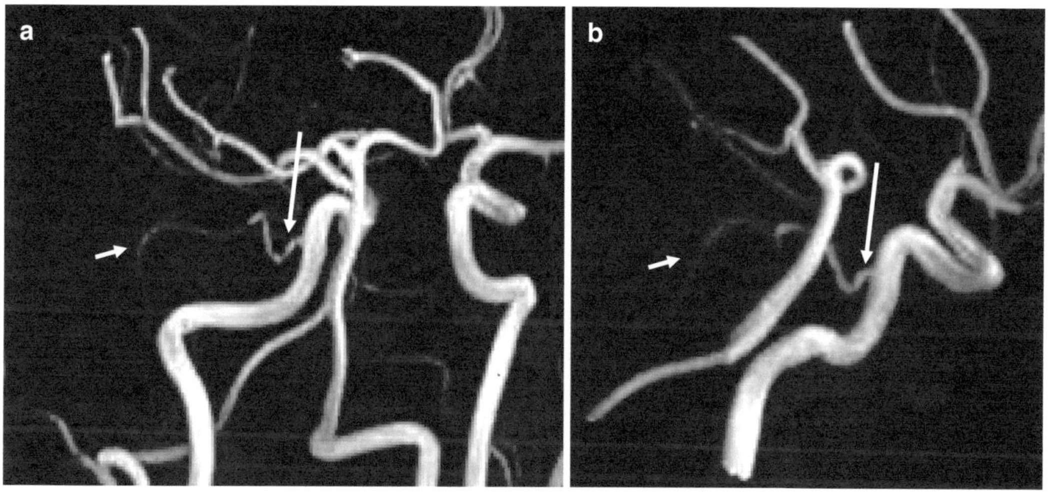

Fig. 5.10 (**a**) Slightly RAO projection of MR angiography and (**b**) lateral projection of a partial MIP image show a small artery arising from the precavernous right ICA (*long arrows*). It takes a course similar to the AICA, indicative of an AICA-type PTA variant (*short arrows*)

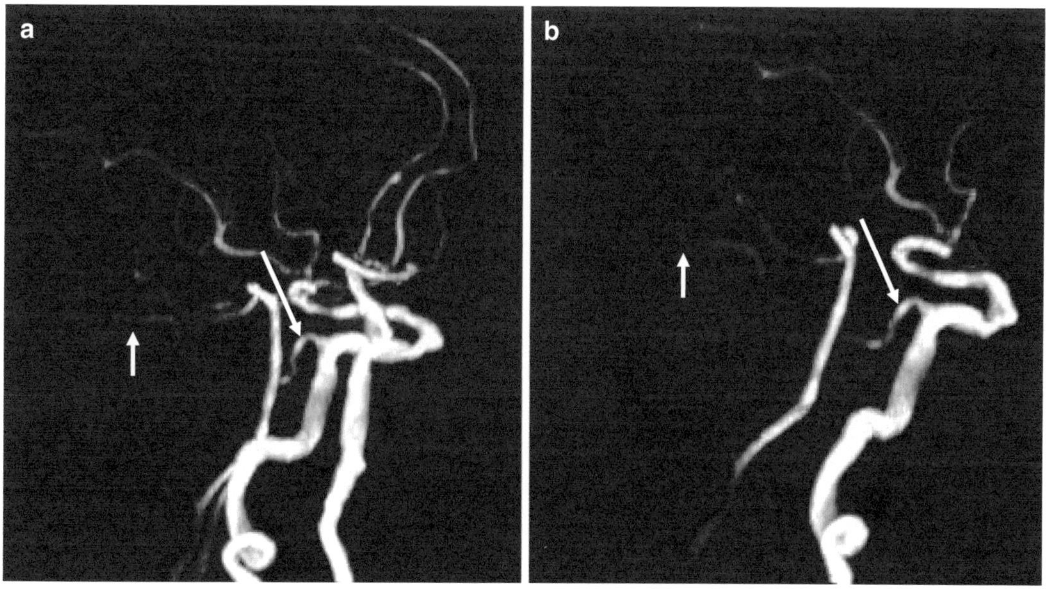

Fig. 5.11 (**a**) Nearly lateral projection of MR angiography and (**b**) lateral projection of partial MIP image show a small artery arising from the cavernous right ICA (*long arrows*). It takes a course similar to the SCA, indicative of an SCA-type PTA variant (*short arrows*)

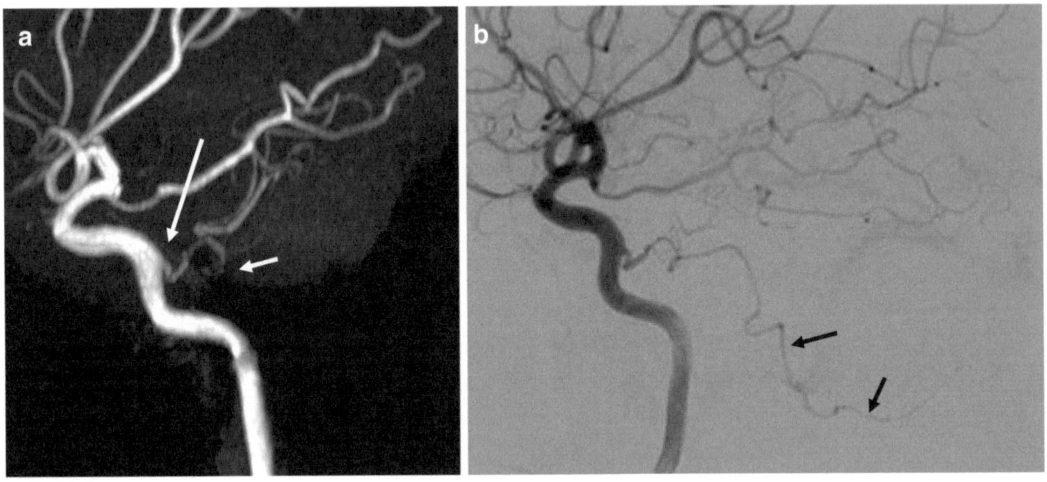

Fig. 5.12 (**a**) Lateral projection of partial MIP MR angiography shows a small artery arising from the cavernous left ICA (*long arrow*). Unfortunately, the distal segment of this artery is not visualized (*short arrow*). MR angiography obtained using a multislab TOF technique cannot demonstrate vessels in which blood flows in the craniocaudal direction. (**b**) Lateral projection of the left internal carotid angiogram shows that this artery takes a course similar to the PICA, indicative of a PICA-type PTA variant (*arrows*)

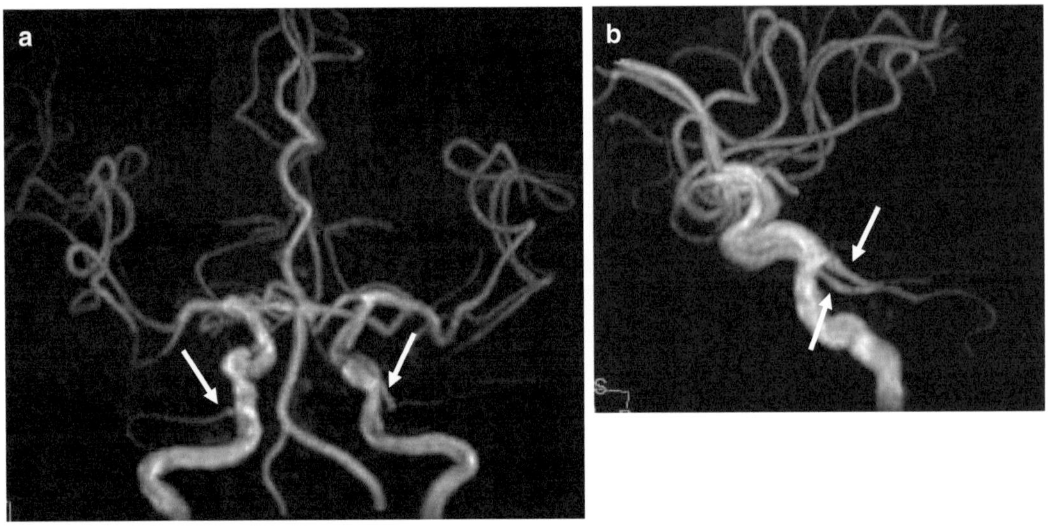

Fig. 5.13 (**a**) A-P projection of MR angiography and (**b**) partial MIP lateral image show AICAs arising from the cavernous ICAs, bilaterally, indicative of bilateral PTA variants (*arrows*)

5.2 Persistent Hypoglossal Artery (PHA) and Its Variants

5.2.1 PHA (Usual Type, Type 1)

The PHA is the second most frequently occurring anastomosis between carotid and vertebrobasilar arterial systems. It arises from the cervical ICA and enters the posterior cranial fossa via the hypoglossal canal (HC). For the definitive diagnosis of the PHA, the anomalous artery must be identified at the HC. The catheter angiographic prevalence of PHA was reported as 0.027% to 0.26% [15], but its CT angiographic prevalence was reported to be 0.29% [16]. The true prevalence may be about 0.1% in the general popula-

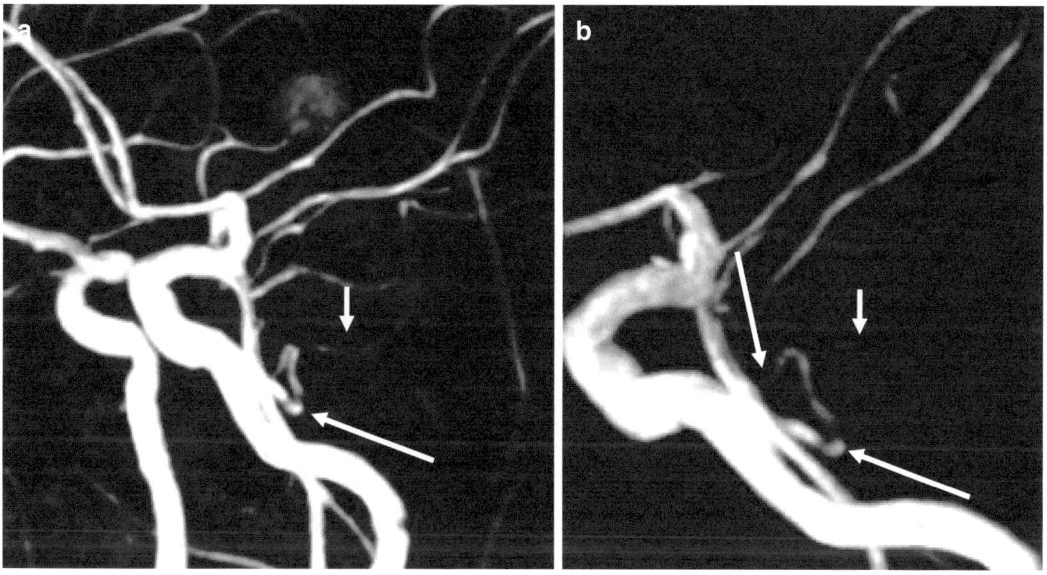

Fig. 5.14 (**a**) LAO projection of MR angiography and (**b**) partial MIP image show small left lateral type PTA (*long arrows*). The left SCA is arising from the PTA (*short arrows*), indicative of another rare PTA variant

tion. The PHA is usually large in caliber, and bilateral VAs are usually aplastic (Fig. 5.15) or hypoplastic (Fig. 5.16). Extremely rarely, a small PHA can be seen with normally developed bilateral VAs (Fig. 5.17). Even more rarely, the PHA occurs bilaterally (Fig. 5.18) [17]. A low origin of the PHA can also be seen (Fig. 5.19) [18].

5.2.2 External Carotid Artery Origin PHA (Type 2)

The PHA extremely rarely arises from the ECA (Figs. 5.20, 5.21) [19]. This type of PHA was proposed to be called type 2 PHA [16]. This anastomosis may be developmentally related to the hypoglossal branch of the APA. Occipital artery arises from some of this type of PHA [20].

5.2.3 PHA Variant (PICA Arising from the ICA Via the Hypoglossal Canal)

Extremely rarely, a small artery arises from the cervical ICA and passes the HC, eventually continuing to the PICA without connection to the VA (Fig. 5.22). This is regarded as a PHA variant [21].

5.3 Ascending Pharyngeal Artery (APA)-PICA Anastomosis

5.3.1 APA-PICA Anastomosis Via the Hypoglossal Canal

Extremely rarely, the hypoglossal branch of the APA supplies the PICA (Fig. 5.23). This variation can be regarded as another type of PHA variant [16]. Because the posterior meningeal artery also can arise from the hypoglossal branch of the APA, it should not be confused with this rare variation.

5.3.2 APA-PICA Anastomosis Via the Jugular Foramen

Extremely rarely, the jugular branch of the APA supplies the PICA (Fig. 5.24) [22, 23]. Because

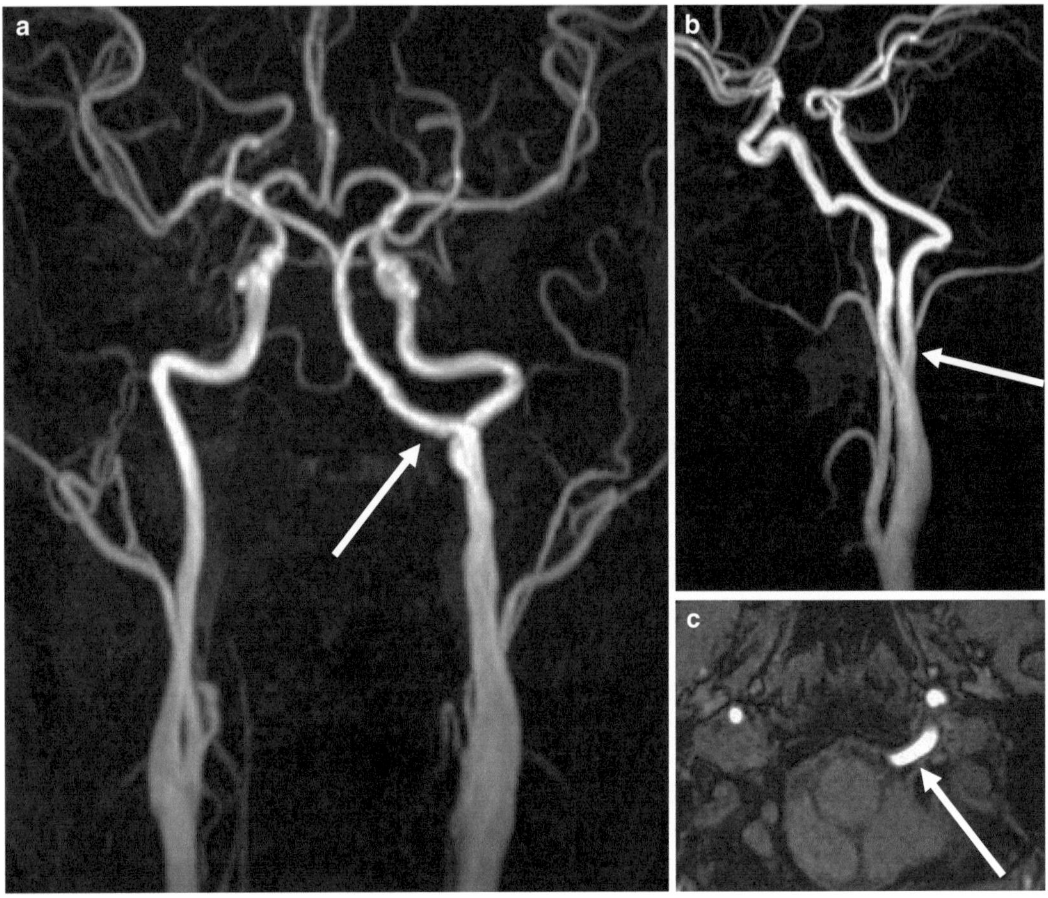

Fig. 5.15 (**a**) A-P projection of MR angiography and (**b**) lateral projection of partial MIP images show a large artery arising from the left cervical ICA (*arrows*). Bilateral VAs are not identified. (**c**) MR angiographic source image shows the artery passing the left HC, indicative of a PHA (*arrow*)

the posterior meningeal artery also can arise from the jugular branch of the APA, it should not be confused with this rare variation. Including this variation, four types of PICA supplied by the carotid system are known (Fig. 5.25) [23].

5.4 APA-Vertebral Artery (VA) Anastomosis Via the Jugular Foramen (Transjugular Artery)

Extremely rarely, congenital anastomosis between the ECA and VA via the JF is seen (Figs. 5.26 and 5.27) [24]. Because the proximal segment of the anomalous artery runs in a similar fashion to the APA, this anastomosis may be developmentally related to the jugular branch of the APA and is called the transjugular artery [25]. The anastomotic artery penetrating the clivus was also reported as the transclival artery [26].

5.5 Type 1 Proatlantal Artery (Persistent Proatlantal Artery)

There are two types of proatlantal artery: type 1 and type 2 [27]. Extremely rarely, a large artery arises from the cervical ICA and ascends to the

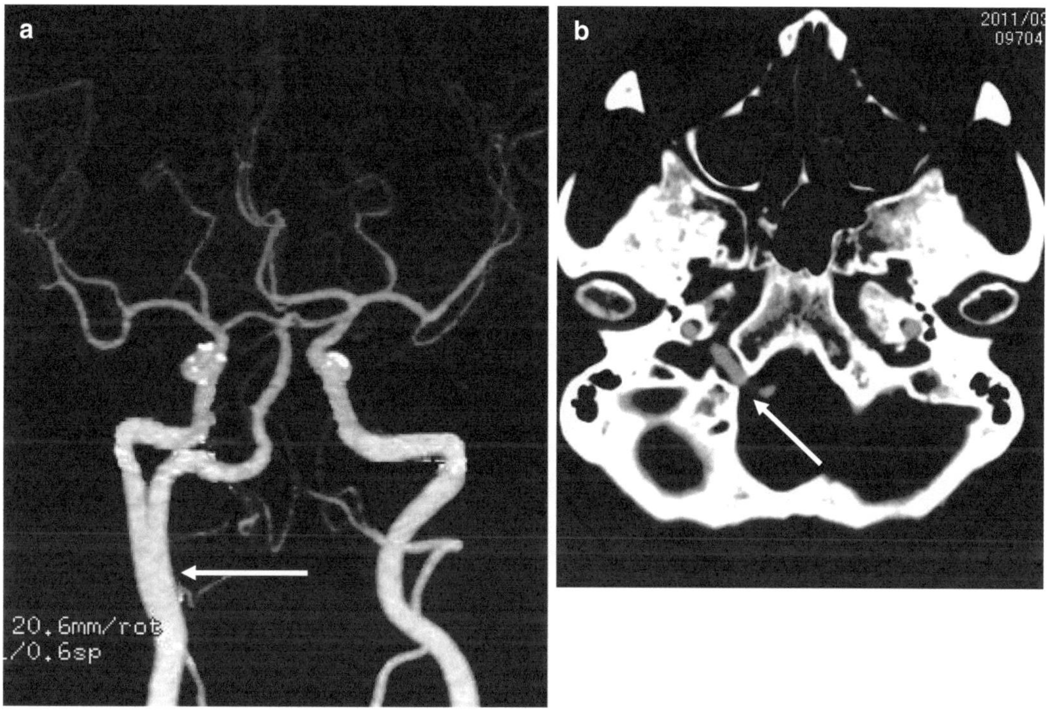

Fig. 5.16 (**a**) A-P projection of CT angiography shows a large artery arising from the right cervical ICA (*arrow*). Bilateral VAs are present but hypoplastic. (**b**) CT angiographic source image shows the artery passing the right HC, indicative of a PHA (*arrow*)

level of the occipitoatlantal space without passing through the TF. It enters the posterior cranial fossa via the anterior wall of the foramen magnum (FM), ultimately continuing to the V4 segment of the VA (Fig. 5.28). This variation is considered to be a persistent proatlantal artery and termed type 1 proatlantal artery. This variation may be associated with vascular abnormalities and variations [28, 29].

5.6 Type 2 Proatlantal Artery (Persistent First Cervical Intersegmental Artery)

Extremely rarely, a large artery arises from the proximal ECA and takes a similar course to the occipital artery and fuses with the distal V3 segment of the VA. Just before entering the posterior cranial fossa via the FM, the distal occipital artery arises (Fig. 5.29). This variation is considered a persistent first cervical intersegmental artery and termed type 2 proatlantal artery [27]. Normally, there are small anastomoses between the occipital artery and VA [30]. If a pressure gradient presents between the occipital artery and VA, these anastomoses subsequently dilate. These postnatal collateral vessels should not be confused with this variation [31]. The association of this variation with PTA was reported [32].

5.7 Persistent Second Cervical Intersegmental Artery

Extremely rarely, congenital anastomosis between the proximal segment of the ECA and proximal V3 segment of the VA is found (Fig. 5.30). The occipital artery can be seen sepa-

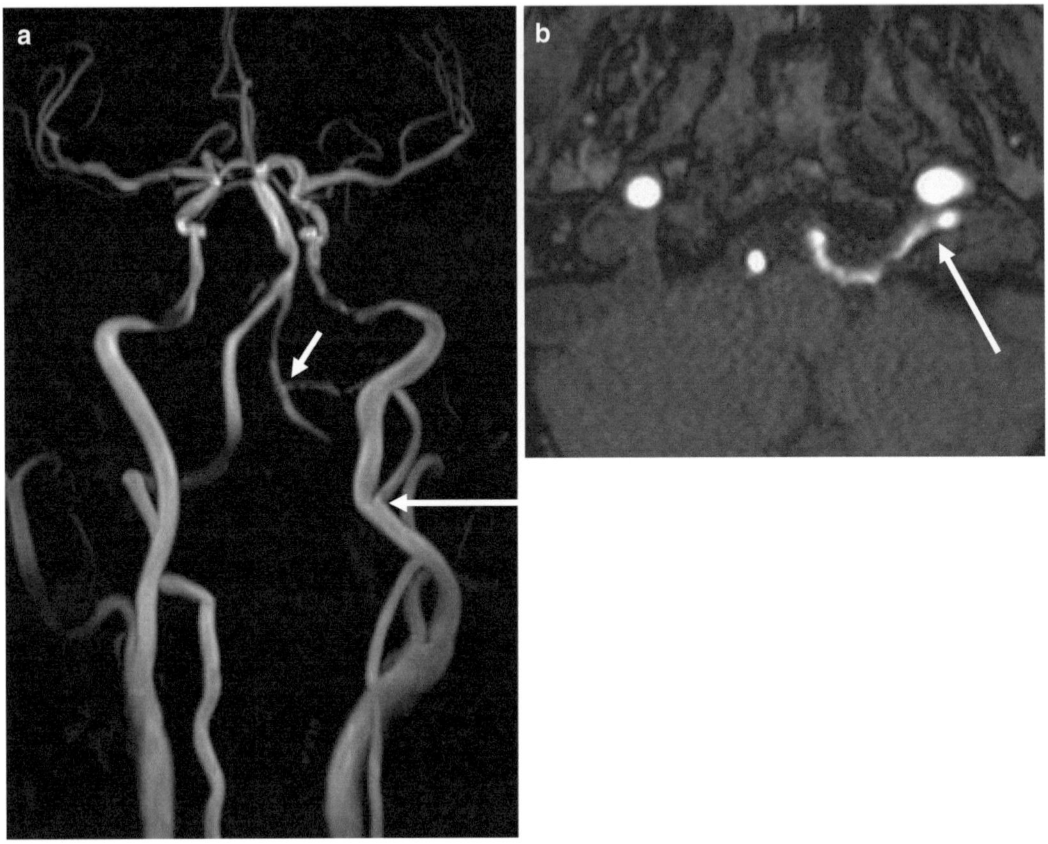

Fig. 5.17 (**a**) A-P projection of MR angiography shows a small artery arising from the left cervical ICA (*long arrow*) and fusing to the V4 segment of the left VA (*short arrow*). The bilateral VAs are normally developed. (**b**) MR angiographic source image shows the artery passing the left HC, indicative of a PHA (*arrow*)

rately. Thus, this is not a type 2 proatlantal artery (persistent first cervical intersegmental artery) and is instead regarded as a persistent second cervical intersegmental artery [33, 34]. Figure 5.31 is a schematic illustration of the development of the four types of anastomotic arteries [35].

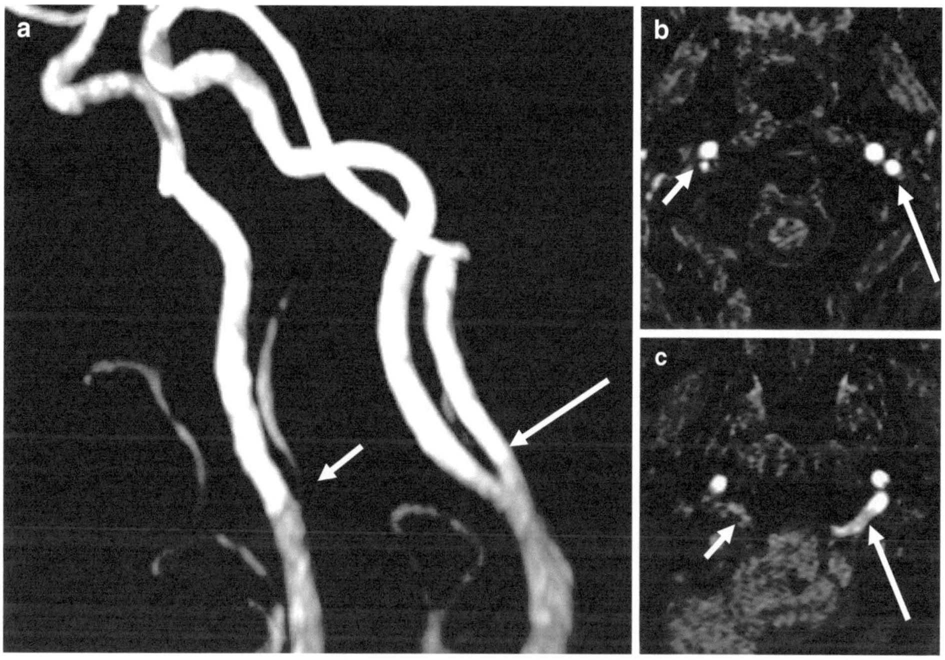

Fig. 5.18 (**a**) LAO projection of MR angiography shows a large artery arising from the left cervical ICA and continuing to the BA (*long arrow*). A small artery also arising from the right cervical ICA (*short arrow*). (**b**) MR angiographic source image at the level of C1 shows the bilateral anomalous arteries ascending dorsolateral to the cervical ICAs (*long and short arrows*). (**c**) MR angiographic source image at the level of the HC shows a large artery passing the left HC (*long arrow*). On the right side, a tiny artery is faintly visualized at the HC, suggesting bilateral PHAs (*short arrow*)

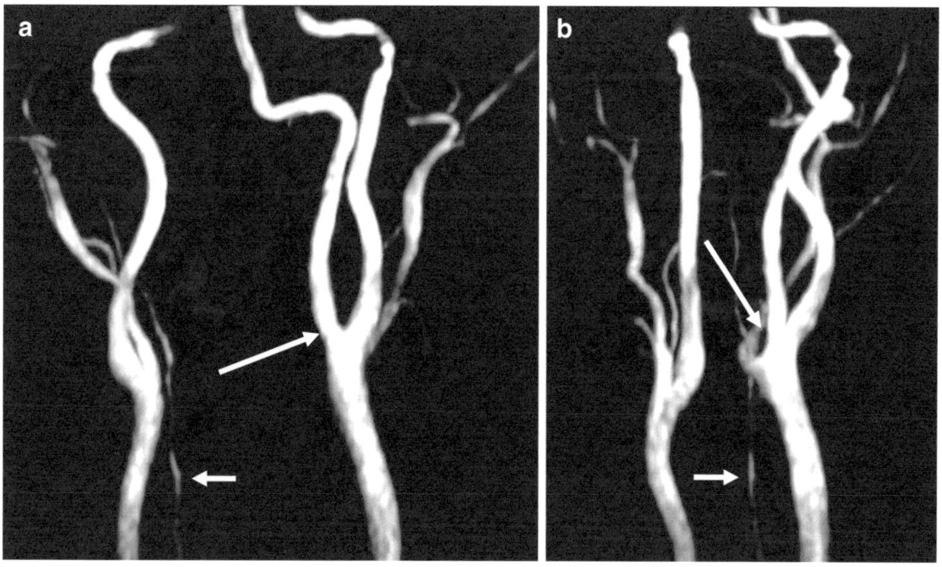

Fig. 5.19 (**a**) A-P and (**b**) LAO projections of MR angiography show a low origin of the large left PHA. Because this patient has slightly high left carotid bifurcation, the PHA arises from just distal to the carotid bifurcation (*long arrows*). Ipsilateral VA is absent, and contralateral VA is hypoplastic (*short arrows*)

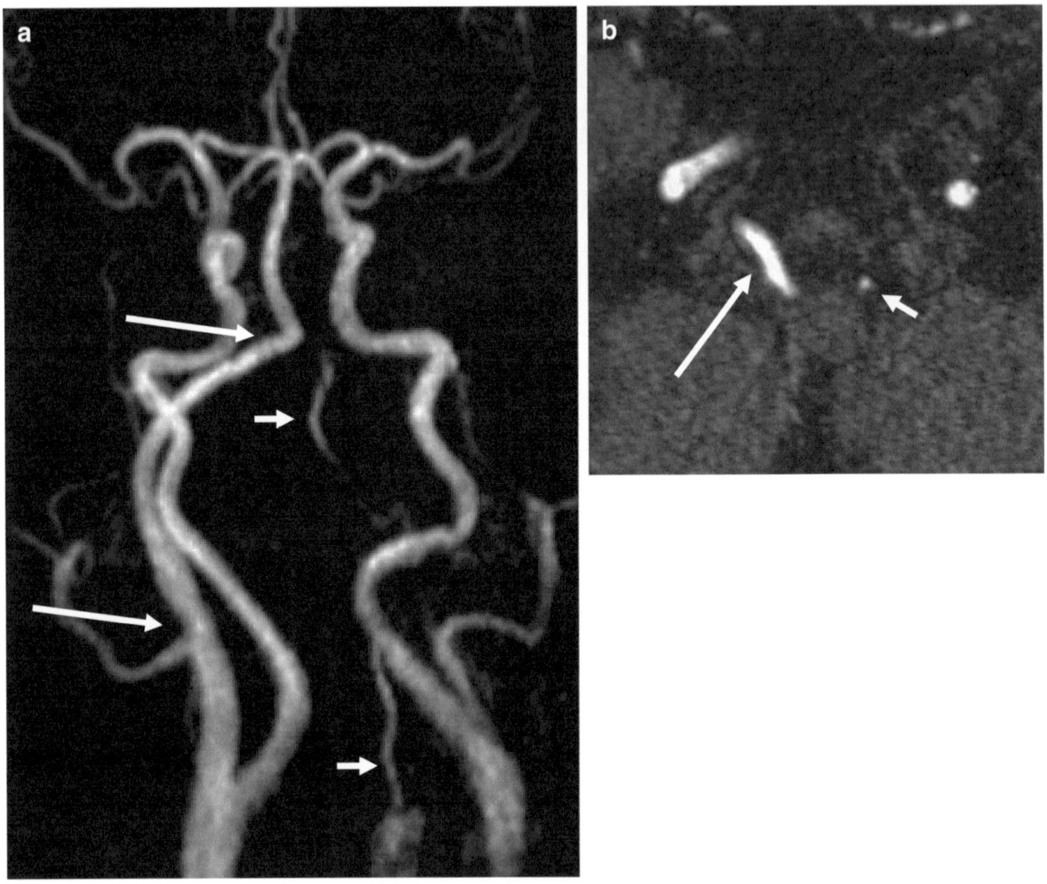

Fig. 5.20 (**a**) A-P projection of MR angiography shows a hyperplastic right ECA and a large anomalous artery arising from it and continuing to the BA (*long arrows*). The right VA is aplastic, and the left VA is hypoplastic (*short arrows*). (**b**) MR angiographic source image shows the artery passing the HC (long arrow), indicative of a PHA of ECA origin. A hypoplastic left VA can be seen (*short arrow*)

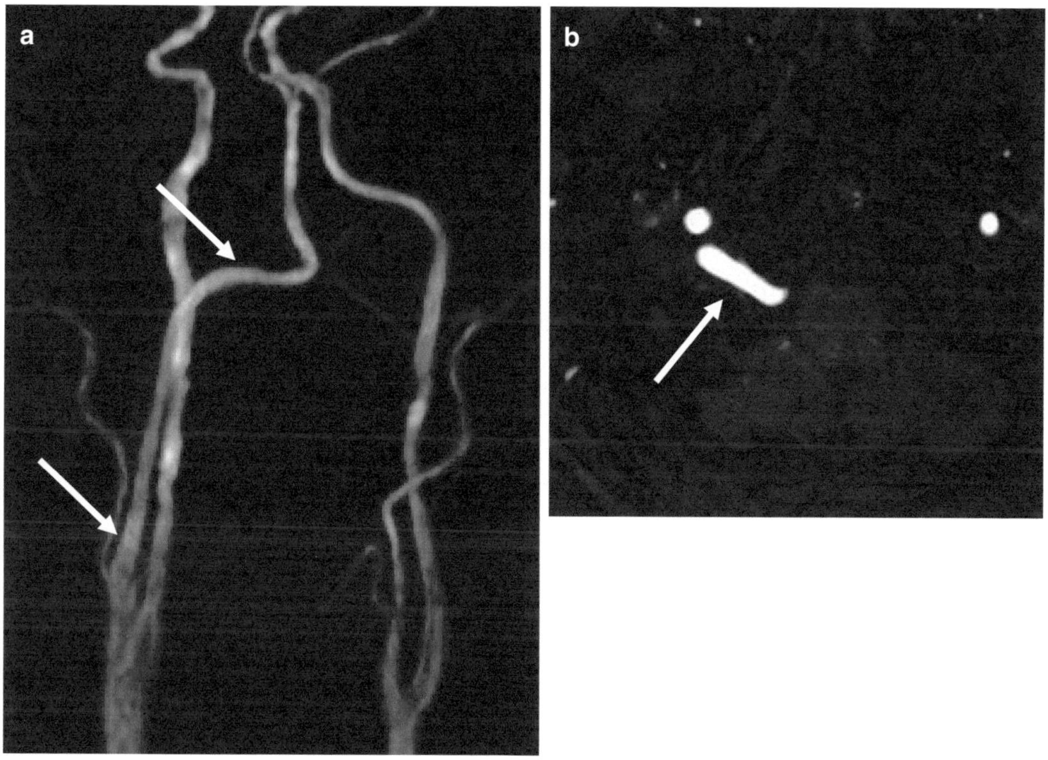

Fig. 5.21 (**a**) LAO projection of MR angiography shows hyperplastic right ECA and a large anomalous artery is arising from it and continuing to the BA (*long arrows*). Bilateral VAs are absent. (**b**) MR angiographic source image shows the artery passing the HC (*arrow*), indicative of a PHA of ECA origin

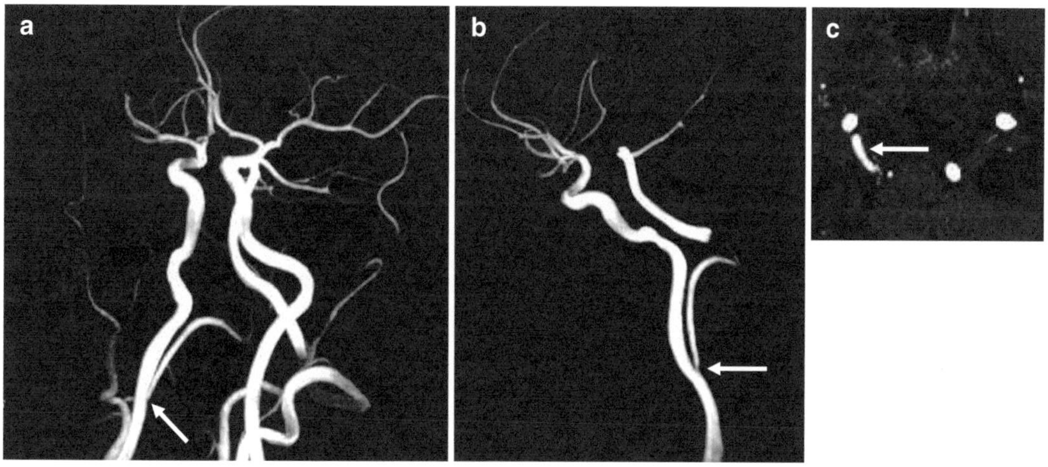

Fig. 5.22 (**a**) Slightly LAO projection of MR angiography and (**b**) partial MIP lateral image show a small artery arising from the cervical segment of the right ICA (*arrow*). (**c**) MR angiographic source image shows the artery passing the HC, but there is no connection to the VA, indicative of a PHA variant (*arrow*)

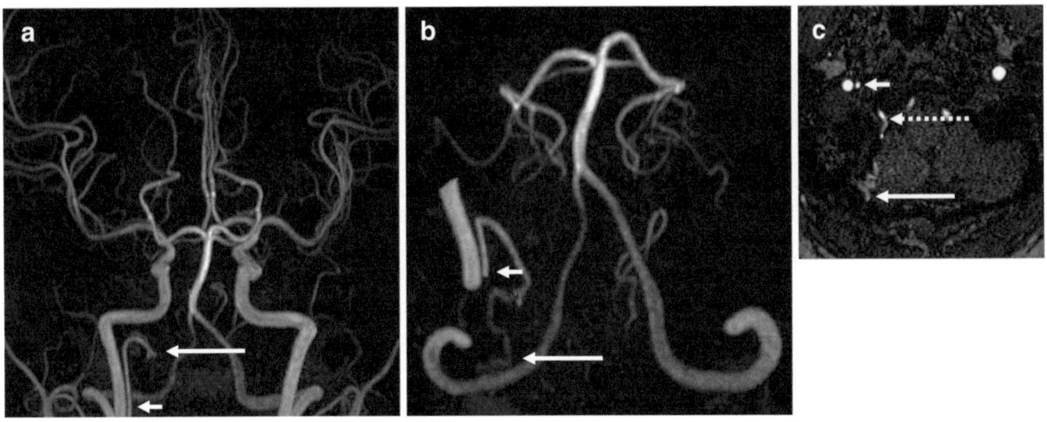

Fig. 5.23 (**a**) A-P projection of MR angiography, (**b**) partial MIP I-S projection and (**c**) MR angiographic source image show a hyperplastic right APA (*short arrows*) supplying the right PICA (*long arrows*). It passes the HC (*dotted arrow*), indicative of an APA-PICA anastomosis via the HC

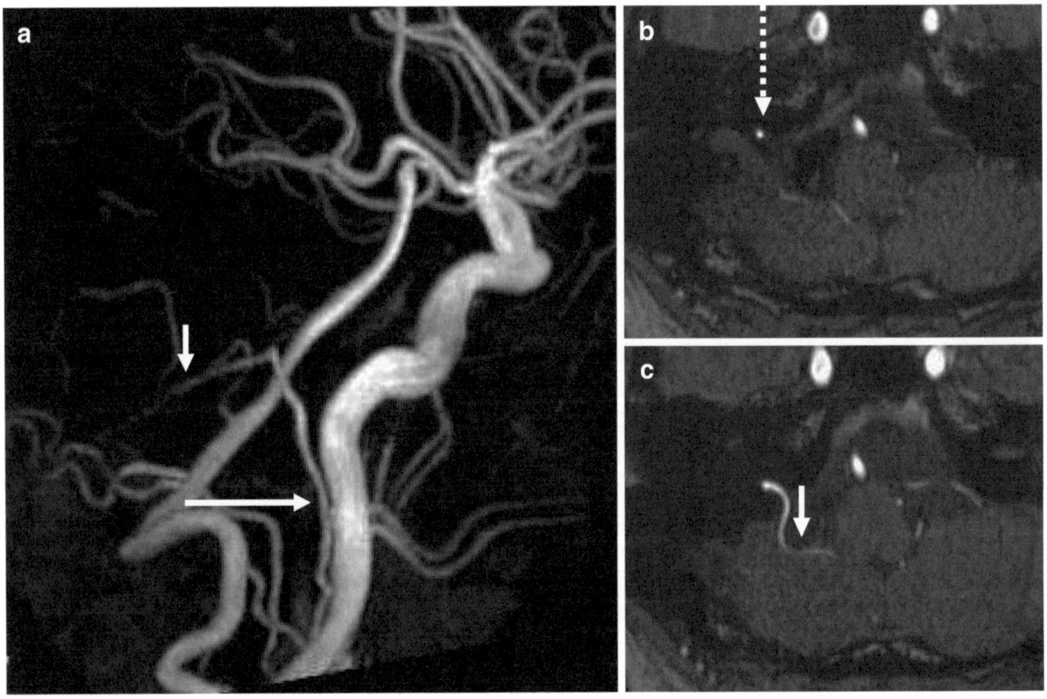

Fig. 5.24 (**a**) Lateral projection of MR angiography and (**b**, **c**) its source images show a hyperplastic right APA (*long arrow*) passing the medial side of the JF pars vascularis (*dotted arrow*) and continuing to the PICA (*short arrows*), indicative of an APA-PICA anastomosis via the JF

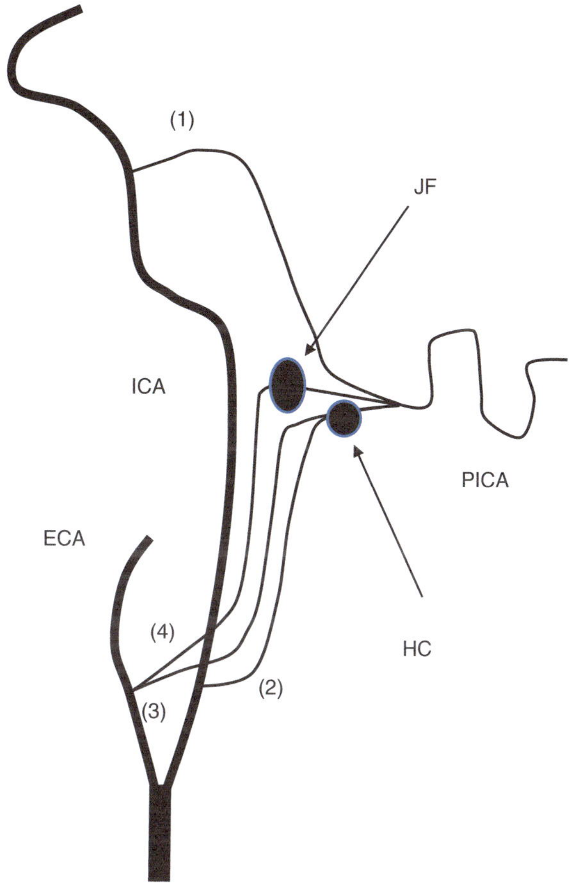

Fig. 5.25 Schematic illustrations of four types of PICA supplied by the carotid system in the lateral projection. (Modified from [23]). (1) PICA-type PTA variant (Sect. 5.1.3), (2) PHA variant (Sect. 5.2.3), (3) APA-PICA anastomosis via the HC (Sect. 5.3.1) and (4) APA-PICA anastomosis via the JF (Sect. 5.3.2). *ECA* external carotid artery, *HC* hypoglossal canal, *ICA* internal carotid artery, *JF* jugular foramen, *PICA* posterior inferior cerebellar artery

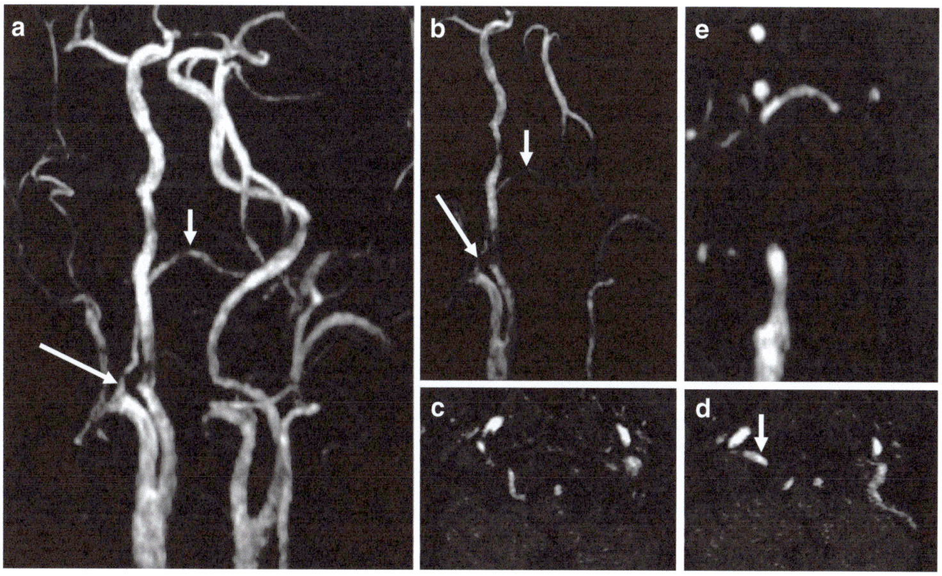

Fig. 5.26 (**a**) LAO projection of MR angiography and (**b**) partial MIP image show an anomalous artery arising from the proximal right ECA (*long arrows*) and continuing to the right VA (*short arrows*). (**c**, **d**) MR angiographic source images and (**e**) its oblique sagittal reformatted image show this artery passing the medial side of the JF pars vascularis, indicative of a transjugular artery (*short arrows*)

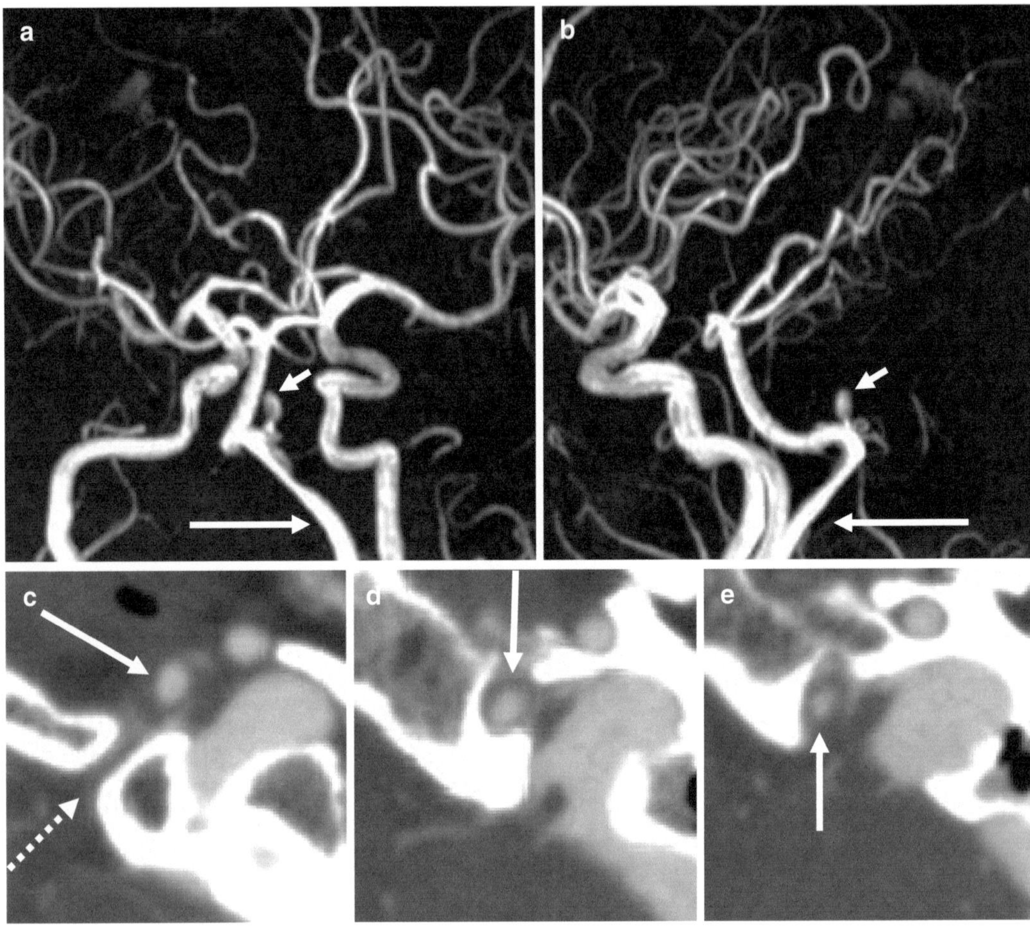

Fig. 5.27 (**a**) Slightly RAO and (**b**) lateral projection of MR angiography show a large anomalous artery taking postero-supero-medial course and continuing to the BA (*long arrows*). This artery arises from the left ECA on CT angiography (not shown). An aneurysm is seen at the proximal left PICA (*short arrows*). (**c**–**e**) CT angiographic source images show this artery passing the canal located medial side of the JF, indicative of a transjugular artery. The *dotted arrow* indicates the HC. (Courtesy of Dr. Kazufumi Kikuchi)

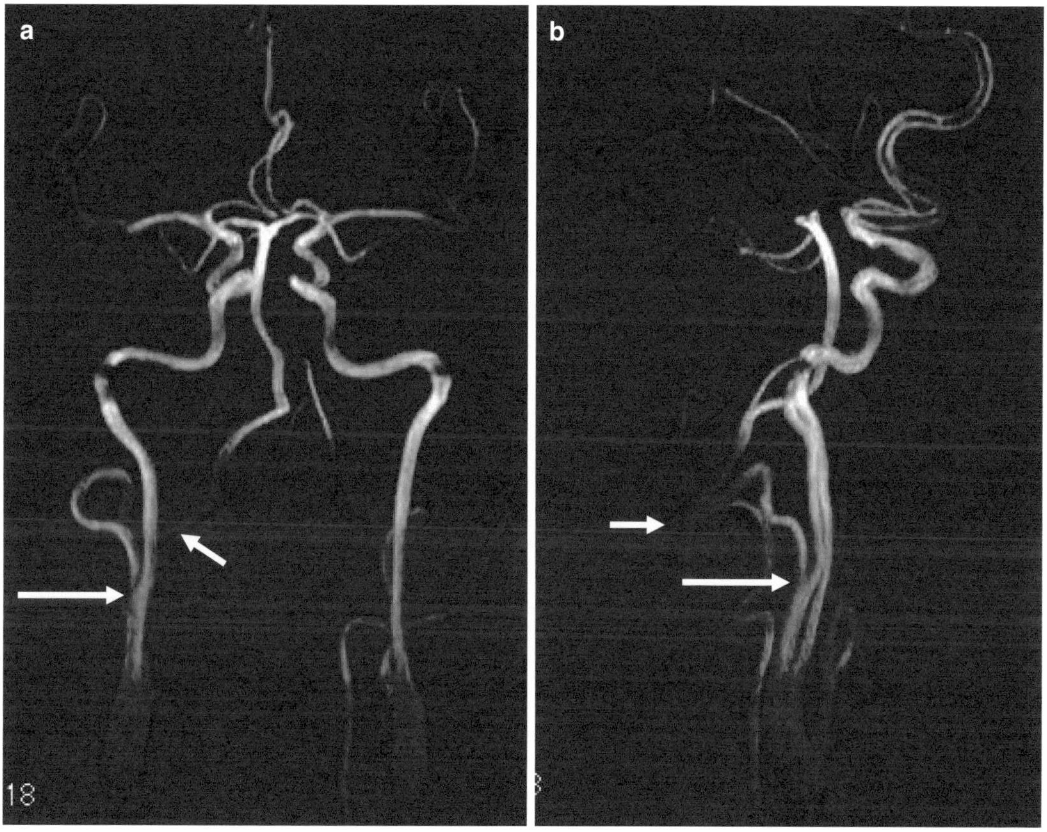

Fig. 5.28 (**a**) A-P and (**b**) lateral projections of MR angiography show a large artery arising from the cervical right ICA (*long arrows*). This artery enters the posterior cranial fossa via the FM (*short arrows*), similar to the level of normal left VA, and continues to the V4 segment of the right VA, indicative of a type 1 proatlantal artery. The proximal right VA is absent

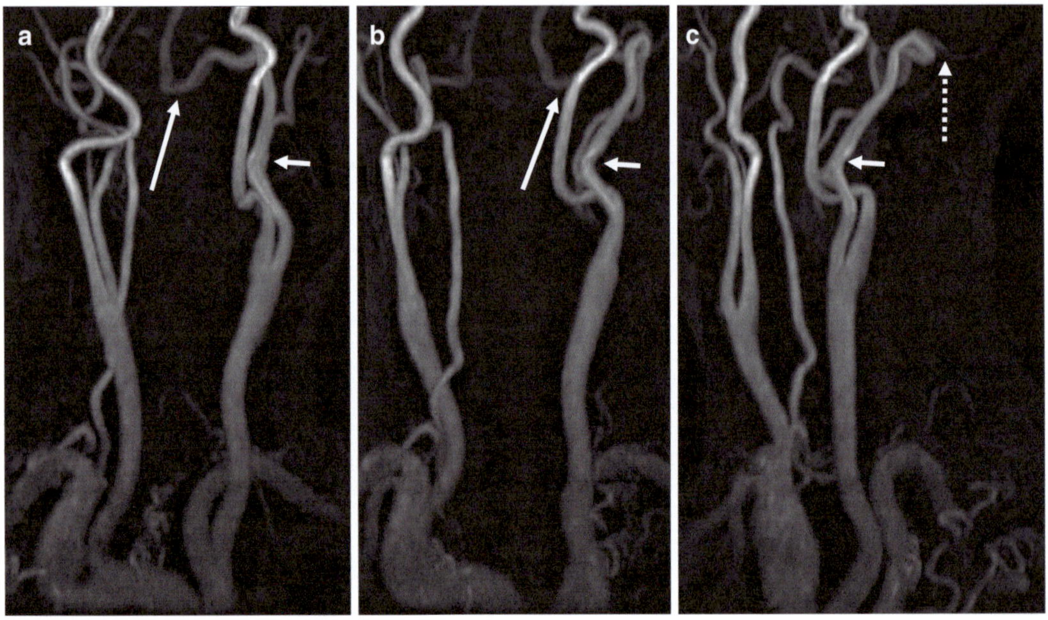

Fig. 5.29 (**a**) Slightly RAO, (**b**) A-P and (**c**) LAO projections of MR angiography show a hyperplastic left ECA and a large anomalous artery arising from its proximal segment (*short arrows*). The artery enters the posterior fossa via the FM (*long arrows*). The left occipital artery arises from this artery before entering the FM (*dotted arrow*), indicative of a type 2 proatlantal artery. The proximal left VA is absent. (Courtesy of Dr. Takashi Yoshiura)

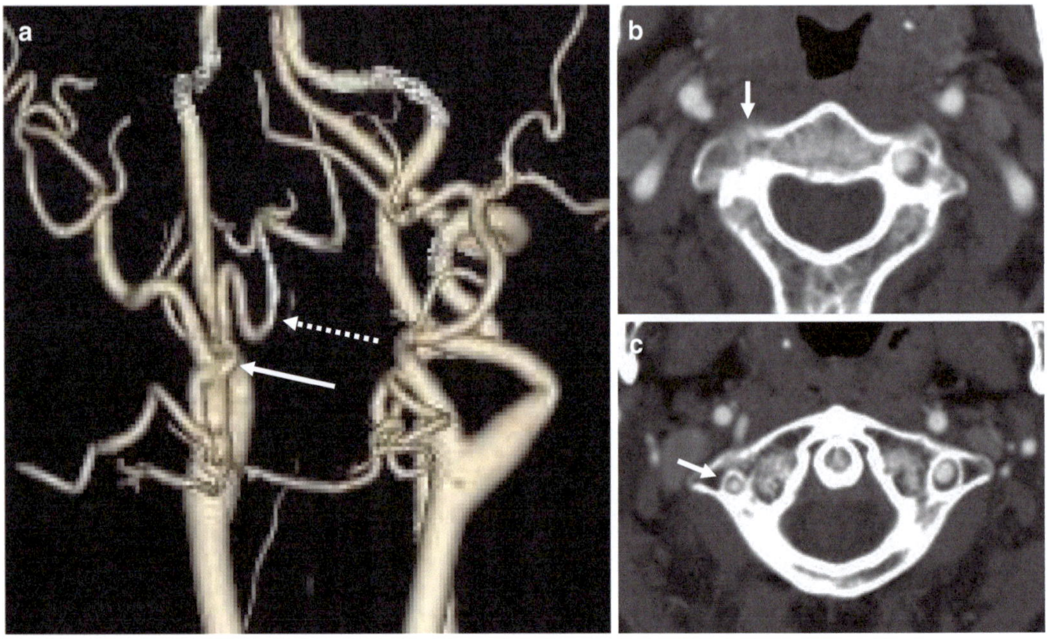

Fig. 5.30 (**a**) LAO projection of CT angiography shows an artery arising from the proximal right ECA (*long arrow*) and continuing to the proximal V3 segment of the right VA (*dotted arrow*). There is no relationship between the occipital artery. (**b**, **c**) CT angiographic source images show an absent right TF of C2 and present right TF of C1 with the VA in the foramen (*short arrows*), indicative of a persistent second cervical intersegmental artery

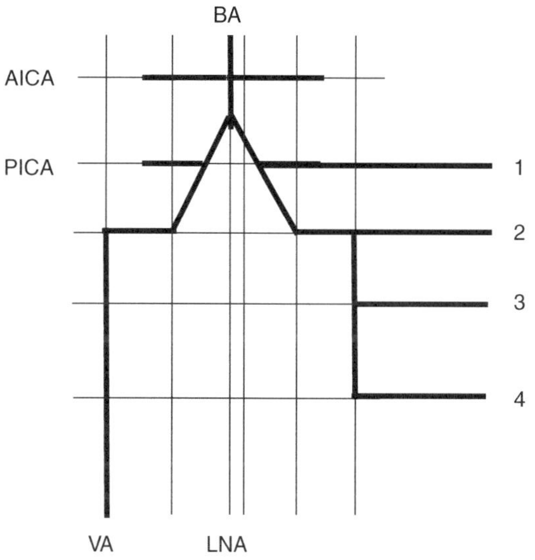

Fig. 5.31 Schematic illustration of the development of anastomotic arteries. (Modified from [35]). Four types of persistent primitive anastomotic artery exist, excluding persistent trigeminal artery. 1: Persistent hypoglossal artery, 2: Type 1 proatlantal artery (Persistent proatlantal artery), 3: Type 2 proatlantal artery (Persistent first cervical intersegmental artery), 4: Persistent second cervical intersegmental artery. *AICA* anterior inferior cerebellar artery, *BA* basilar artery, *LNA* longitudinal neural artery, *PICA* posterior inferior cerebellar artery, *VA* vertebral artery

References

1. Uchino A. Carotid-vertebrobasilar anastomosis: magnetic resonance and computed tomographic angiographic demonstration. Jpn J Radiol. 2019;37:565–78.
2. Saltzman GF. Patent primitive trigeminal artery studied by cerebral angiography. Acta Radiol. 1959;51:329–36.
3. Weon YC, Choi SH, Hwang JC, Shin SH, Kwon W-J, Kang BS. Classification of persistent primitive trigeminal artery (PPTA): a reconsideration based on MRA. Acta Radiol. 2011;52:1043–51.
4. O'uchi E, O'uchi T. Persistent primitive trigeminal arteries (PTA) and its variant (PTAV): analysis of 103 cases detected in 16,415 cases of MRA over 3 years. Neuroradiology. 2010;52:1111–9.
5. Salas E, Ziyal IM, Sekhar LN, Wright DC. Persistent trigeminal artery: an anatomic study. Neurosurgery. 1998;43:557–61.
6. Okada Y, Shima T, Nishida M, Yamada T, Yamane K, Okita S, Kagawa R. Bilateral persistent trigeminal arteries presenting with brain-stem infarction. Neuroradiology. 1992;34:283–6.
7. Bhattacharya JJ, Lamin S, Thammaroj J. Otic or mytic? AJNR Am J Neuroradiol. 2004;25:160–2.
8. Uchino A, Saito N, Kurita H, Ishihara S. Persistent trigeminal artery arising from the arterial ring/fenestration of the cavernous segment of the internal carotid artery. Surg Radiol Anat. 2012;34:651–4.
9. Uchino A, Saito N, Okada Y, Kozawa E, Mizukoshi W, Inoue K, Takahashi M. Persistent trigeminal artery and its variants on MR angiography. Surg Radiol Anat. 2012;34:271–6.
10. Uchino A, Ohno H, Kondo R, Ishihara S. Medial type persistent trigeminal artery associated with a saccular aneurysm at its trunk. Surg Radiol Anat. 2021;43:433–6.
11. Uchino A, Kato A, Takase Y, Kudo S. Persistent trigeminal artery variants detected by MR angiography. Eur Radiol. 2000;10:1801–4.
12. Uchino A. Bilateral persistent trigeminal artery variants diagnosed by MR angiography. Cerebellum. 2011;10:745–7.
13. Uchino A, Neki H, Yamane F. Right persistent trigeminal artery variant (PTAV) and tiny left PTA associated with bilateral ophthalmic arteries arising from the cavernous segments of the internal carotid arteries. Surg Radiol Anat. 2017;39:1279–83.
14. Uchino A, Sawada A, Takase Y, Kudo S, Koizumi T. Moyamoya disease associated with an anterior inferior cerebellar artery arising from a persistent trigeminal artery. Eur Radiol. 2002;12(Suppl 3):S14–7.
15. Brismar J. Persistent hypoglossal artery, diagnostic criteria. Report of a case. Acta Radiol Diagn. (Stockh) 1976;17:160–6.
16. Uchino A, Saito N, Okada Y, Kozawa E, Nishi N, Mizukoshi W, Inoue K, Nakajima R, Takahashi M. Persistent hypoglossal artery and its variants diagnosed by CT and MR angiography. Neuroradiology. 2013;55:17–23.
17. Ozawa M, Uchino A, Saito N, Maruyama H. Bilateral persistent hypoglossal arteries: a case report and literature review. Surg Radiol Anat. 2019;41:1083–5.
18. Suzuki S, Uchino A, Numaguchi Y. Low origin of the persistent hypoglossal artery associated with high carotid bifurcation: a case report. Surg Radiol Anat. 2020;42:1081–3.
19. Nakamura M, Kobayashi S, Yoshida T, Kamagata M, Sasaki T. Persistent external carotid-vertebrobasilar anastomosis via the hypoglossal canal. Neuroradiology. 2000;42:821–3.
20. Yamamoto R, Mori N, Nakae Y, Tanaka F, Johkura K. Anomalous anastomosis between the external carotid artery and vertebrobasilar artery via the hypoglossal canal: a case report and review of literature. Surg Radiol Anat. 2019;41:849–52.
21. Uchino A, Suzuki C. Variant of a persistent hypoglossal artery supplying only the posterior inferior cerebellar artery diagnosed by magnetic resonance angiography: a case report. Surg Radiol Anat. 2018;40:807–10.
22. Uchino A, Suzuki C. Posterior inferior cerebellar artery supplied by the jugular branch of the ascending pharyngeal artery diagnosed by MR angiography: report of two cases. Cerebellum. 2011;10:204–7.

23. Uchino A, Ohno H, Kondo R, Ishihara S. Ascending pharyngeal artery-posterior inferior cerebellar artery anastomosis via the jugular foramen: a case report and literature review. Surg Radiol Anat. 2021;43:1019–22.
24. Ranchod AI, Gora S, Swartz RN, Andronikou S, Mngomezulu V. A rare carotid-basilar anastomosis traversing the jugular foramen: origin and clinical implications. Interv Neuroradiol. 2011;17:347–50.
25. Vezeridis AM, Hoffman BJ, Chen JY, Imbesi SG. The transjugular artery: a rare variant carotid-basilar anastomosis. Neurographics. 2017;7:195–8.
26. Kirkland JD, Dahlin BC, O'Brien WT. The transclival artery: a variant persistent carotid-basilar arterial anastomosis not previously reported. J Neurointerv Surg. 2017;9:e11.
27. Lasjaunias P, Théron J, Moret J. The occipital artery. Anatomy—normal arteriographic aspects—embryological significance. Neuroradiology. 1978;15:31–7.
28. Basekim CC, Silit E, Mutlu H, Pekkafali MZ, Ozturk E, Kizilkaya E. Type I proatlantal artery with bilateral absence of the external carotid arteries. AJNR Am J Neuroradiol. 2004;25:1619–21.
29. Saito N, Uchino A, Ishihara S. Complex anomalies of type 1 proatlantal intersegmental artery and aortic arch variations. Surg Radiol Anat. 2013;35:177–80.
30. Uchino A. Cervical arterial collateral network (Letter). AJNR Am J Neuroradiol. 2006;27:1161.
31. Purkayastha S, Gupta AK, Varma R, Kapilamoorthy TR. Proatlantal intersegmental arteries of external carotid artery origin associated with Galen's vein malformation. AJNR Am J Neuroradiol. 2005;26:2378–83.
32. Uchino A, Saito N, Inoue K. Type 2 proatlantal intersegmental artery associated with persistent trigeminal artery diagnosed by MR angiography. Surg Radiol Anat. 2012;34:773–6.
33. Uchino A, Saito N, Kurita H. Anastomosis of the external carotid artery and the V3 segment of the vertebral artery (presumed persistent second cervical intersegmental artery) diagnosed by CT angiography. Surg Radiol Anat. 2018;40:233–6.
34. Uchino A, Saito N, Kohyama S. Persistent second cervical intersegmental artery diagnosed by MR angiography. Radiol Case Rep. 2019;14:967–70.
35. Lasjaunias P, Berenstein A, ter Brugge KG. The pharyngo-occipital system. In: Lasjaunias P, Berenstein A, ter Brugge KG, editors. Surgical neuroangiography. Vol. 1. Clinical vascular anatomy and variations. 2nd ed. Berlin: Springer; 2001. p. 165–224.

Variations of the Origin of the Ophthalmic Artery (OphA)

6

Abstract

This chapter includes (1) Ophthalmic artery arising from the cavernous internal carotid artery (Persistent dorsal ophthalmic artery), (2) Double ophthalmic arteries arising from the internal carotid artery, (3) Ophthalmic artery arising from the middle meningeal artery, (4) Double ophthalmic arteries arising from the internal carotid artery and middle meningeal artery, and (5) Ophthalmic artery arising from the anterior cerebral artery. There are 7 figures and 1 illustration.

Ophthalmic artery arising from the middle meningeal artery is not uncommon and is particularly dangerous during catheter intervention in the external carotid artery territory.

Keywords

External carotid artery · Internal carotid artery · Middle meningeal artery · Ophthalmic artery

6.1 OphA Arising from the Cavernous ICA

Normally, the OphA arises from the supraclinoid ICA and enters the orbit via the optic canal (OC). Rarely, the OphA originates from the cavernous ICA and enters the orbit via the superior orbital fissure (SOF) instead of the OC (Fig. 6.1). During early gestation, there are primitive dorsal and ventral OphAs; the dorsal OphA usually regresses, while the ventral OphA remains and forms a normal OphA. If the situation is reversed and the ventral OphA disappears and the dorsal OphA remains, this variation may be formed. Lasjaunias et al. [1] attributed this variation to a persistent dorsal OphA. The inferolateral trunk of the ICA has a tiny branch that runs towards the SOF. Should the ventral OphA regress, this tiny artery enlarges for collateral circulation and serves as an aberrant OphA that originates from the cavernous ICA. Komiyama [2] indicated this anomalous OphA should not be called a persistent dorsal OphA, as a dorsal OphA that persists passes through the OC rather than the SOF. Although this variation was traditionally termed "persistent dorsal OphA" [3], this name may not be adequate for this variation. Recently, this anomalous origin is believed to be due to the persistence and enlargement of the lateral branch of the primitive maxillary artery [4]. Its MR angiographic prevalence was reported to be 0.42% per OphA [5], and there is a tendency toward right-side predominance. Extremely rarely, it can be seen bilaterally (Fig. 6.2). This type of OphA also rarely arises from the carotid siphon, distal to the usual point but proximal to the normal arising point (Fig. 6.3).

A. Uchino, *Atlas of the Supraaortic Craniocervical Arterial Variations*,
https://doi.org/10.1007/978-981-16-6803-6_6

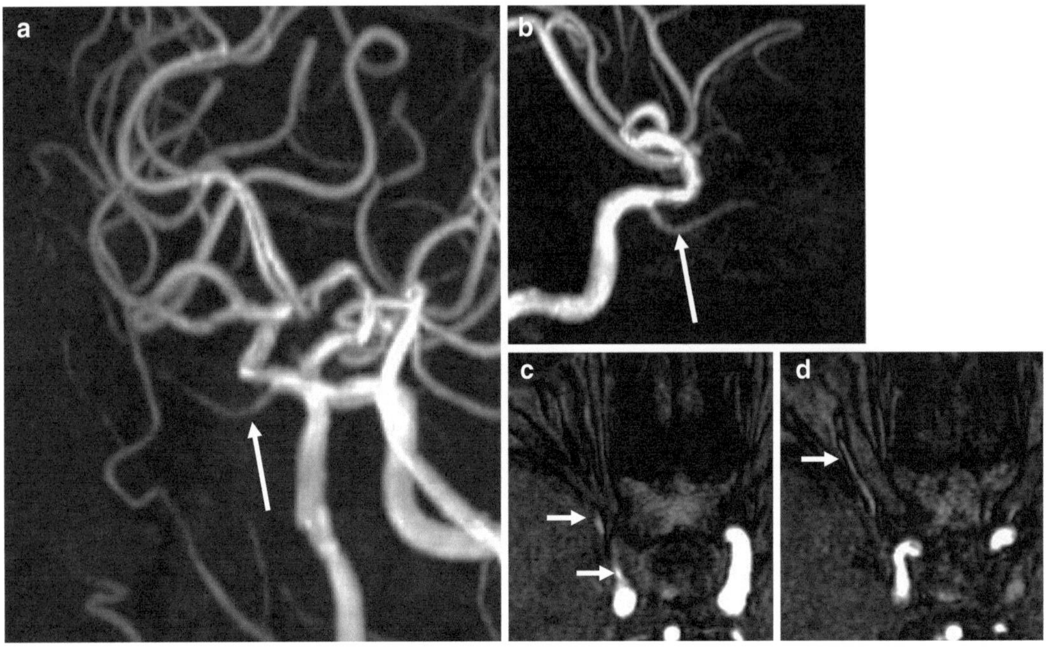

Fig. 6.1 (**a**) LAO projection of MR angiography and (**b**) partial MIP lateral image show the right OphA arising from the cavernous ICA (*long arrows*), so-called persistent dorsal OphA. (**c**, **d**) MR angiographic source images show the artery entering the orbit via the SOF (*short arrows*), not the OC

6.2 Double OphAs Arising from the ICA

Extremely rarely, two small OphAs arise from the cavernous and supraclinoid ICAs (Fig. 6.4) [6, 7]. That arising from the cavernous ICA is the same variation as described in Sect. 6.1, while that arising from the supraclinoid ICA is the normal OphA that mainly supplies the central retinal artery.

6.3 OphA Arising from the Middle Meningeal Artery (MMA)

The OphA arises relatively frequently from the MMA. Its MR angiographic prevalence was reported to be 1.45% per OphA [5]. There is right-side predominance, and the bilateral type is not rare (Fig. 6.5). This common variation is important during transarterial embolization or infusion chemotherapy in the ECA territory, as ischemic complications of the central retinal artery or retinal damage may be seen [8].

6.4 Double OphAs Arising from the ICA and MMA

Rarely, in the case of MMA origin OphA (Sect. 6.3), a normally originating small OphA can be seen (Fig. 6.6) [5]. The ICA origin OphA mainly supplies the central retinal artery. Because the ICA origin OphA is a tiny artery, some may not be identified on MR angiography. Using a 3-Tesla scanner, careful observation of source images is required for the identification of this variation.

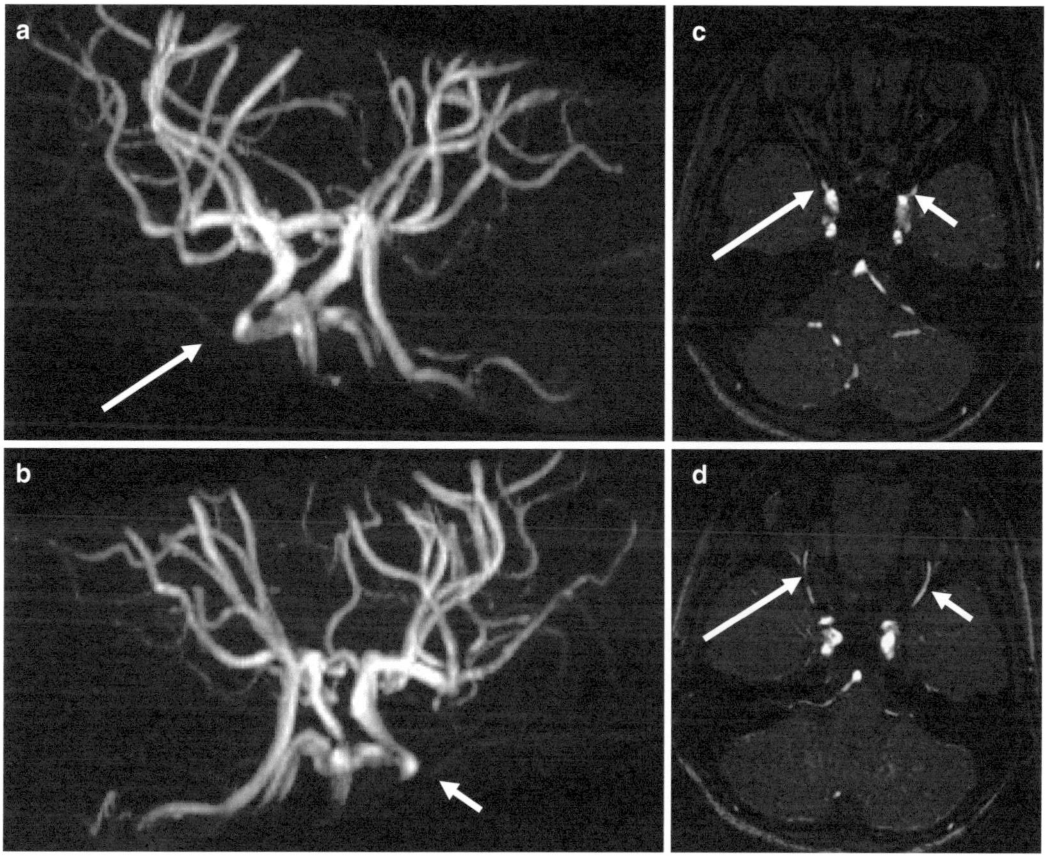

Fig. 6.2 (**a**) LAO and (**b**) RAO projections of MR angiography show bilateral OphAs arising from the cavernous segments of the ICAs (*long and short arrows*). (**c**, **d**) MR angiographic source images show the arising points of the OphAs at the cavernous ICAs and passing points at the SOFs (*long and short arrows*)

6.5 OphA Arising from the Anterior Cerebral Artery (ACA)

Extremely rarely, the OphA arises from the A1 segment of the ACA (Fig. 6.7) [9]. According to Padget [10], the ventral OphA arises from the cranial branch of the primitive ICA and migrates caudally to the normal position of the origin of the OphA. The OphA of ACA origin may be the result of a failure of this caudal migration. Most patients previously reported having this variation were identified during catheter angiography or surgery [11]. Because this vessel is a tiny artery that adopts an anteroinferior course, identification of this variation on MR angiography may be difficult. The fronto-orbital artery, which supplies the inferior surface of the frontal lobe, should not be confused with this rare variation [12].

Figure 6.8 is a schematic illustration of OphA origin and proximal course variations.

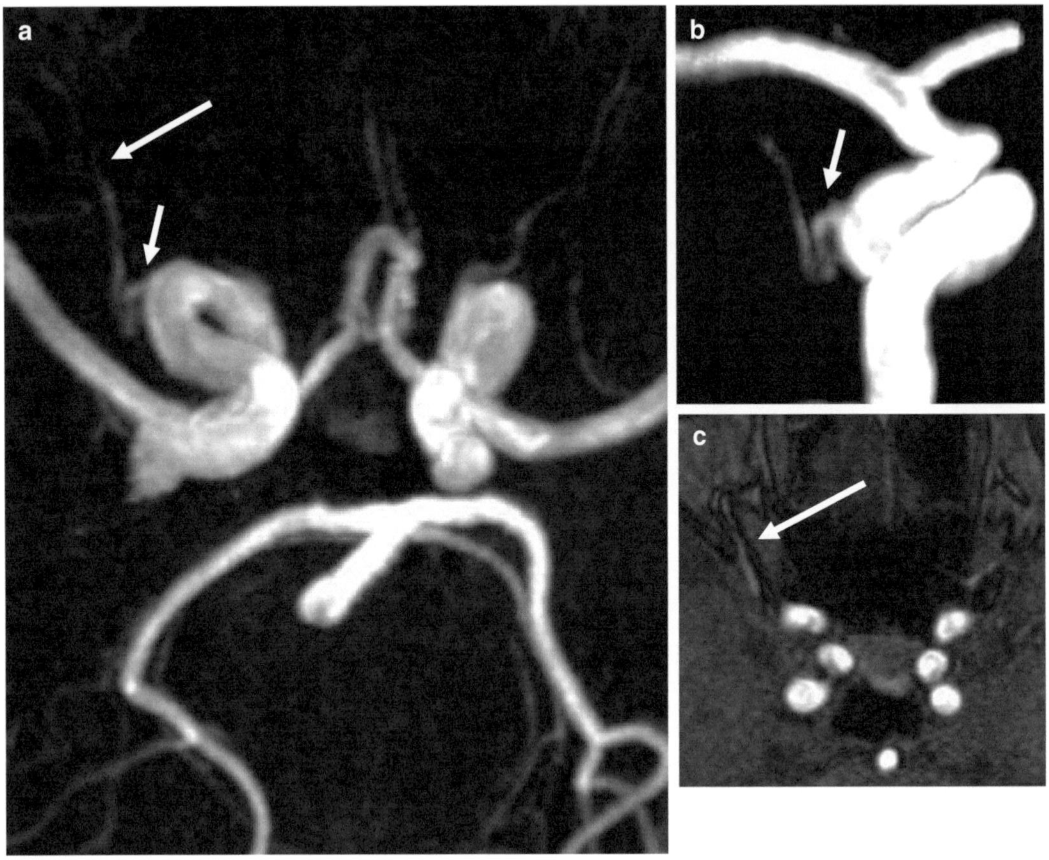

Fig. 6.3 (**a**) I-S and (**b**) LAO projections of partial MIP MR angiography show the right OphA arising from the carotid siphon (*short arrows*). The left OphA arises normally. (**c**) MR angiographic source image shows the right OphA passing through the SOF (*long arrows*), not the OC

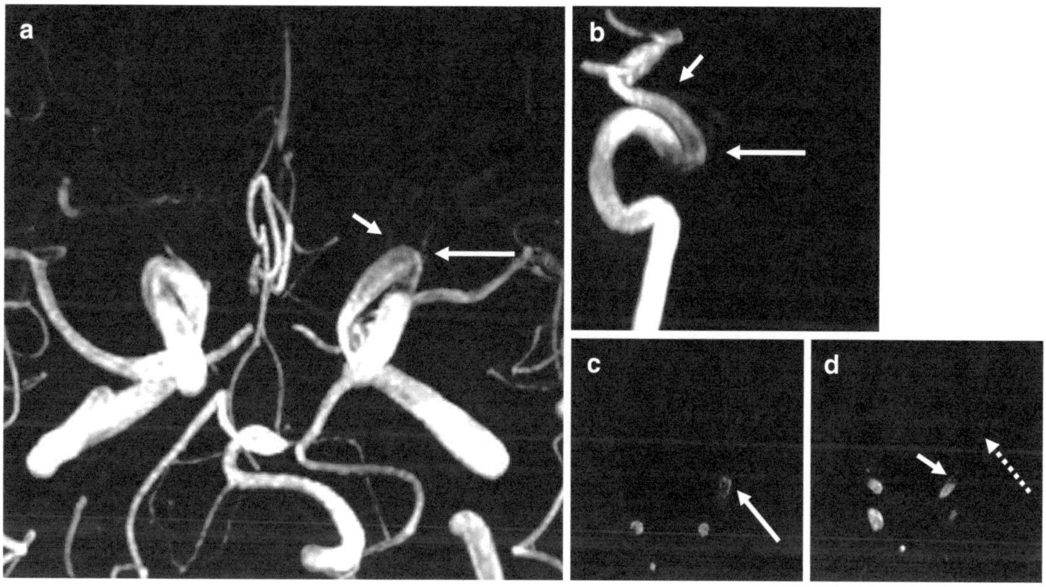

Fig. 6.4 (**a**) I-S projection of MR angiography and (**b**) partial MIP right lateral image show two small left OphAs arising from the cavernous (*long arrow*) and supraclinoid (*short arrow*) segments of the ICA. (**c**, **d**) MR angiographic source images show arising points of both OphAs (*long and short arrows*) and passing point of the cavernous ICA origin OphA in the SOF (*dotted arrow*)

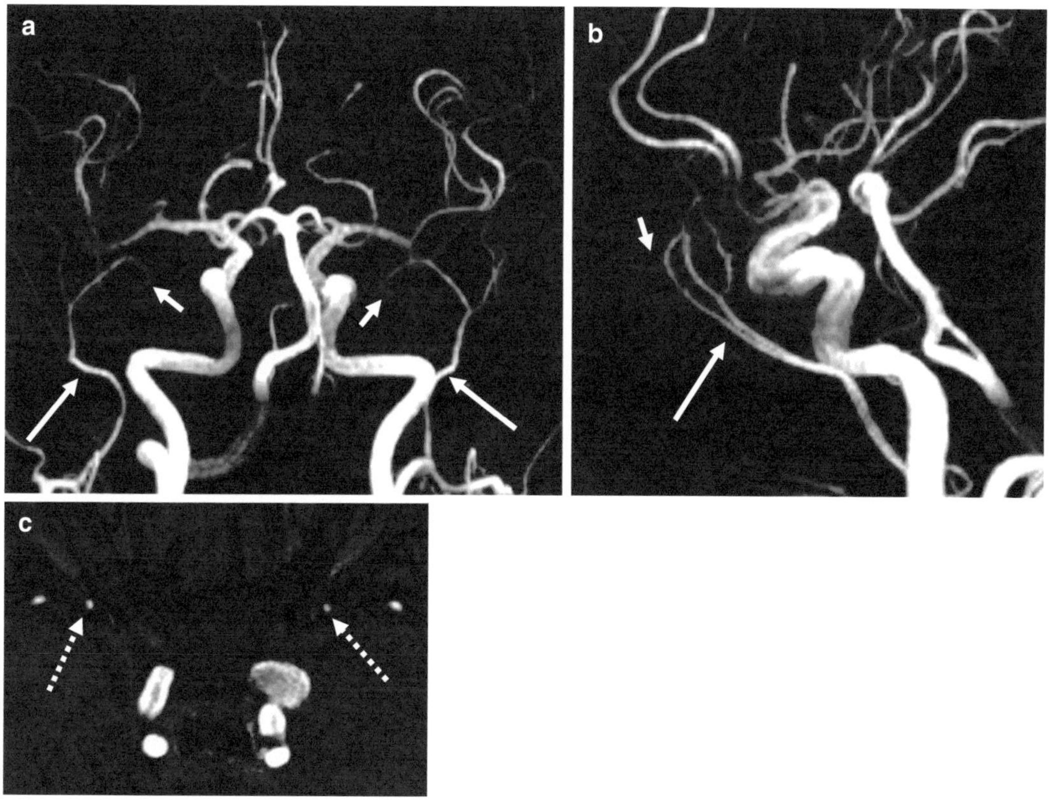

Fig. 6.5 (**a**) A-P and (**b**) lateral projections of MR angiography show bilateral hyperplastic MMAs (*long arrows*). The bilateral OphAs arise from the MMAs (*short arrows*) instead of the ICAs. (**c**) MR angiographic source image shows the bilateral OphAs in the SOF (*dotted arrows*). There is an aneurysm at the left cavernous ICA

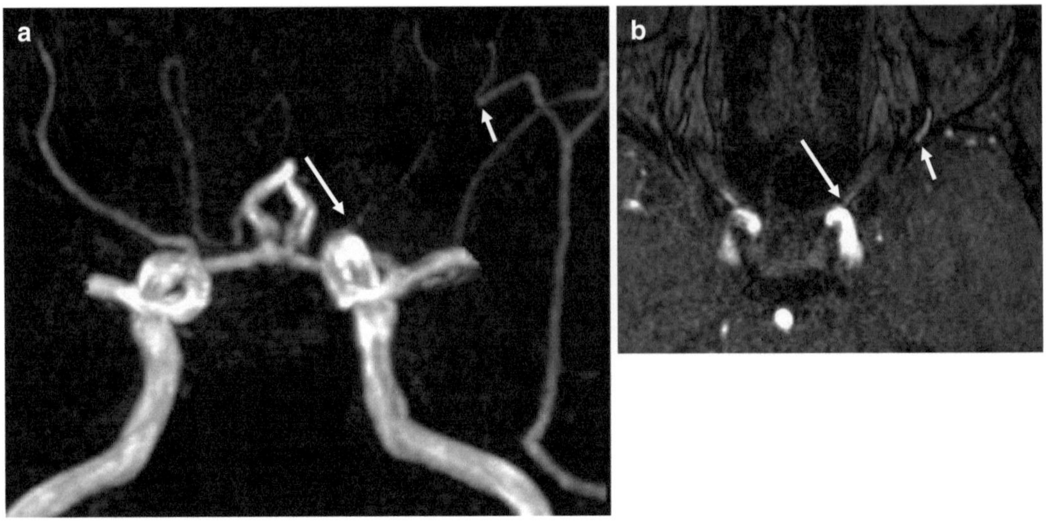

Fig. 6.6 (**a**) Partial MIP I-S projection of MR angiography and (**b**) its source image show a normally arising tiny left OphA (*long arrows*) and another artery arising from the left MMA that enters the orbit via the SOF (*short arrows*)

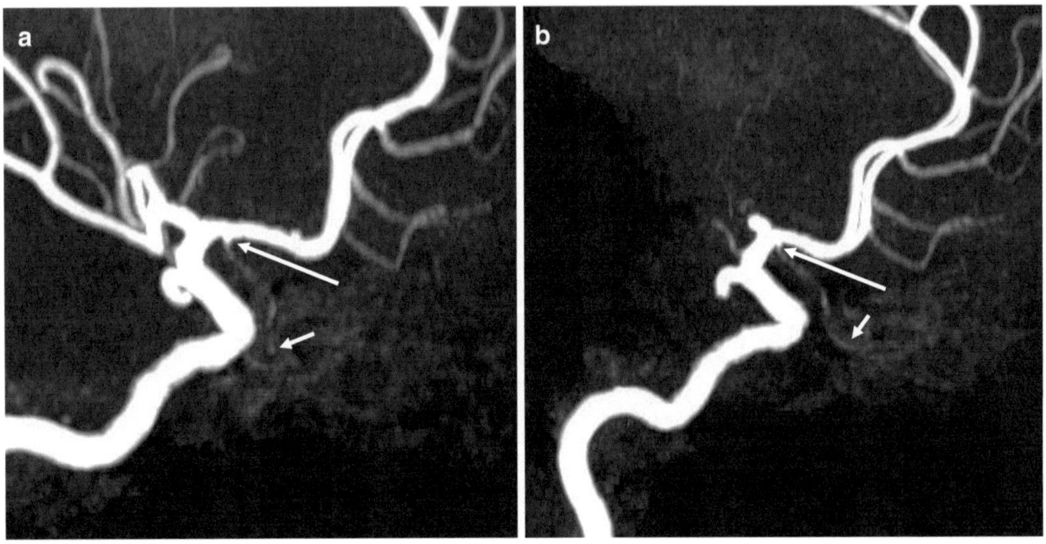

Fig. 6.7 (**a**) RAO projection and (**b**) lateral projection of partial MIP MR angiography show a tiny artery arising from the proximal A1 segment of the right ACA (*long arrows*). The artery takes an anteroinferior course and reaches the level of the optic canal (*short arrows*)

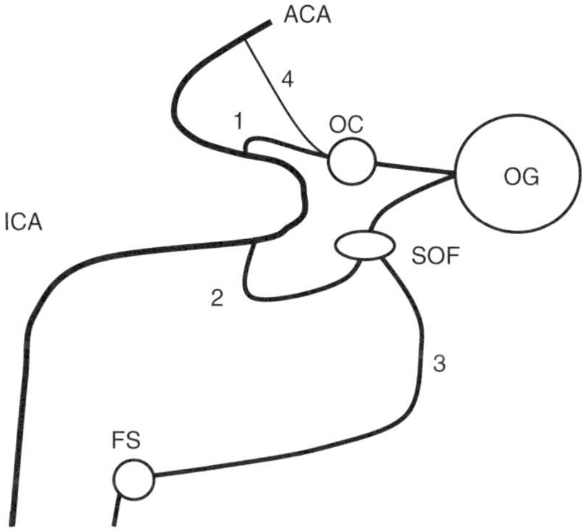

Fig. 6.8 Schematic illustration of the OphA variations in lateral projection. (Modified from [9]). 1: Normally originating OphA, 2: OphA arising from the cavernous ICA, 3: OphA arising from the MMA, 4: OphA arising from the A1 segment of the ACA. *ACA* anterior cerebral artery, *FS* foramen spinosum, *ICA* internal carotid artery, *OC* optic canal, *OG* optic globe, *SOF* superior orbital fissure

References

1. Lasjaunias P, Moret J, Mink J. The anatomy of the inferolateral trunk (ILT) of the internal carotid artery. Neuroradiology. 1977;13:215–20.
2. Komiyama M. Embryology of the ophthalmic artery: a revised concept. Interv Neuroradiol. 2009;15:363–8.
3. Fiore DL, Pardatscher K, Fiore D, Zuccarello M, Iraci G. Persistent dorsal ophthalmic artery. Report of a case with associated fibromuscular hyperplasia of the extracranial internal carotid artery and multiple cerebral aneurysms. Neurochirurgia (Stuttgart). 1981;24:106–8.
4. Bertelli E, Regoli M, Bracco S. An update on the variations of the orbital blood suply and hemodynamic. Surg Radiol Anat. 2017;39:485–96.
5. Uchino A, Saito N, Takahashi M, Kozawa E, Mizukoshi W, Nakajima R, Okano N. Persistent dorsal ophthalmic artery and ophthalmic artery arising from the middle meningeal artery diagnosed by MR angiography at 3 T. Surg Radiol Anat. 2013;35:775–82.
6. Uchino A, Saito N, Kurita H, Ishihara S. Double ophthalmic arteries arising from the internal carotid artery. Surg Radiol Anat. 2013;35:173–5.
7. Agarwal N, Singh PL, Karimib RJ, Gandhi CD, Prestigiacomo CJ. Persistent vestige of dorsal ophthalmic artery: a case report. J Neurointerv Surg. 2013;5:e25.
8. Watanabe A, Hirano K, Ishii R. Dural caroticocavernous fistula with both ophthalmic arteries arising from middle meningeal arteries. Neuroradiology. 1996;38:806–8.
9. Uchino A, Saito N, Ikeda S, Ishihara S. Ophthalmic artery arising from the anterior cerebral artery diagnosed by MR angiography. Surg Radiol Anat. 2015;37:1009–12.
10. Padget DH. The development of the cranial arteries in the human embryo. Contrib Embryol. 1948;32:205–61.
11. Li Y, Horiuchi T, Yako T, Ishizaka S, Hongo K. Anomalous origin of the ophthalmic artery from the anterior cerebral artery. Neurol Med Chir (Tokyo). 2011;51:579–81.
12. Indo M, Oya S, Tanaka M, Matsui T. High incidence of ICA anterior wall aneurysms in patients with an anomalous origin of the ophthalmic artery: possible relevance to the pathogenesis of aneurysm formation. J Neurosurg. 2014;120:93–8.

7 Variations of the Posterior Communicating Artery (PCoA), Proximal Posterior Cerebral Artery (PCA), and Anterior Choroidal Artery (AChA)

Abstract

This chapter includes (1) P1 aplasia and hypoplasia of the PCA (Fetal-type PCA), (2) Extremely long PCoA and P1 segment of the PCA, (3) Duplicate origin of the PCoA, (4) PCA branch arising from the PCoA, (5) Hyperplastic AChA (Accessory PCA, Replaced PCA), (6) Duplication of the PCA, (7) Duplicate origin of the PCA, (8) Fenestration of the PCA, (9) Early bifurcation of the PCA, (10) Artery of Percheron, and (11) Infundibular dilatation of the PCoA, AChA and hypoplastic P1 segment of the PCA. There are 21 figures and 2 illustrations.

There are many variations in this area. They play important role in collateral circulation. They can represent cerebral ischemia due to unique blood flow.

Keywords

Anterior choroidal artery · Artery of Percheron · Posterior cerebral artery Posterior communicating artery

7.1 P1 Aplasia and Hypoplasia of the PCA (Fetal-Type PCA)

The circle of Willis (CW) is an anastomotic arterial ring that connects the bilateral carotid systems (anterior circulation) and the vertebrobasilar system (posterior circulation), thus providing a potential source of collaterals in the case of arterial occlusion or aplasia. It was reported that normal and complete CW was found in only 60% of 150 Indian cadavers [1]. Using MR angiography, complete CW was found in only 42% of 150 volunteers [2]. If the P1 segment of the PCA is absent, the PCA originates directly from the supraclinoid ICA and is called fetal-type PCA (Figs. 7.1 and 7.2). According to Avci et al. [3], approximately 10% of the PCoA is absent, and a fetal-type PCA (P1 aplasia) is seen in approximately 10% of patients.

7.2 Extremely Long PCoA and P1 Segment of the PCA

The P1 segment of the PCA extends from the basilar tip to the junction with the PCoA. The PCoA arises from the supraclinoid ICA. It is usually short with a small diameter and fuses with the P1-P2 junction of the PCA. A report of a microsurgical anatomic study described PCoA lengths ranging from 5.0 to 18.0 mm (average 12.0 mm) [4]. When the PCoA fuses with the distal segment of the PCA, forming an extremely long PCoA and extremely long P1 segment of the PCA (Fig. 7.3) [5, 6]. Figure 7.4 shows a schematic illustration of this variation.

A. Uchino, *Atlas of the Supraaortic Craniocervical Arterial Variations*,
https://doi.org/10.1007/978-981-16-6803-6_7

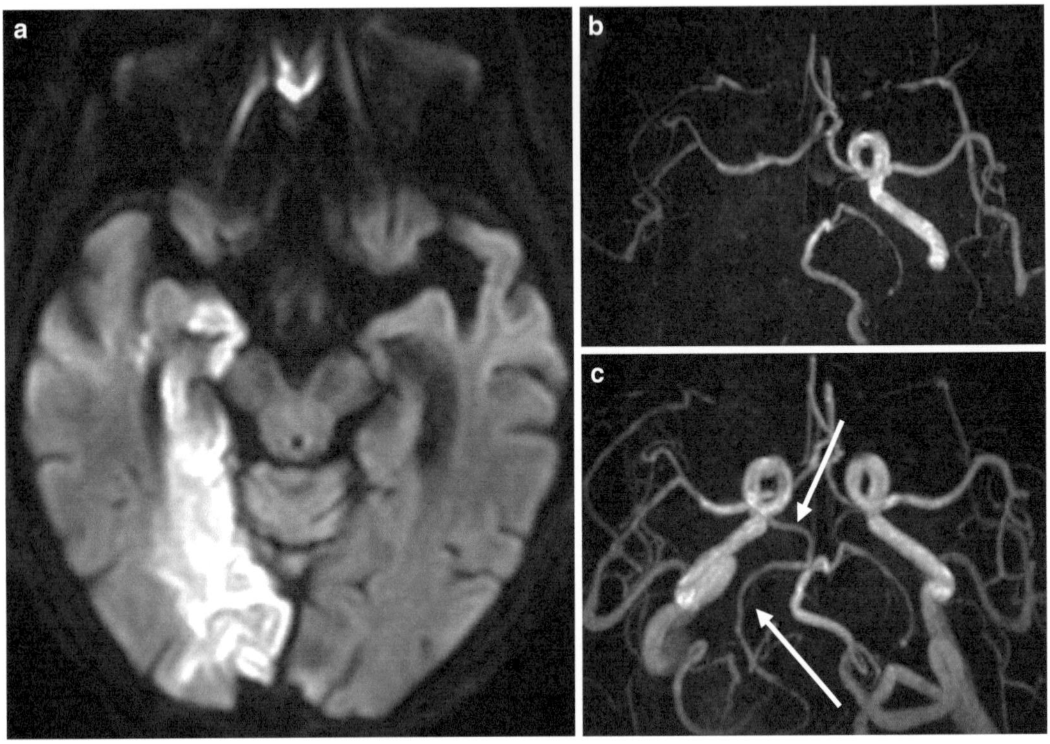

Fig. 7.1 (**a**) Diffusion-weighted MR imaging shows acute infarction of the right PCA territory. (**b**) I-S projection of MR angiography shows total occlusion of the right ICA and right PCA. The right MCA is well visualized by collateral circulation via the ACoA. (**c**) I-S projection of MR angiography obtained immediately after thrombectomy shows complete recanalization of the right ICA and right PCA. The right PCA is arising from the ICA, which is indicative of a fetal-type PCA (*arrows*)

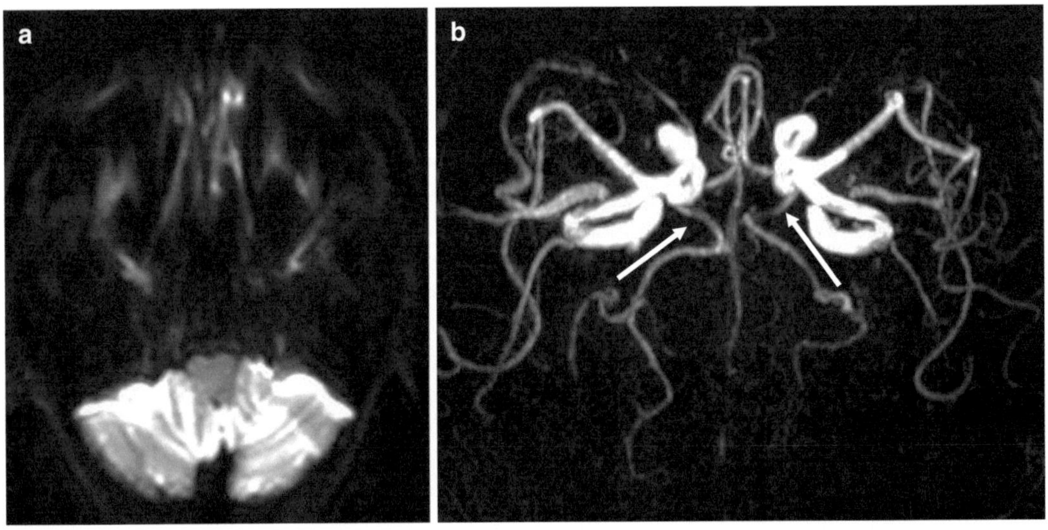

Fig. 7.2 (**a**) Diffusion-weighted MR imaging shows acute infarction of the bilateral cerebellar hemispheres. There is no infarction in the occipital lobes (not shown). (**b**) I-S projection of MR angiography shows complete occlusion of the vertebrobasilar system. The bilateral PCAs are patent because of the fetal type (*arrows*)

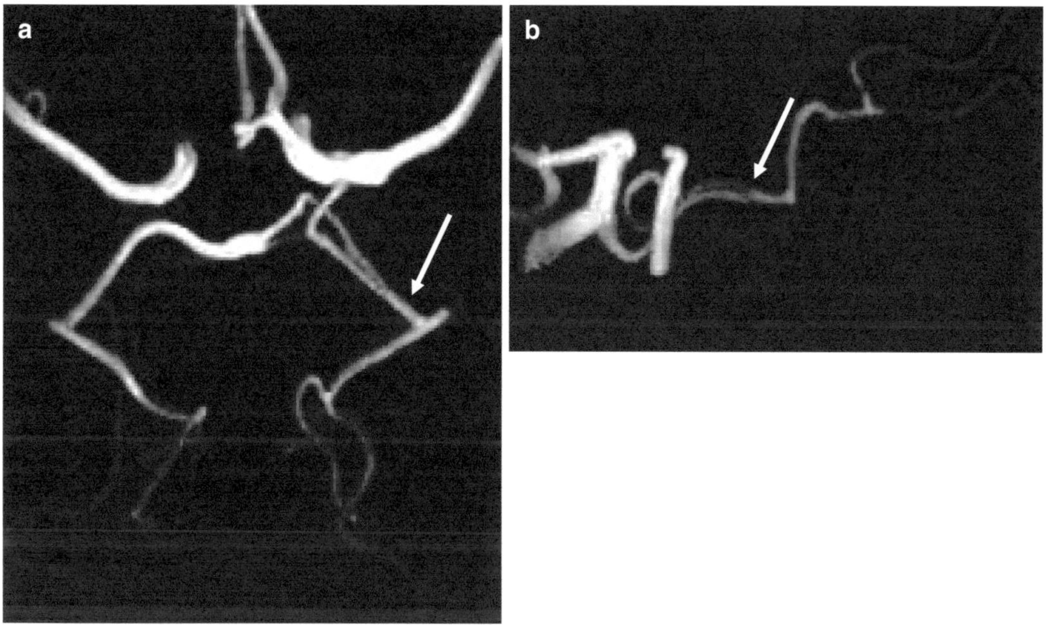

Fig. 7.3 (**a**) I-S and (**b**) lateral projections of partial MIP MR angiography show the left PCoA arising from the normal point and fusing with the PCA at its posterior ambient (P2P) segment (*arrows*), forming an extremely long PCoA and extremely long precommunicating (P1) segment of the PCA

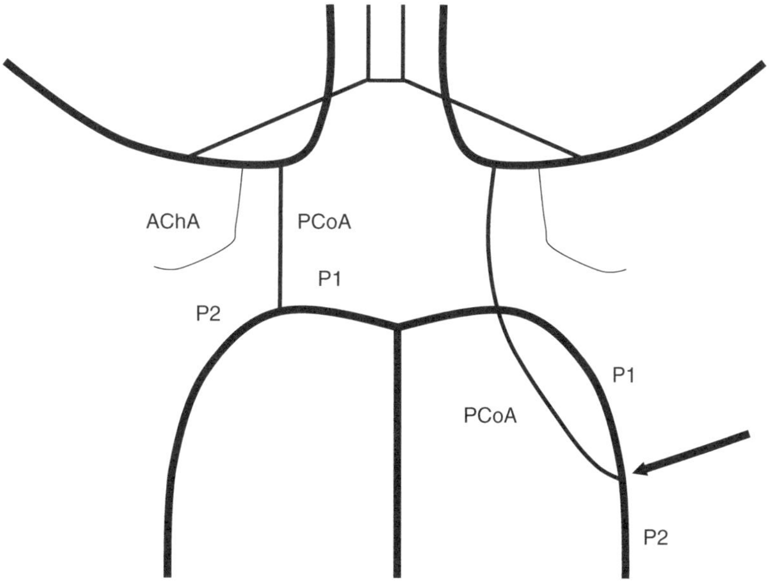

Fig. 7.4 Schematic illustration of an extremely long left PCoA and P1 segment of the left PCA. (Modified from [5]). *AChA* anterior choroidal artery, *PCoA* posterior communicating artery, *P1* precommunicating (interpeduncular) segment, *P2* crural and ambient segments

7.3 Duplicate Origin of the PCoA

When two branches of the PCoA arise separately from the supraclinoid segment of the ICA and quickly fuse to form an arterial ring, a PCoA of duplicate origin occurs (Fig. 7.5) [7]. This variation has been confused with fenestration. Schematic illustration of three types of arterial ring at the ICA-PCoA junction is shown in Fig. 7.6.

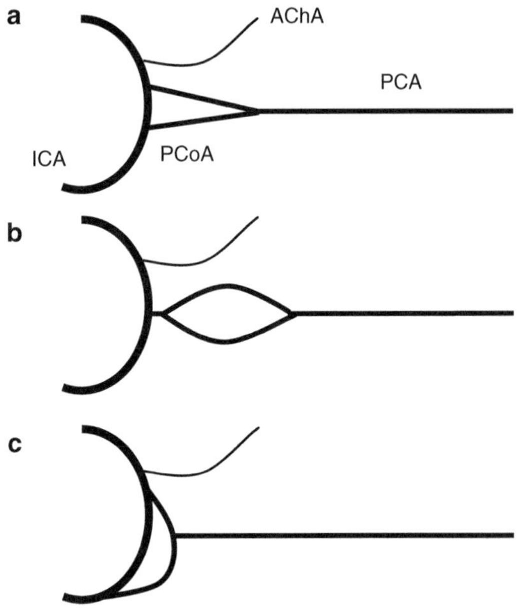

Fig. 7.6 Schematic illustration of three types of arterial ring at the ICA-PCoA junction. (Modified from [7]). (**a**) Duplicate origin of the PCoA, (**b**) PCoA fenestration, (**c**) PCoA arising from the ICA fenestration. *AChA* anterior choroidal artery, *ICA* internal carotid artery, *PCA* posterior cerebral artery, *PCoA* posterior communicating artery

7.4 PCA Branch Arising from the PCoA

A microsurgical anatomic study demonstrates several tiny perforating arteries arising from the PCoA [8]. Extremely rarely, MR angiography detects a large artery, one of the branches of the PCA, arising from the PCoA (Fig. 7.7) [9]. Because the temporal branch arises as the first branch of the PCA, this anomalous artery is the temporal branch.

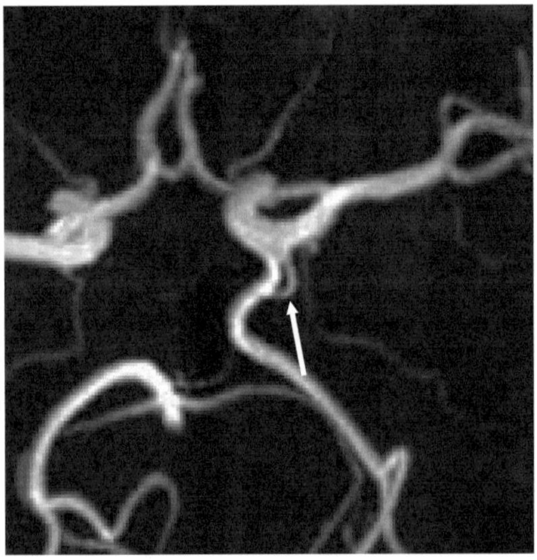

Fig. 7.5 I-S projection of partial MIP MR angiography shows fetal-type left PCA. A small artery is also arising from the ICA and fuses together soon, indicating the duplicate origin of the PCoA (*arrow*)

7.5 Hyperplastic AChA (Accessory PCA, Replaced PCA)

One of the branches of the PCA relatively frequently arises from the AChA, a variation of the AChA described as hyperplastic AChA. The prevalence of this variation on catheter angiography was reported to be 2.3% [10]. On the other hand, the prevalence of this variation on MR angiography was reported to be 0.55%—only a quarter of the prevalence on catheter angiography study [11]. This discrepancy between the prevalence of catheter and MR angiography studies may be due to the low spatial resolution of MR angiography. This variation can also be regarded as an accessory PCA (Figs. 7.8, 7.9 and 7.10) [11]. The temporal branch is most frequently supplied by this variation. If the entire branches of the PCA arise from

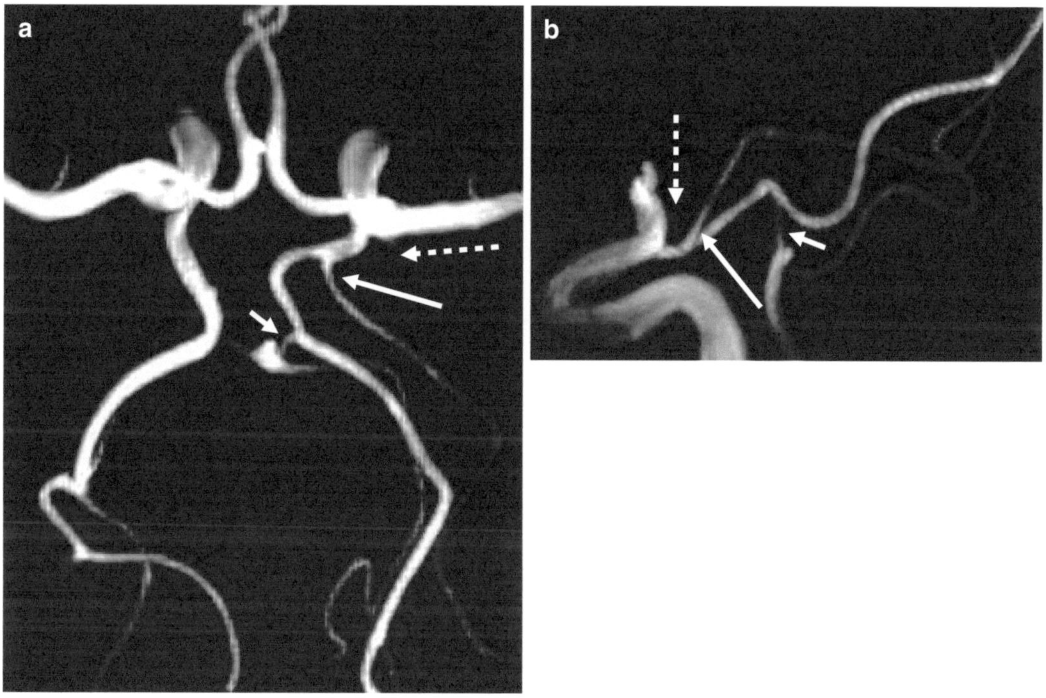

Fig. 7.7 (**a**) I-S and (**b**) lateral projections of partial MIP MR angiography show the temporal branch of the left PCA arising from the left PCoA (*long arrows*). The P1 segment of the left PCA is present but hypoplastic (*short arrows*). The left AChA is identified as a tiny artery (*dotted arrows*)

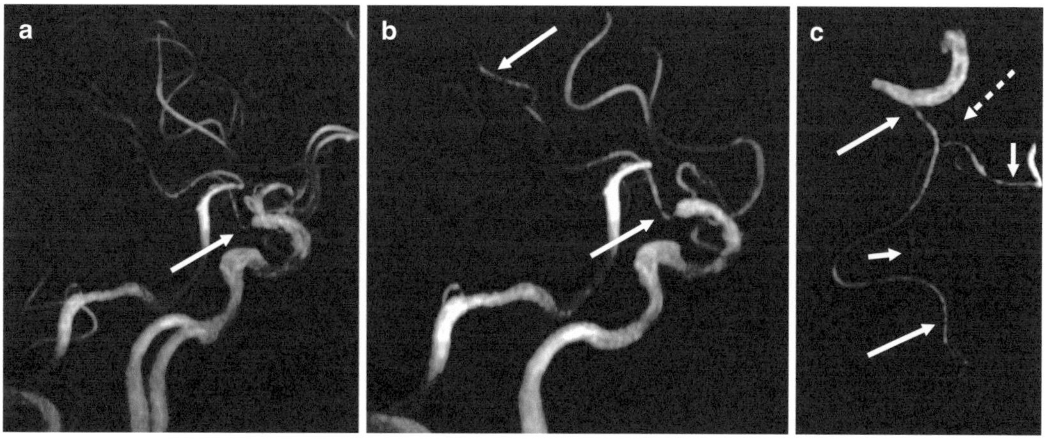

Fig. 7.8 (**a**) Lateral projection of MR angiography and (**b**, **c**) partial MIP images show a large artery arising from the right ICA and supplying the parieto-occipital branch of the PCA (*long arrows*). The small right PCA arises from the BA and supplies the temporal branch (*short arrows*). There is a tiny right PCoA (*dotted arrow*). Thus, the large artery can be diagnosed as a hyperplastic AChA (accessory PCA)

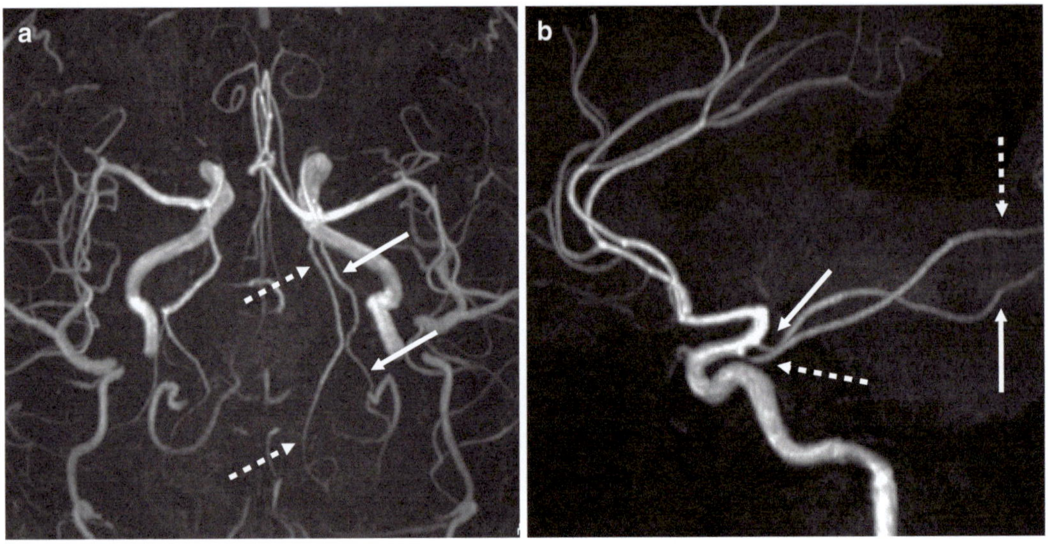

Fig. 7.9 (**a**) I-S projection of MR angiography and (**b**) partial MIP lateral image show two PCAs arising from the left ICA. The distally originating artery is not the PCA but the hyperplastic AChA (accessory PCA) and supplies the temporal branch of the PCA (*arrows*). The proximally originating artery is a fetal-type PCA and supplies the parieto-occipital branch (*dotted arrows*)

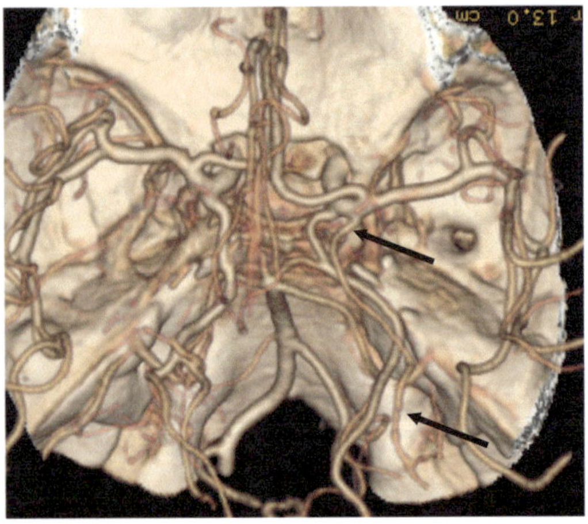

Fig. 7.10 S-I projection of CT angiography shows hyperplastic right AChA (accessory right PCA) supplying the temporal branch of the right PCA (*arrows*)

the AChA, it can be regarded as a replaced PCA (Fig. 7.11) [11, 12]. This rare condition has been reported as transposition of the AChA and PCoA [13]; however, the name seems inadequate.

7.6 Duplication of the PCA

Extremely rarely, duplication of the PCA is found. For differentiation from the hyperplastic AChA, identification of a normal tiny AChA arising from the ICA distal to the PCoA is necessary (Fig. 7.12) [11].

7.7 Duplicate Origin of the PCA

Rarely, an artery arises from the distal BA and fuses with the P1 segment of the PCA, forming a triangular arterial ring. This variation is not a true fenestration but a duplicate origin (Figs. 7.13 and 7.14) [14]. A high prevalence (2.35%) of P1 duplication was reported in a cadaver study [1]. This may have been attributable to the superiority of anatomical dissection to MR angiography in the detection of tiny arterial variations.

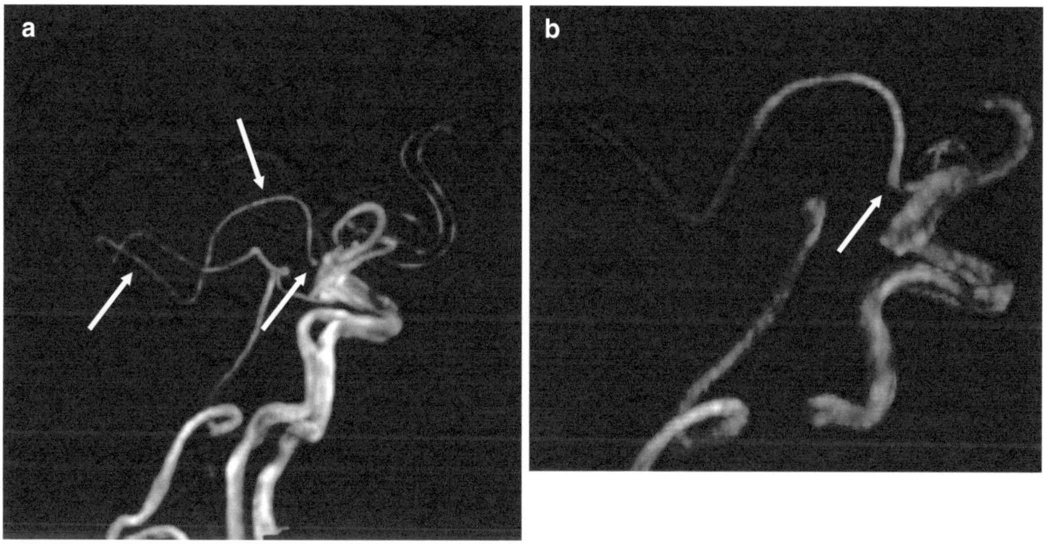

Fig. 7.11 (**a**) Lateral projection of MR angiography and (**b**) partial MIP image show a large artery arising from the terminal segment of the right ICA and supplying the entire branches of the right PCA (*arrows*). There is no PCoA, and no PCA arises from the BA. Thus, the large artery can be diagnosed as a hyperplastic AChA (replaced PCA)

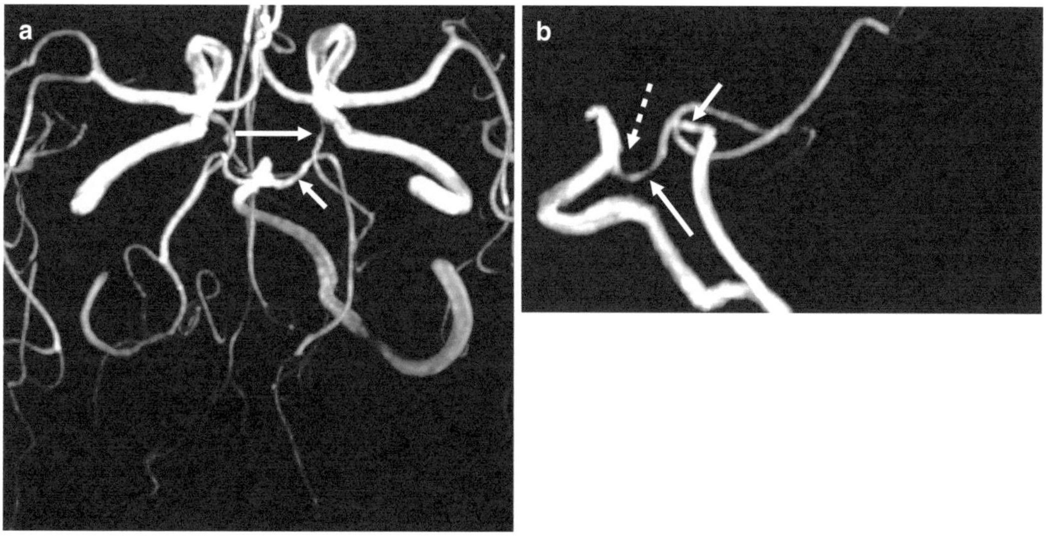

Fig. 7.12 (**a**) I-S projection of MR angiography and (**b**) partial MIP lateral image show the left PCoA-temporal branch of the PCA (*long arrows*) and the left P1-parietooccipital branch of the PCA (*short arrows*). These two arteries do not fuse with each other. The tiny left AChA is normally identified (*dotted arrow*), indicating that this is not a hyperplastic AChA but a duplication of the PCA

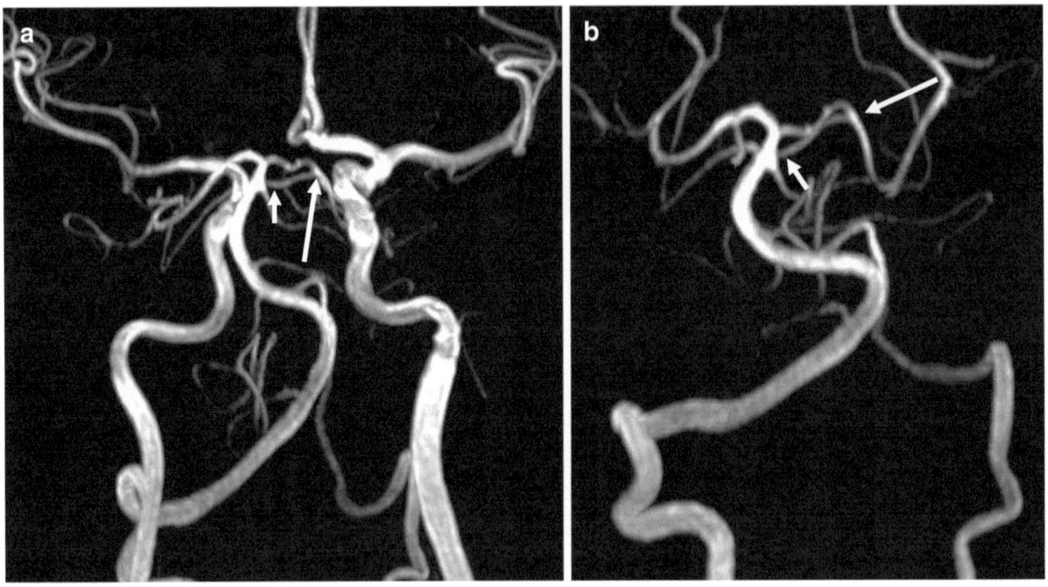

Fig. 7.13 (**a**) A-P projection of MR angiography and (**b**) partial MIP AS-PI projection image show an artery arising from the left side of the distal BA (*short arrows*) and fusing with the long P1 segment of the left PCA (*long arrows*), forming a large triangular arterial ring, indicative of a duplicate origin of the PCA

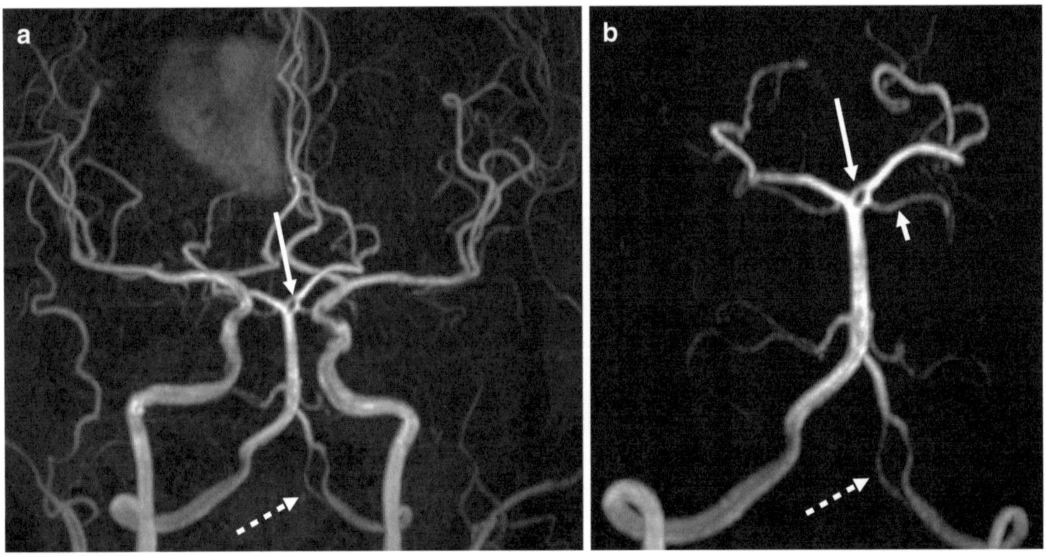

Fig. 7.14 (**a**) A-P projection of MR angiography and (**b**) partial MIP image show a small arterial ring at the BA-left PCA junction (*long arrow*), indicative of a duplicate origin of the left PCA. The left SCA arises from the arterial ring (*short arrow*) (Sect. 12.10). There is a fenestration at the V4 segment of the left VA (*dotted arrows*) (Sect. 10.3.2)

7.8 Fenestration of the PCA

According to a microsurgical anatomic study, 1 of 100 (1%) patients had a fenestration of the PCA [15]. On a large MR angiography series, the prevalence of the PCA fenestration was reported to be 0.34%, which is not so rare [11]. They are usually observed at the P1 and P2 segments (Figs. 7.15, 7.16, 7.17 and 7.18). PCA fenestration itself has little clinical significance, but extremely rarely, an aneurysm may occur at the proximal end of the PCA fenestration [16].

Superimposition of the anterior circulation may prevent the observation of PCA fenestration on A-P projections, and the superimposition of the bilateral PCAs and SCAs may prevent the identification of PCA fenestration on lateral projections. Thus, PCA fenestrations may be easily

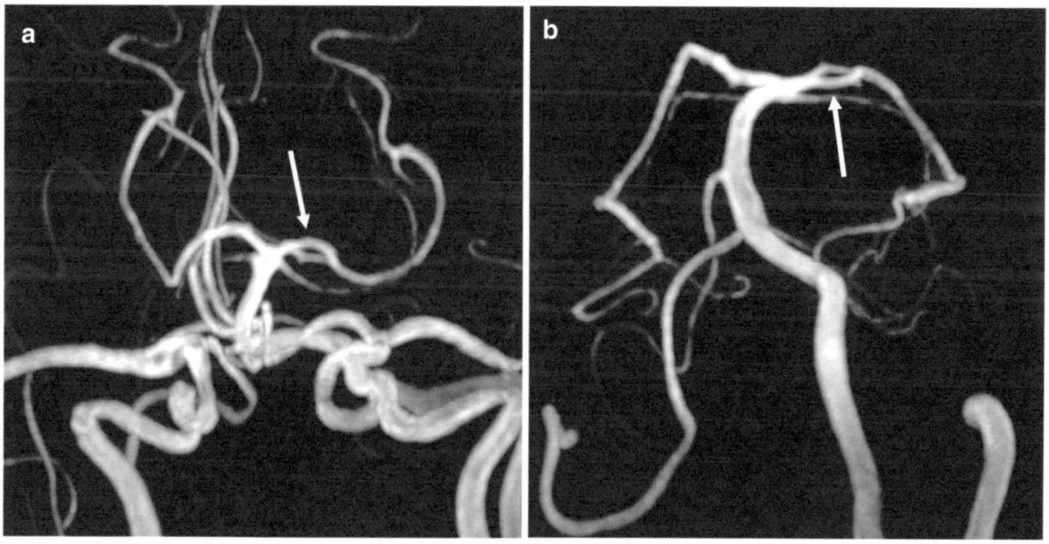

Fig. 7.15 (**a**) AS-PI projection of MR angiography and (**b**) partial MIP straight A-P projection image show a small fenestration at the P1 segment of the left PCA (*arrows*)

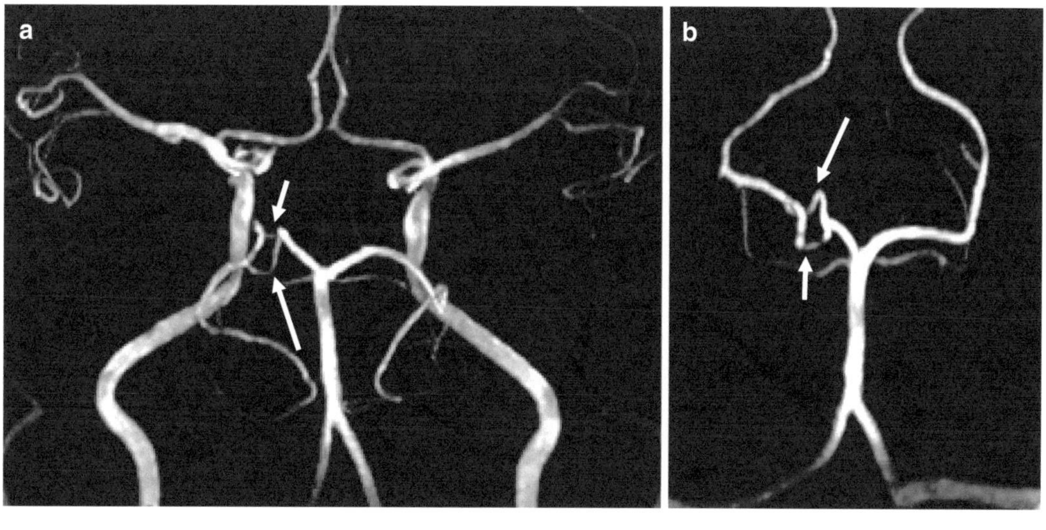

Fig. 7.16 (**a**) AI-PS projection of MR angiography and (**b**) partial MIP AS-PI projection image show a large fenestration at the proximal P2 segment of the right PCA (*long and short arrows*)

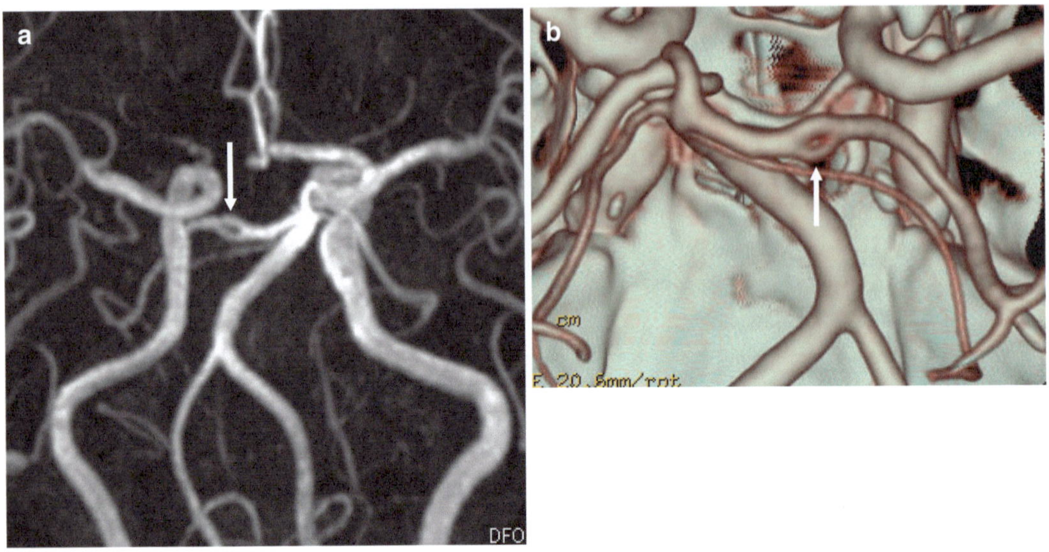

Fig. 7.17 (**a**) AI-PS projection of MR angiography and (**b**) S-I projection of CT angiography show a small fenestration at the proximal P2 segment of the right PCA (*arrows*)

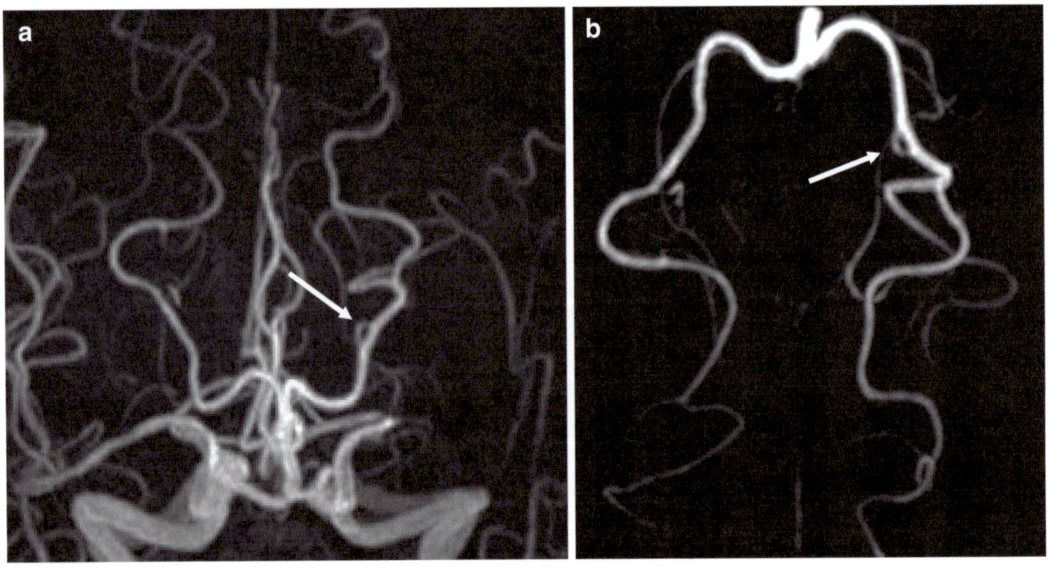

Fig. 7.18 (**a**) AS-PI projection of MR angiography and (**b**) I-S projection of a partial MIP image show a small fenestration at the distal P2 segment of the left PCA (*arrows*)

overlooked on routine catheter angiography. A misinterpretation of MR angiography of crossing arterial branches as a fused vessel may result in a misdiagnosis of fenestration. Partial MIP MR angiography is useful for the detection and confirmation of this variation.

7.9 Early Bifurcation of the PCA

The first large cortical branch of the PCA is the anterior temporal artery, and it usually arises from the P2-P3 junction. Rarely, the PCA is bifurcated at the P1 segment, P1-P2 junction, or proximal

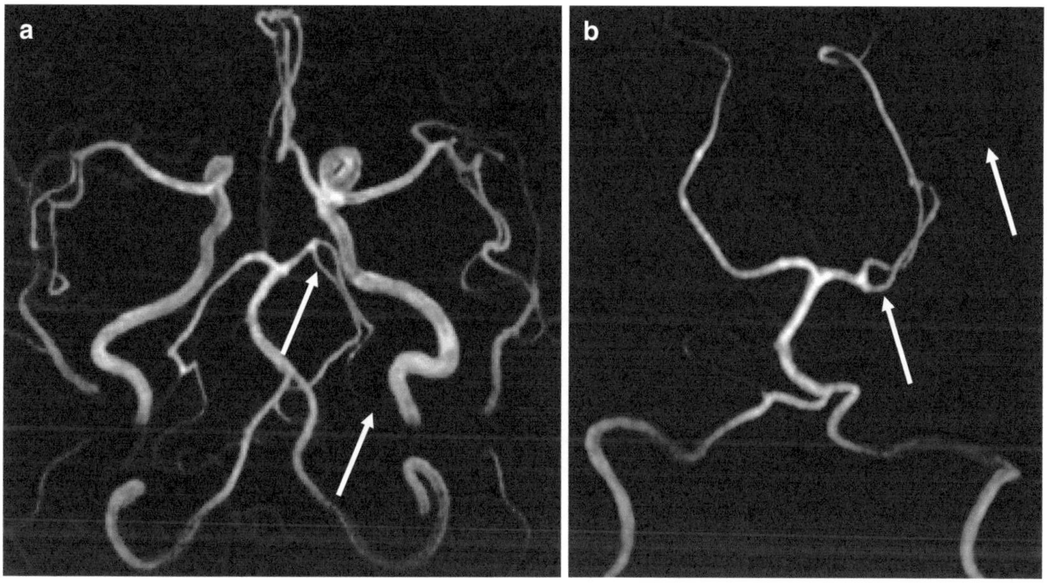

Fig. 7.19 (**a**) I-S projection of MR angiography and (**b**) partial MIP AS-PI projection image show the left temporal branch arising from the P1-P2 junction of the left PCA, which is indicative of an early bifurcation (*arrows*)

P2A segment, a variation regarded as early bifurcation (Fig. 7.19) [15]. The prevalence of this variation on MR angiography was reported to be 0.34% [11].

7.10 Artery of Percheron

The artery of Percheron is a rare anatomical variation wherein a single thalamic perforating artery arises from the P1 segment of the PCA and supplies the rostral midbrain and bilateral paramedian thalami. When this artery is occluded, infarctions will develop in these characteristic areas [17]. Because this artery is small in size and is surrounded by larger arteries, it may be frequently overlooked on MR angiography. Partial MIP images are useful for the identification of this variation (Fig. 7.20).

7.11 Infundibular Dilatation of the PCoA, AChA, and Hypoplastic P1 Segment of the PCA

Infundibular dilatation (ID) is frequently seen at the origin of the PCoA. A funnel-shaped origin of the PCoA continues from the ID apex to the PCA. When this triangular-shaped widening is <3 mm in diameter, it can be called PCoA-ID (Fig. 7.21). Currently, PCoA-ID is considered a normal anatomic variation, and the majority of PCoA-IDs are stable. However, some PCoA-IDs can evolve into aneurysms and they may rupture [18]. According to an anatomical study [19], there were no cases of ID in fetuses. Therefore, ID develops postnatally and is probably due to the influence of hemodynamic factors or hypertension. The PCoA-ID is usually asymptomatic itself, however, it rarely causes oculomotor nerve palsy [20].

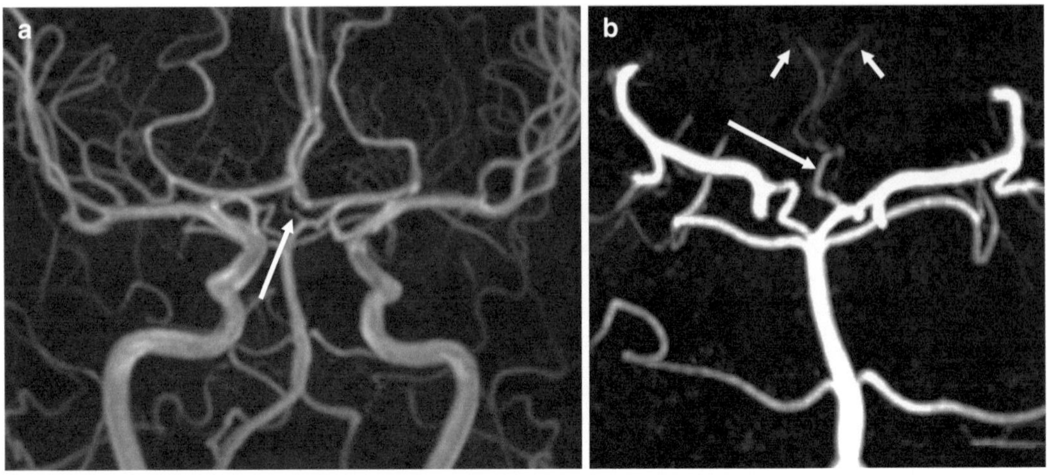

Fig. 7.20 (**a**) A-P projection of MR angiography and (**b**) partial MIP image show a large perforating artery arising from the P1 segment of the left PCA (*long arrows*). This artery is supplying the bilateral thalami (*short arrows*), indicative of an artery of Percheron

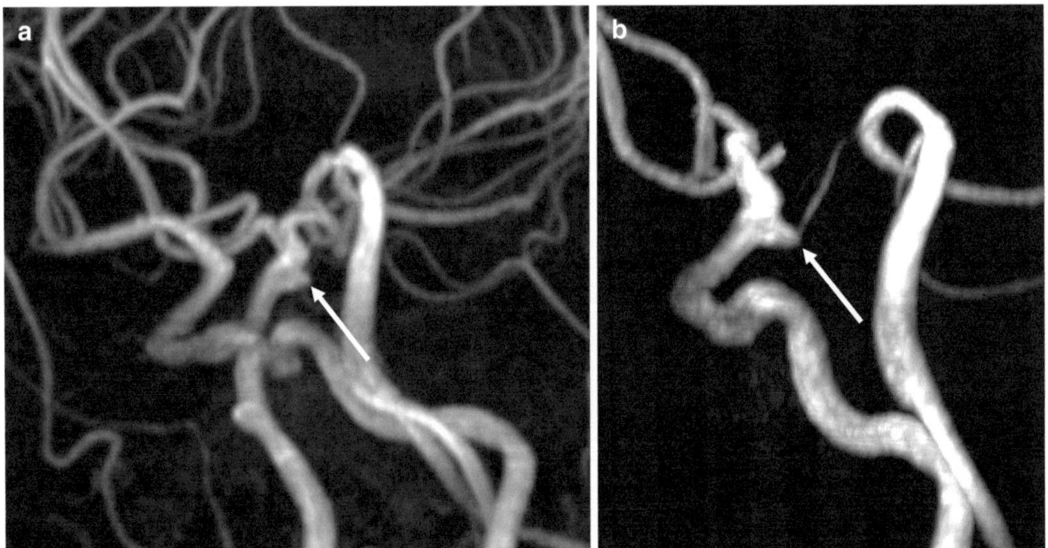

Fig. 7.21 (**a**) LAO projection of MR angiography suggests a small aneurysm at the supraclinoid left ICA (*arrow*). (**b**) Partial MIP image shows that the suggested small aneurysm is ID of the left PCoA, because it has a triangular shape and the PCoA arises from the apex (*arrow*)

ID can also be seen at the origins of the AChA (Fig. 7.22) and at the origin of the hypoplastic P1 segment of the PCA (Fig. 7.23). These IDs should not be misinterpreted as tiny aneurysms. For differentiation of ID from aneurysm, both partial MIP and reformatted source images are useful.

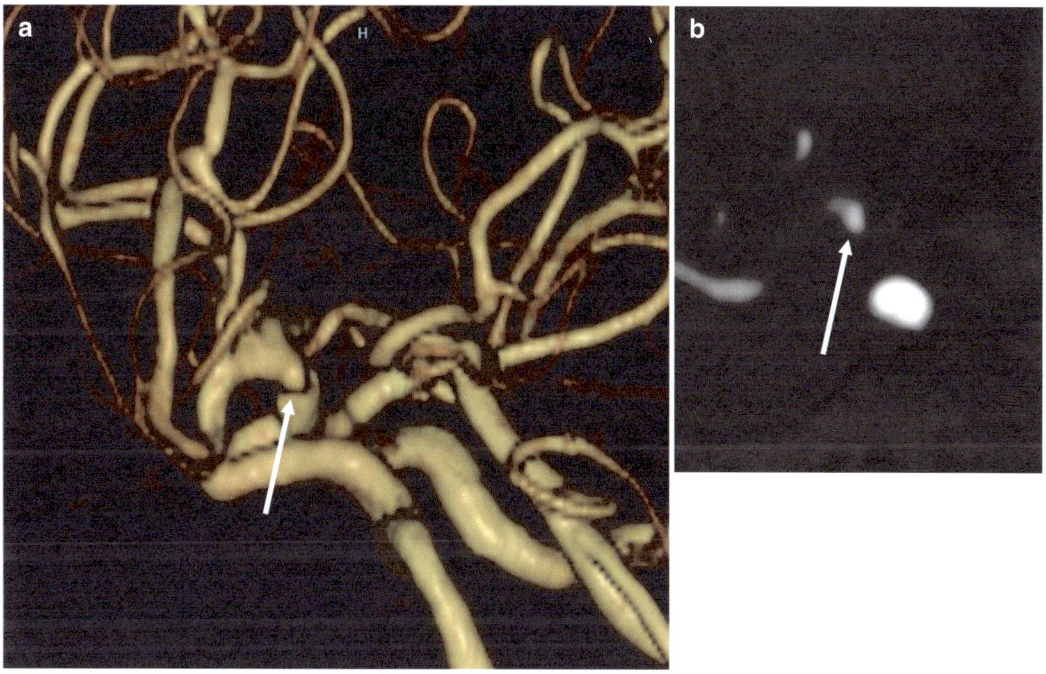

Fig. 7.22 (**a**) LPO projection of VR image of MR angiography shows an aneurysmal dilatation at the supraclinoid left ICA (*arrow*). (**b**) Reformatted source image shows the AChA arising from the apex of the dilatation, which is indicative of an ID of the AChA (*arrow*)

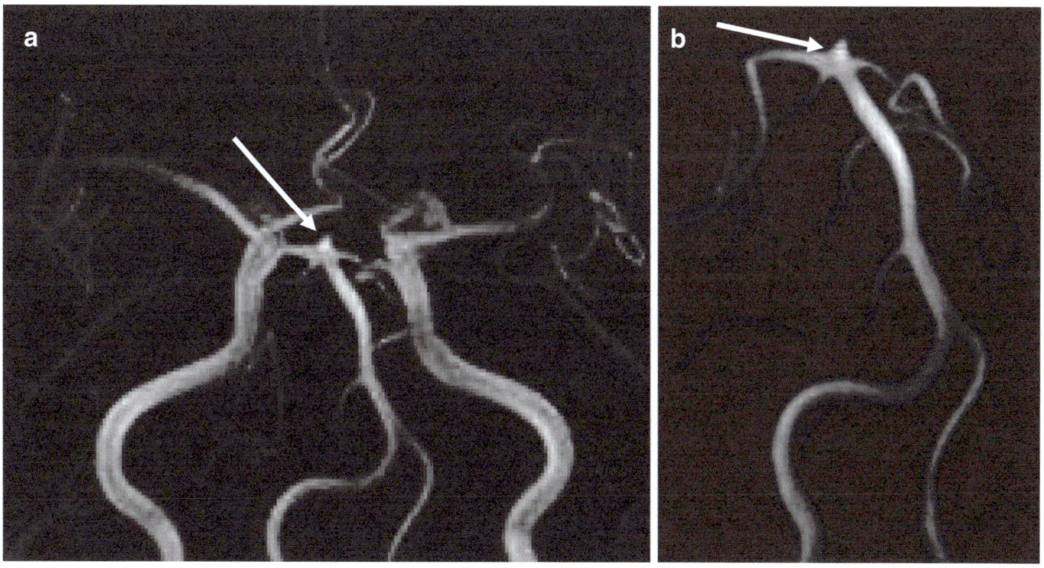

Fig. 7.23 (**a**) AI-PS projection of MR angiography and (**b**) partial MIP image show a hypoplastic P1 segment of the left PCA with ID at its origin (*arrows*)

References

1. Gunnal SA, Farooqui MS, Wabale RN. Anatomical variations of the circulus arteriosus in cadaveric humans. Neurol Res Int. 2014;2014:687281.
2. Krabbe-Hartkamp MJ, van der Grond J, de Leeuw FE, de Groot JC, Algra A, Hillen B, Breteler MM, Mali WP. Circle of Willis: morphologic variation on three-dimensional time-of-flight MR angiograms. Radiology. 1998;207:103–11.
3. Avci E, Bademci G, Oztürk A. Posterior communicating artery: from microsurgical, endoscopic and radiological perspective. Minim Invasive Neurosurg. 2005;48:218–23.
4. Gibo H, Lenkey C, Rhoton AL Jr. Microsurgical anatomy of the supraclinoid portion of the internal carotid artery. J Neurosurg. 1981;55:560–74.
5. Uchino A, Suzuki C, Tanaka M. Extremely long posterior communicating artery diagnosed by MR angiography: report of two cases. Surg Radiol Anat. 2015;37:565–8.
6. Uchino A, Ehara T, Kurita H. Hypoplasia of the internal carotid artery with associated fenestration and extremely long P1 segment of the ipsilateral posterior cerebral artery diagnosed by MR angiography. Surg Radiol Anat. 2019;41:707–11.
7. Uchino A, Kamiya K, Suzuki C. Duplicate origin of the posterior communicating artery diagnosed by magnetic resonance angiography. Surg Radiol Anat. 2013;35:741–3.
8. Gabrovsky N. Microanatomical bases for intraoperative division of the posterior communicating artery. Acta Neurochir. 2002;144:1205–11.
9. Uchino A, Suzuki C. Temporal branch of the posterior cerebral artery arising from the posterior communicating artery diagnosed by MR angiography. Surg Radiol Anat. 2016;38:153–5.
10. Takahashi S, Suga T, Kawata Y, Sakamoto K. Anterior choroidal artery: angiographic analysis of variations and anomalies. AJNR Am J Neuroradiol. 1990;11:719–29.
11. Uchino A, Saito N, Takahashi M, Okano N, Tanisaka M. Variations of the posterior cerebral artery diagnosed by MR angiography at 3 tesla. Neuroradiology. 2016;58:141–6.
12. Uchino A, Kamide T, Kurita H. Replaced posterior cerebral artery (PCA): origin of all branches of the PCA from the anterior choroidal artery diagnosed by MR angiography. Surg Radiol Anat. 2019;41:703–5.
13. Moyer DJ, Flamm ES. Anomalous arrangement of the origins of the anterior choroidal and posterior communicating arteries. Case report. J Neurosurg. 1992;76:1017–8.
14. Matsuda M, Uchino A, Saito N, Neki H, Kohyama S, Yamane F. Duplicate origin and extremely long P1 segment of the posterior cerebral artery diagnosed by MR angiography. Surg Radiol Anat. 2017;39:699–702.
15. Caruso G, Vincentelli F, Rabehanta P, Giudicelli G, Grisoli F. Anomalies of the P1 segment of the posterior cerebral artery: early bifurcation or duplication, fenestration, common trunk with the superior cerebellar artery. Acta Neurochir. 1991;109:66–71.
16. Iwashita T, Tanaka Y, Hongo K, Koyama Ji J, Koyama T, Nitta J. Aneurysm originating from the fenestration of the posterior cerebral artery: case report. Neurosurgery. 2002;50:881–4.
17. Arauz A, Patiño-Rodríguez HM, Vargas-González JC, Arguelles-Morales N, Silos H, Ruiz-Franco A, Ochoa MA. Clinical spectrum of artery of Percheron infarct: clinical-radiological correlations. J Stroke Cerebrovasc Dis. 2014;23:1083–8.
18. Lee W, Han HJ, Kim J, Choi JY, Park KY, Kim YB, Chung J. Ruptured infundibular dilatation of the posterior communicating artery. Acta Neurochir (Wien). 2021;163:797–803.
19. Vlajković S, Vasović L, Trandafilović M, Jovanović I, Ugrenović S, Dorđević G. Infundibular dilatation of the posterior communicating artery in a defined population. Ann Anat. 2015;197:50–8.
20. Fukami S, Akimoto J, Fukuhara H, Kohno M. Microvascular decompression for oculomotor nerve palsy due to compression by infundibular dilatation of posterior communicating artery. World Neurosurg. 2018;119:142–5.

Variations of the Proximal Middle Cerebral Artery (MCA)

8

Abstract

This chapter includes (1) Duplicated MCA, (2) Two types of accessory MCA, (3) Duplicate origin of the MCA, (4) Fenestration of the MCA, and (5) Early bifurcation of the MCA. There are 18 figures and 1 illustration.

The M1 segment of the MCA shows numerous variations, which are not uncommon. These play important role in collateral circulation and aneurysm formation.

Keywords

Duplicate origin · Duplication · Fenestration Middle cerebral artery

8.1 Duplicated MCA

There are five types of variations in the proximal MCA (Fig. 8.1) [1]. A duplicated MCA is a smaller artery that arises from the ICA just proximal to the carotid bifurcation. This artery usually supplies the anterior temporal lobe (Fig. 8.2) [2]. The reported prevalence on MR angiography is 2.1% [3]. At the origin of the duplicated MCA, an aneurysm can be seen (Fig. 8.3) [4]. Extremely rarely, a duplicated MCA arises from the origin of the hyperplastic AChA (Fig. 8.4) [5].

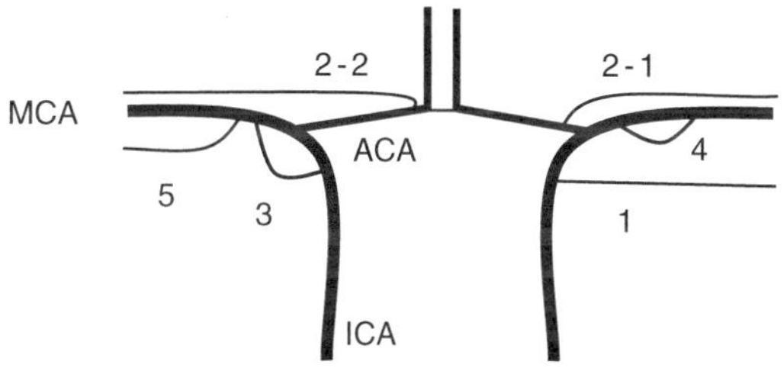

Fig. 8.1 Schematic illustration of five types of MCA variations in A-P projections. (Modified from [1]). 1: Duplicated MCA, 2–1: Proximal A1 origin accessory MCA, 2–2: Distal A1 or A1-A2 junction origin accessory MCA, 3: Duplicate origin of the MCA, 4: Fenestration of the MCA, 5: Early bifurcation of the MCA. *ACA* anterior cerebral artery, *ICA* internal carotid artery, *MCA* middle cerebral artery

8.2 Accessory MCA

8.2.1 Proximal A1 Origin Accessory MCA

A small branch of the MCA arising from the ACA is called an accessory MCA, and it usually supplies the anterior frontal lobe [2]. The prevalence of this variation on MR angiography was reported to be 1.2% [3]. There are two types according to the point at which it arises.

A proximal A1 origin accessory MCA should be differentiated from a duplicated MCA (Fig. 8.5). The carotid bifurcation is the junction

A. Uchino, *Atlas of the Supraaortic Craniocervical Arterial Variations*,
https://doi.org/10.1007/978-981-16-6803-6_8

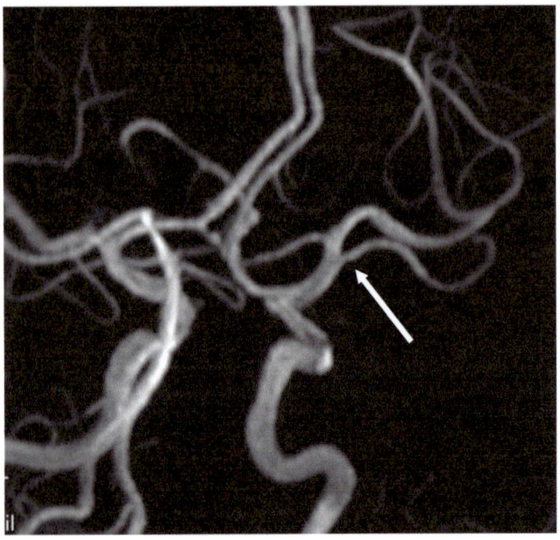

Fig. 8.2 Slightly RAO projection of MR angiography shows a small artery arising from the supraclinoid segment of the left ICA (*arrow*). This duplicated MCA continues to the temporal branch

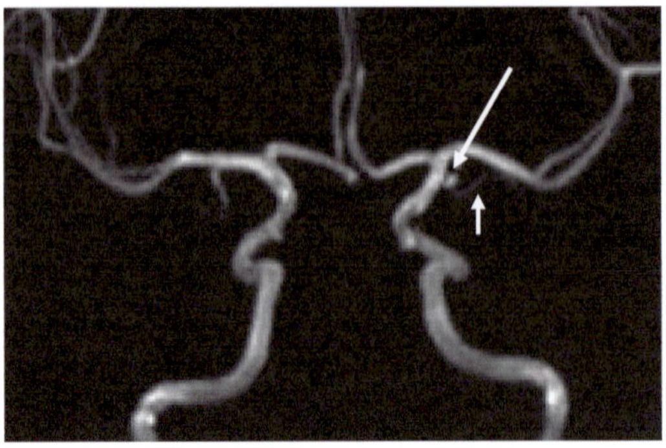

Fig. 8.3 A-P projection of partial MIP MR angiography shows a small aneurysm at the supraclinoid segment of the left MCA (*long arrow*). From the neck of the aneurysm, a small artery arises and runs laterally (*short arrow*), which is indicative of a duplicated MCA, not an AChA

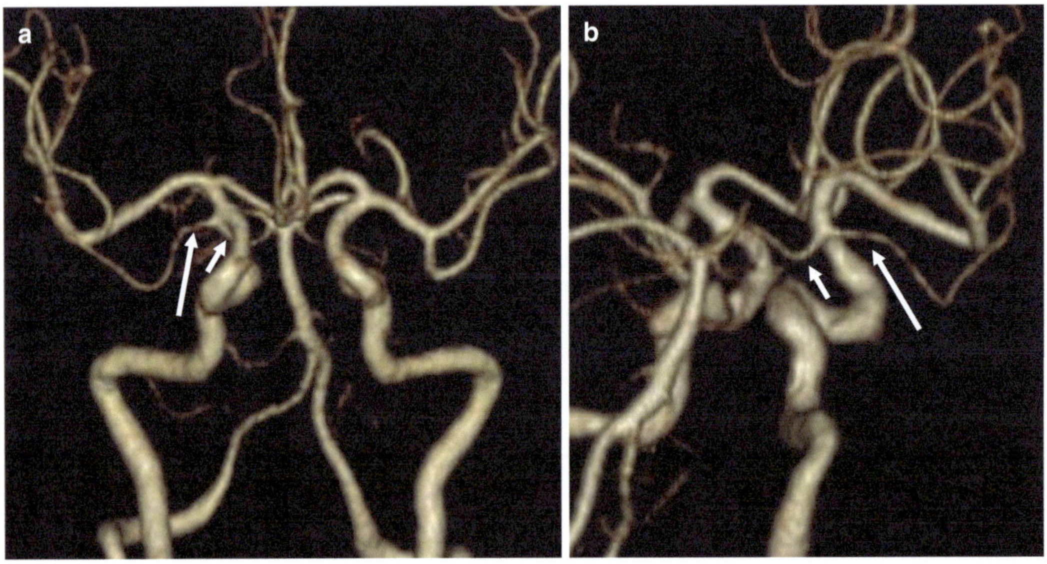

Fig. 8.4 (**a**) A-P and (**b**) RPO projections of CT angiography show a duplicated right MCA (*long arrows*). This anomalous artery has a common trunk with a hyperplastic AChA (*short arrows*)

of the ICA, larger MCA, and ACA. If there are two equally sized MCA branches, it is difficult to distinguish an accessory MCA from a duplicated MCA. In the case of ICA occlusion, the accessory MCA can reserve blood flow to the frontal lobe (Fig. 8.6).

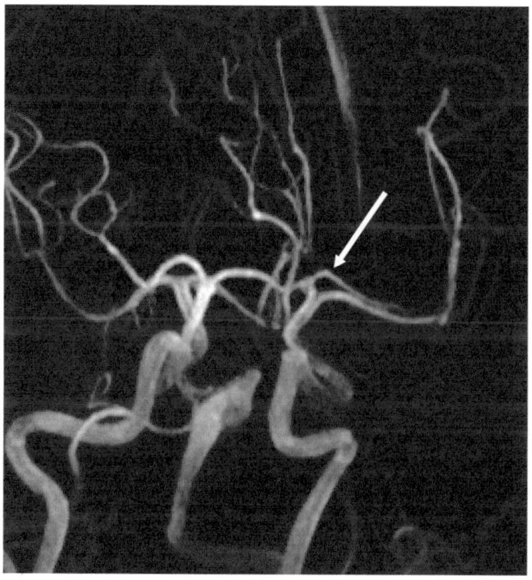

Fig. 8.5 Slightly RAO projection of MR angiography shows a small artery arising from the proximal A1 segment of the left ACA, which is indicative of an accessory MCA, not a duplicated MCA (*arrow*)

8.2.2 Distal A1 or A1-A2 Junction Origin Accessory MCA

An accessory MCA arising from the distal A1 or A1-A2 junction is relatively rare [2]. Because of superimposition with the A1 segment of the ACA and the M1 segment of the MCA, this type of variation may be easily overlooked on routine MIP MR angiography images. VR images are useful for the detection and confirmation of this variation (Fig. 8.7). The recurrent artery of Heubner, which is small and supplies basal ganglia, should not be confused with this variation [6]. This variation can be seen bilaterally (Fig. 8.8).

8.3 Duplicate Origin of the MCA

Duplicate origin of the MCA is relatively rare and has been misdiagnosed or confused as the fenestration of the proximal M1 segment of the MCA and fenestration of the terminal segment of the ICA [7]. The condition is not a true fenestration and occurs when a smaller MCA branch arises from the terminal segment of the ICA (Figs. 8.9 and 8.10) or from the A1 segment of

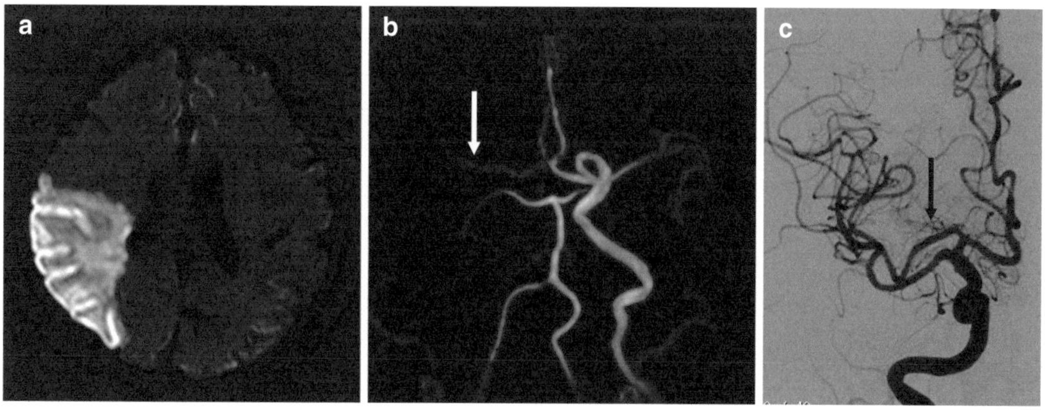

Fig. 8.6 (**a**) Diffusion-weighted MR imaging shows right parietal lobe infarction. The right frontal lobe is not involved. (**b**) AI-PS projection of MR angiography shows right ICA occlusion. The right MCA is visualized by flow via the ACoA, but it is small in caliber (*arrow*). (**c**) A-P projection of right internal carotid angiography immediately after thrombectomy reveals that the MCA shown in (**b**) is a proximal A1 origin accessory MCA (*arrow*)

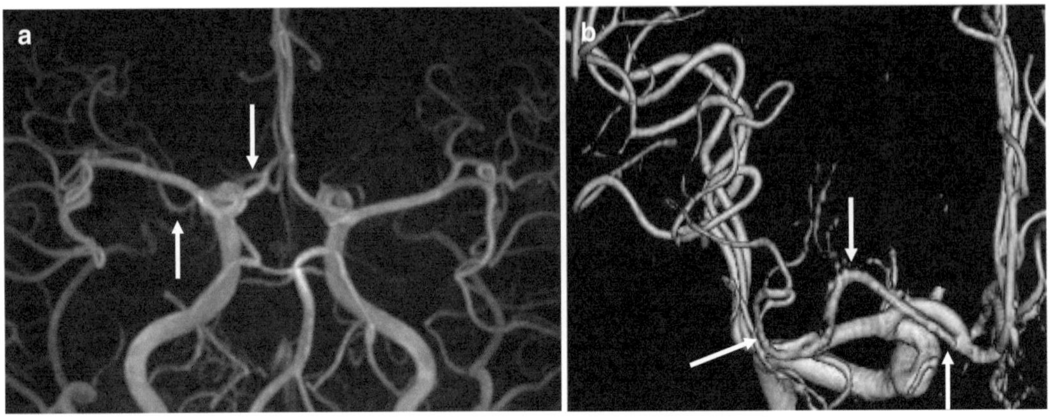

Fig. 8.7 (**a**) AI-PS projection of MR angiography shows a small artery arising from the A1-A2 junction of the right ACA and running along A1 and M1 (*arrows*). (**b**) S-I projection of a partial VR image clearly demonstrates the artery running above A1 and M1, which is indicative of an accessory MCA (*arrows*)

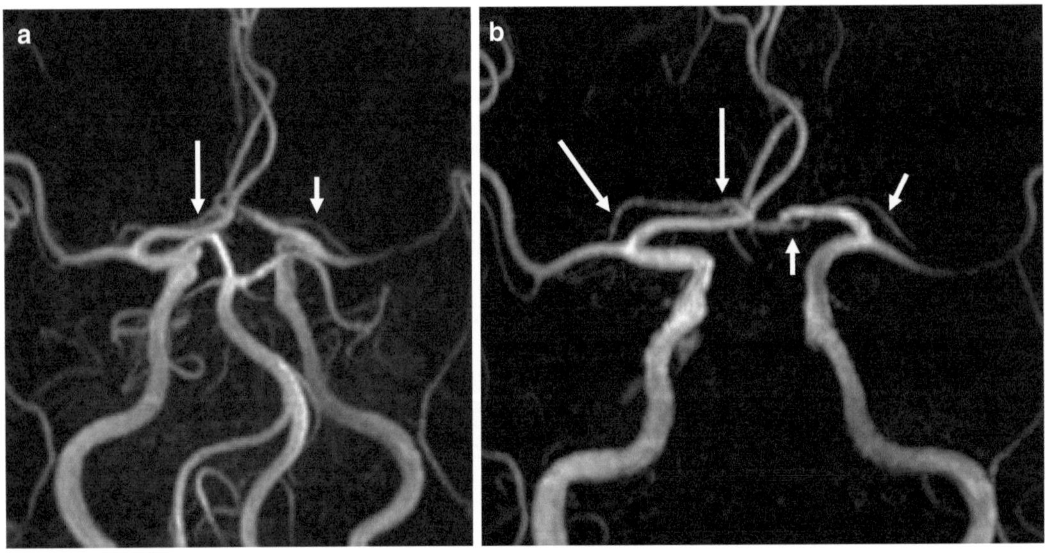

Fig. 8.8 (**a**) A-P projection of MR angiography and (**b**) partial MIP image show a right accessory MCA arising from the A1-A2 junction (*long arrows*) and a left accessory MCA arising from the distal A1 segment (*short arrows*)

the ACA (Fig. 8.11) and fuses with the main MCA branch to form the distal M1 segment of the MCA, forming an arterial ring. Its prevalence on MR angiography was reported to be 0.11% [8]. Clinically, an important difference between duplicate origin and fenestration of the MCA is the potential collateral circulation available from the inferior branch in the case of saddle embolism occlusion of only the superior branch when the vessel has a duplicate origin.

8.4 Fenestration of the MCA

True fenestration of the MCA is slightly rarer than the duplicate origin of the MCA. Its prevalence on MR angiography was reported to be 0.09% [8]. MCA fenestration is usually small and located at the proximal M1 segment, and from the fenestrated M1 segment, the early branching temporopolar artery frequently arises (Figs. 8.12 and 8.13) [9]. Rarely, an

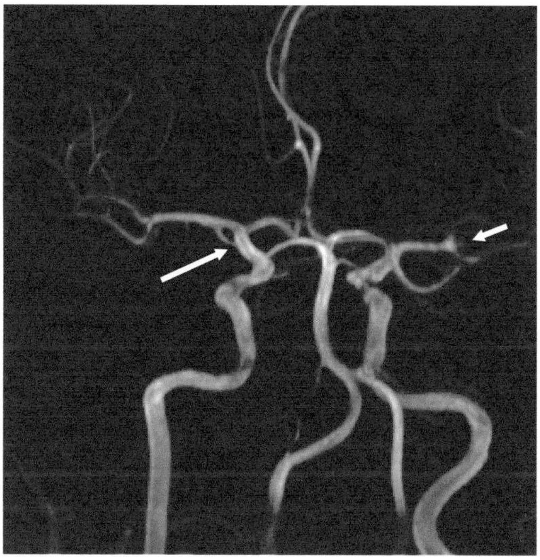

Fig. 8.9 A-P projection of MR angiography shows a small artery arising from the terminal segment of the right ICA and fusing with the main MCA soon, forming a small arterial ring (*long arrow*), indicative of a duplicate origin of the MCA, not a fenestration. The *short arrow* indicates an aneurysm of the left MCA

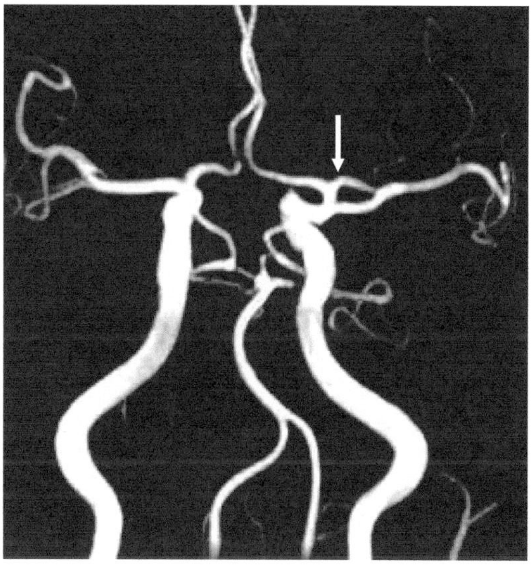

Fig. 8.11 AI-PS projection of MR angiography shows a slightly small artery arising from the proximal A1 segment of the left ACA and fusing with the main MCA, forming a large arterial ring (*arrow*), indicative of a duplicate origin of the MCA, not a fenestration

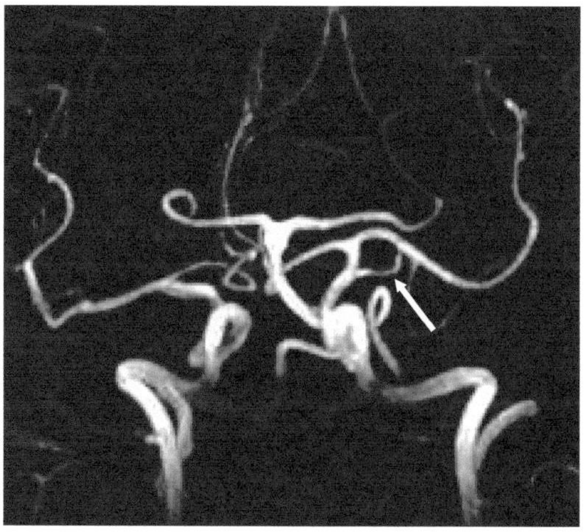

Fig. 8.10 AS-PI projection of MR angiography shows a small artery arising from the supraclinoid segment of the left ICA and fusing with the main MCA, forming a large arterial ring (*arrow*), indicative of a duplicate origin of the MCA, not a fenestration

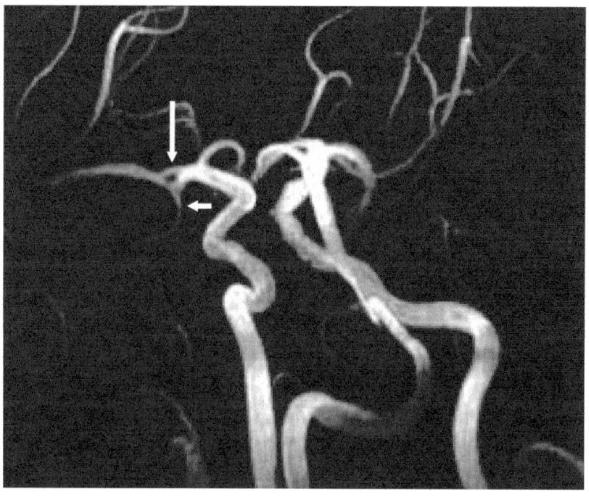

Fig. 8.12 LAO projection of MR angiography shows a small fenestration at the proximal M1 segment of the right MCA (*long arrow*). The right temporopolar artery arises from the fenestrated segment (*short arrow*)

aneurysm can be seen at the proximal end of the fenestration (Fig. 8.13) [10]. MCA fenestration also can be seen at the mid-M1 segment (Fig. 8.14), distal M1 segment (Fig. 8.15), and M2 origin (Fig. 8.16). Superimposition of the M2 branches should not be confused with MCA fenestration of the M2 segment. Fenestrations of the M2 segment may be easily overlooked due to the superimposition of branches.

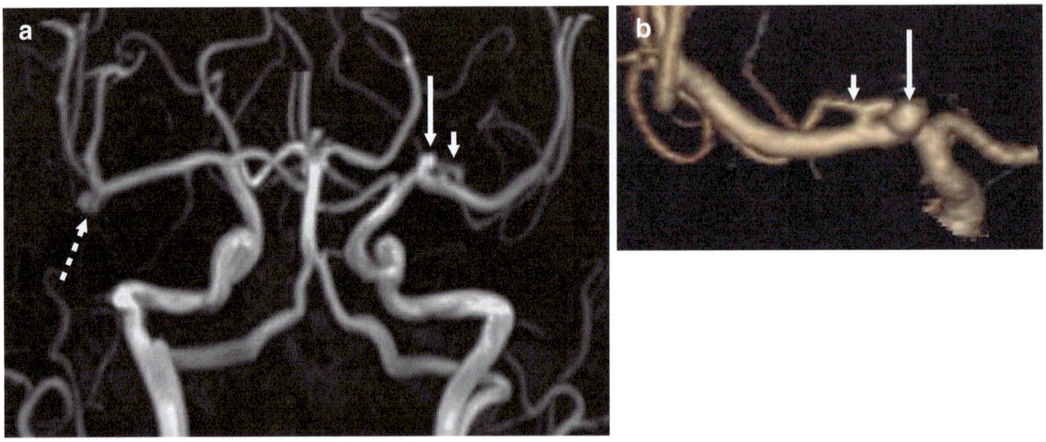

Fig. 8.13 (**a**) A-P projection of MR angiography and (**b**) P-A projection of a partial VR image show an aneurysm at the proximal M1 segment of the left MCA (*long arrows*). There is a small fenestration at the left proximal M1, and the aneurysm is located at the proximal end of the fenestration. The left temporopolar artery arises from the fenestrated segment (*short arrows*). Another aneurysm is seen at the right MCA bifurcation (*dotted arrow*)

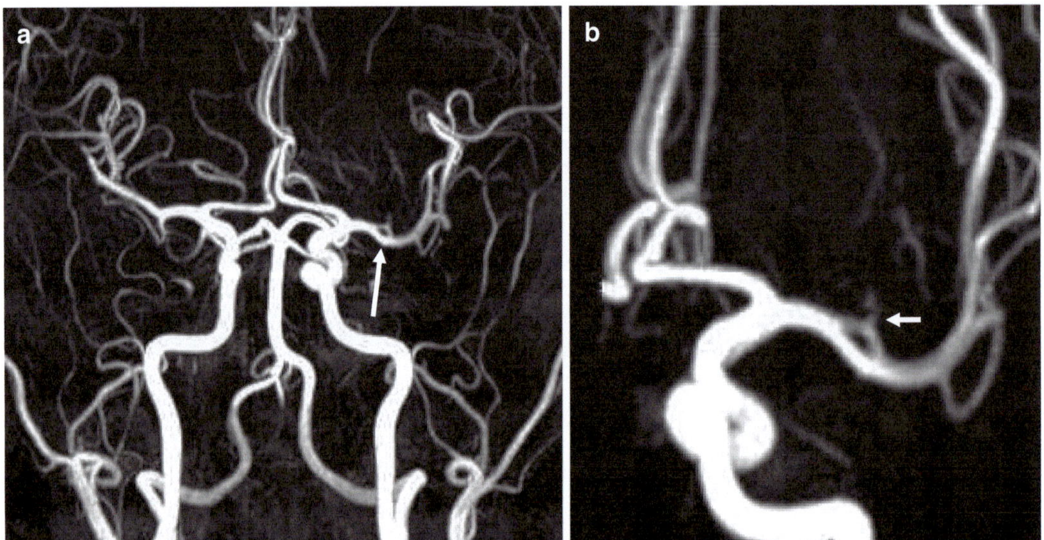

Fig. 8.14 (**a**) A-P projection of MR angiography and (**b**) partial MIP image show a fenestration at the mid-M1 segment of the left MCA (*long arrow*). The left lateral lenticulostriate artery arises from the fenestrated segment (*short arrow*)

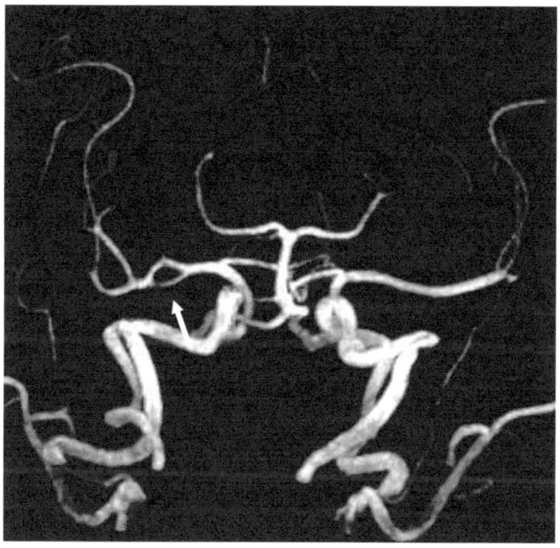

Fig. 8.15 AS-PI projection of MR angiography shows a relatively large fenestration at the distal M1 segment of the right MCA (*arrow*)

8.5 Early Bifurcation of the MCA

Bifurcation of the MCA within one centimeter of its origin is called early bifurcation [11]. It is frequently observed, and the inferior smaller branch usually supplies the temporal lobe (Fig. 8.17), as it does in the case of a duplicated MCA. This variation can rarely be seen in association with the duplicate origin of the MCA (Fig. 8.18). MCA sometimes trifurcates instead of bifurcates. Early trifurcation of the MCA is rarely seen (Fig. 8.19).

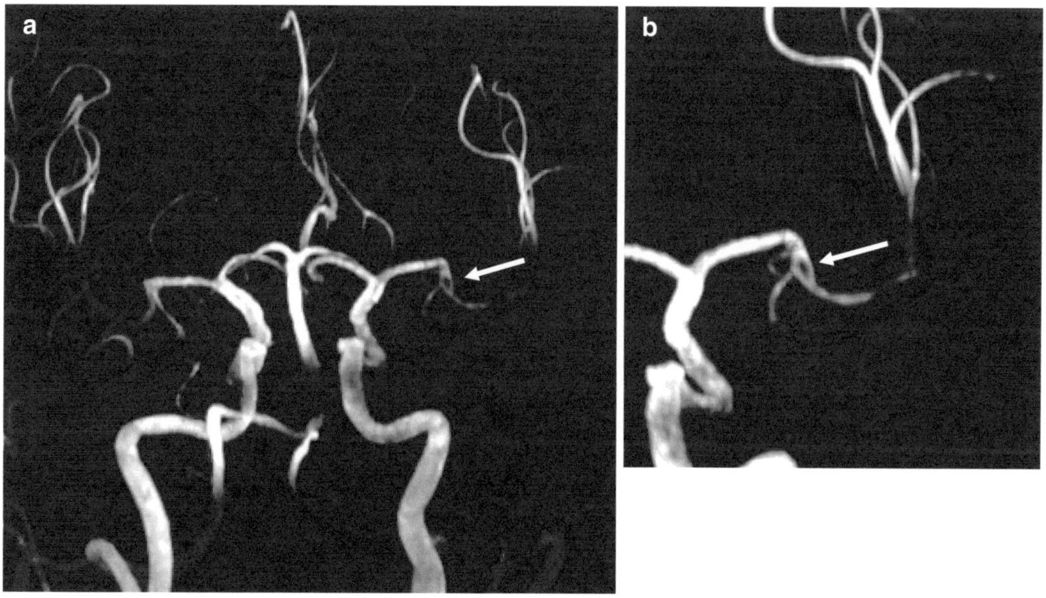

Fig. 8.16 (**a**) A-P projection of MR angiography and (**b**) partial MIP image show a small fenestration at the origin of the M2 segment of the left MCA (*arrows*)

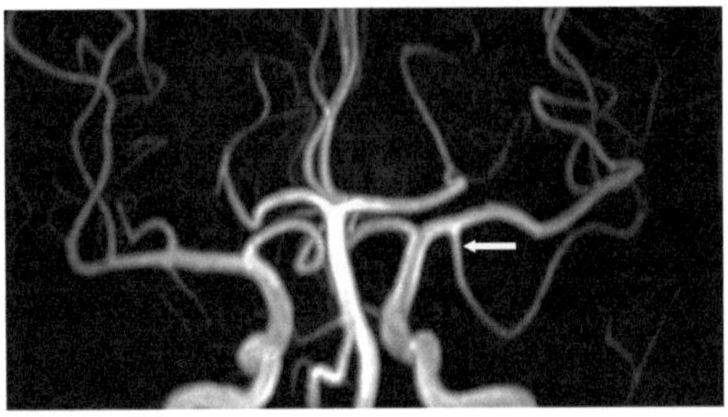

Fig. 8.17 AS-PI projection of MR angiography shows that the temporal branch of the left MCA arises from the extreme proximal M1 segment (*arrow*), indicative of an early bifurcation of the MCA

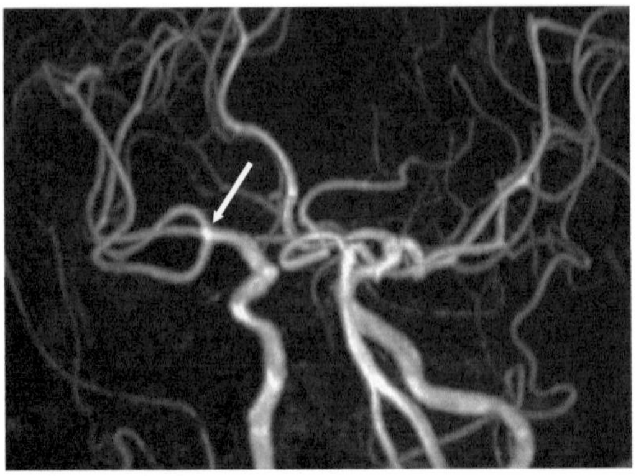

Fig. 8.19 Slightly LAO projection of MR angiography shows an early trifurcated right MCA (*arrow*). The distance between the carotid bifurcation and MCA trifurcation is 6 mm

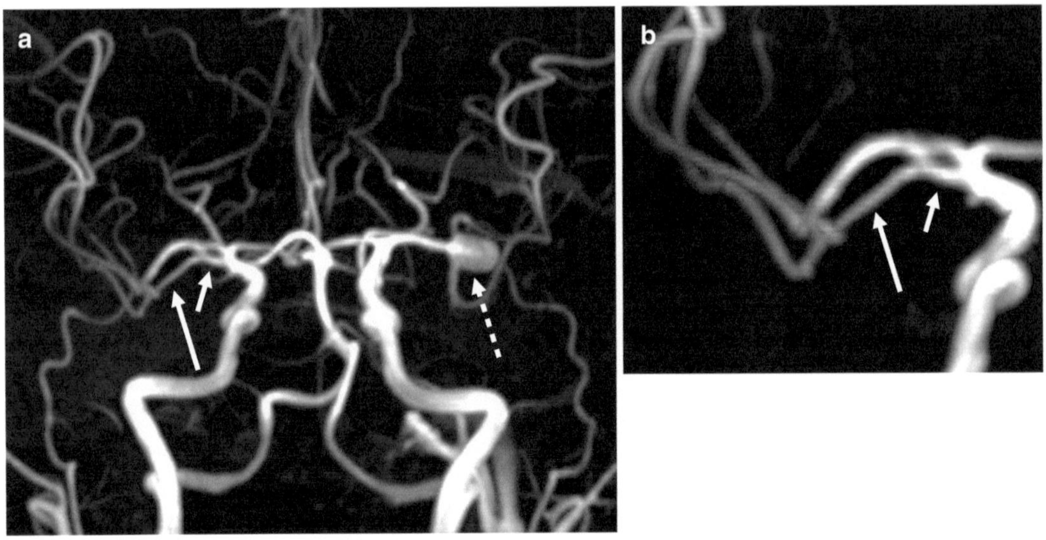

Fig. 8.18 (**a**) A-P projection of MR angiography and (**b**) partial MIP image show duplicate origin of the right MCA (*short arrows*) (Sect. 8.3) from which the temporal branch arises (*long arrows*). An aneurysm of the left MCA can be observed (*dotted arrow*)

References

1. Uchino A. Cerebral arterial variations and anomalies diagnosed by MR angiography. In: Takahashi S, editor. Neurovascular imaging. MRI and microangiography. 1st ed. London: Springer; 2010. p. 197–239.
2. Komiyama M, Nakajima H, Nishikawa M, Yasui T. Middle cerebral artery variations: duplicated and accessory arteries. AJNR Am J Neuroradiol. 1998;19:45–9.
3. Uchino A, Kato A, Takase Y, Kudo S. Middle cerebral artery variations detected by magnetic resonance angiography. Eur Radiol. 2000;10:560–3.
4. Fujimoto K, Hashimoto H, Uchiyama Y, Maekawa H, Shida Y, Nakagawa I. Duplicated middle cerebral artery aneurysms treated by coil embolization; a report of two cases and literature review. J Stroke Cerebrovasc Dis. 2021;30:105773.
5. Uchino A, Ito S, Kurita H, Tanaka M. Duplicated middle cerebral artery arising from the origin of the hyperplastic anterior choroidal artery that mimicked aneurysm on routine MR angiography. Neuroradiol J. 2016;29:106–9.
6. Takahashi S, Hoshino F, Uemura K, Takahashi A, Sakamoto K. Accessory middle cerebral artery: is it a variant form of the recurrent artery of Heubner? AJNR Am J Neuroradiol. 1989;10:563–8.
7. Rennert J, Ullrich WO, Schuierer G. A rare case of supraclinoid internal carotid artery (ICA) fenestration in combination with duplication of the middle cerebral artery (MCA) originating from the ICA fenestration and an associated aneurysm. Clin Neuroradiol. 2013;23:133–6.
8. Uchino A, Saito N, Okada Y, Nakajima R. Duplicate origin and fenestration of the middle cerebral artery on MR angiography. Surg Radiol Anat. 2012;34:401–4.
9. Gailloud P, Albayram S, Fasel JH, Beauchamp NJ, Murphy KJ. Angiographic and embryologic considerations in five cases of middle cerebral artery fenestration. AJNR Am J Neuroradiol. 2002;23:585–7.
10. Yamaguchi S, Ito O, Suzuki S. Coil embolization of a ruptured aneurysm arising from a middle cerebral artery fenestration: case report. Neurol Med Chir (Tokyo). 2010;50:213–6.
11. Teal JS, Rumbaugh CL, Bergeron RT, Segall HD. Anomalies of the middle cerebral artery: accessory artery, duplication, and early bifurcation. Am J Roentgenol Radium Ther Nucl Med. 1973;118:567–75.

Variations of the Proximal Anterior Cerebral Artery (ACA), Including Anterior Communicating Artery (ACoA)

9

Abstract

This chapter includes (1) Unilateral A1 aplasia, (2) Carotid-ACA anastomosis (Infraoptic course of ACA), (3) Persistent primitive olfactory artery, (4) Duplicate origin of the ACA, (5) Fenestration of the ACA, (6) Distal A1 duplication, (7) Azygos (unpaired) ACA, (8) Bihemispheric (asymmetric) ACA, (9) Triple ACA (Accessory ACA), and (10) ACoA duplication, partial duplication, and true fenestration. There are 30 figures and 4 illustrations.

Both carotid-ACA anastomosis and persistent primitive olfactory artery are rare but important variations because they are dangerous during surgery of the suprasellar region and midline anterior skull base.

Keywords

Anterior cerebral artery · Anterior communicating artery · Carotid-anterior cerebral artery anastomosis · Persistent primitive olfactory artery

9.1 Unilateral A1 Aplasia of the ACA

Unilateral A1 aplasia is frequently observed. Its prevalence on MR angiography is reported to be 6.7% [1]. However, acquired occlusion or extreme hypoplasia of the A1 segment cannot be distinguished from A1 aplasia on MR angiography.

An ACA-ACoA junction aneurysm frequently occurs in patients with contralateral A1 aplasia or hypoplasia due to hemodynamic stress (Fig. 9.1) [2]. In patients with unilateral A1 aplasia, the contralateral A1 segment is as large as the MCA. Thus, a thrombus may enter into the hyperplastic A1 more frequently in comparison to a normally-sized A1, resulting in a high incidence of ACA territory embolic infarction (Fig. 9.2) [3].

9.2 Carotid-ACA Anastomosis (Infraoptic Course of ACA)

Rarely, an anomalous artery arises from the medial wall of the ophthalmic segment of the ICA, courses cranially through the space between the optic nerves, and anastomoses with the A1-A2 junction of the ACA. This rare cerebral arterial variation is called carotid-ACA anastomosis or infraoptic course of ACA. Because this artery is not the true A1, and some patients have a coexisting normally positioned A1 segment of the ACA, the name carotid-ACA anastomosis seems to be better than infraoptic course of ACA.

There is a right-sided predominance [4]. Its prevalence on MR angiography was reported to be 0.086% [5]. Wong et al. [6] classified 4 types.

A. Uchino, *Atlas of the Supraaortic Craniocervical Arterial Variations*,
https://doi.org/10.1007/978-981-16-6803-6_9

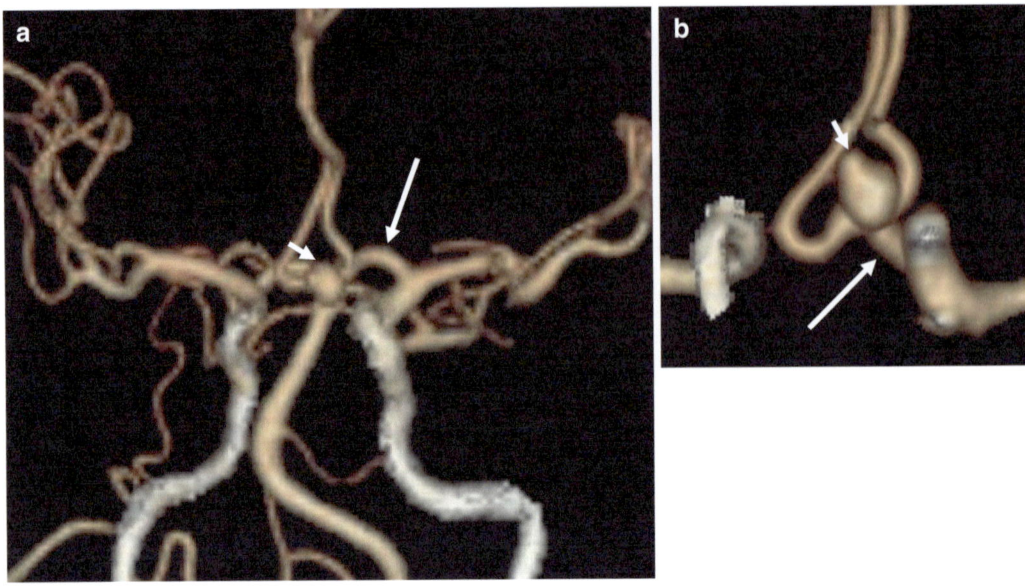

Fig. 9.1 (**a**) A-P projection of CT angiography and (**b**) partial VR image show a large A1 segment of the left ACA (*long arrows*). A ruptured aneurysm is seen at the left ACA-ACoA junction (*short arrows*). The A1 segment of the right ACA cannot be identified

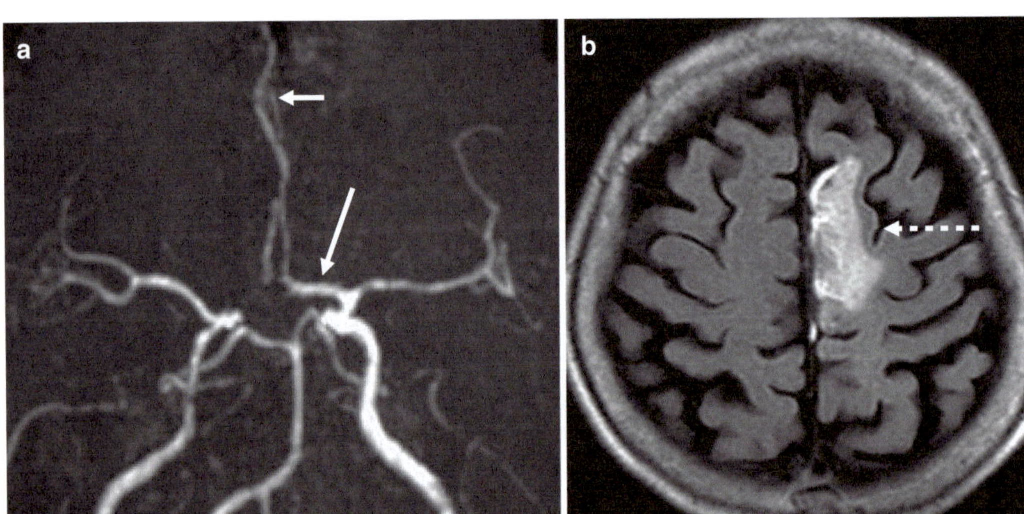

Fig. 9.2 (**a**) AI-PS projection of MR angiography shows a large A1 segment of the left ACA (*long arrow*). The A2 segment of the left ACA is narrow and the distal segment is occluded (*short arrow*). The contralateral A1 segment cannot be identified. (**b**) FLAIR MR image shows an infarction in the distal left ACA territory (*dotted arrow*), suggesting thrombo-embolic infarction

A schematic illustration of the 3 main types is shown in Fig. 9.3. In type 1, there are bilateral normal A1 segments of the ACAs (Fig. 9.4), type 2 has no ipsilateral normal A1 segment (Fig. 9.5), and type 3 has no bilateral normal A1 segments (Fig. 9.6). Although the reason is unclear, this variation is extremely rarely seen on the left side (Fig. 9.7) [7]. This variation can

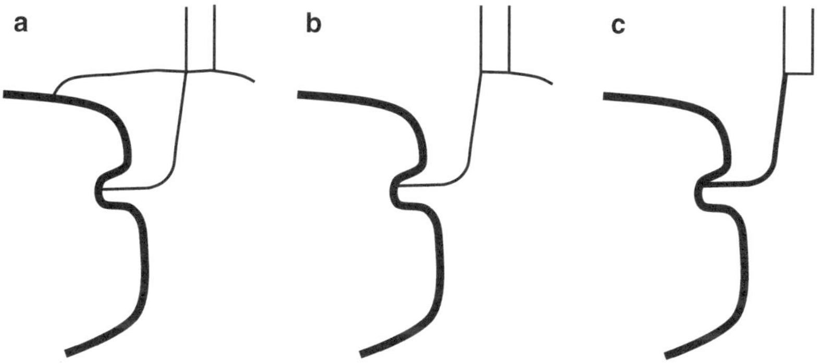

Fig. 9.3 Schematic illustrations of Wong's three main types of carotid-ACA anastomosis. (Modified from [6]). **a**: Type 1, with bilateral normal A1 segments of the ACA. **b**: Type 2, with no ipsilateral A1 segment. **c**: Type 3, with no bilateral A1 segments

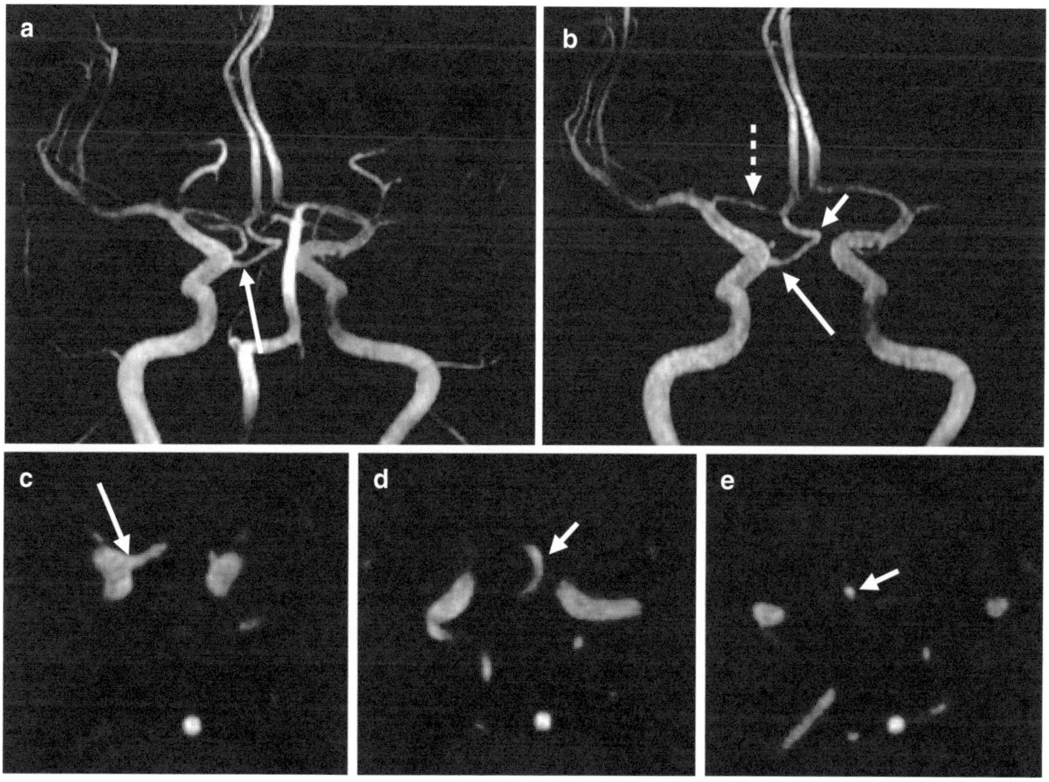

Fig. 9.4 (**a**) A-P projection of MR angiography, (**b**) partial MIP image, and (**c**–**e**) MR angiographic source images show an anomalous artery arising from the medial wall of the ophthalmic segment of the right ICA (*long arrows*) and running cranially through the space between the optic nerves (*short arrows*). An ipsilatetral A1 is present (*dotted arrow*), indicative of a type 1 carotid-ACA anastomosis

also be seen bilaterally, and it is frequently associated with OphA variations (Figs. 9.8 and 9.9) [8, 9]. This variation is also associated with other variations (Figs. 9.6 and 9.10) [10]. The association of this variation with the tetralogy of Fallot was reported with other arterial variations [11, 12].

Carotid-ACA anastomosis is clinically significant because its presence increases the risk for aneurysm formation at the A1-A2-ACoA complex. Hemodynamic stress related to the anastomotic artery may play an important role. Surgery in the suprasellar region via the anterior cranial fossa may be dangerous.

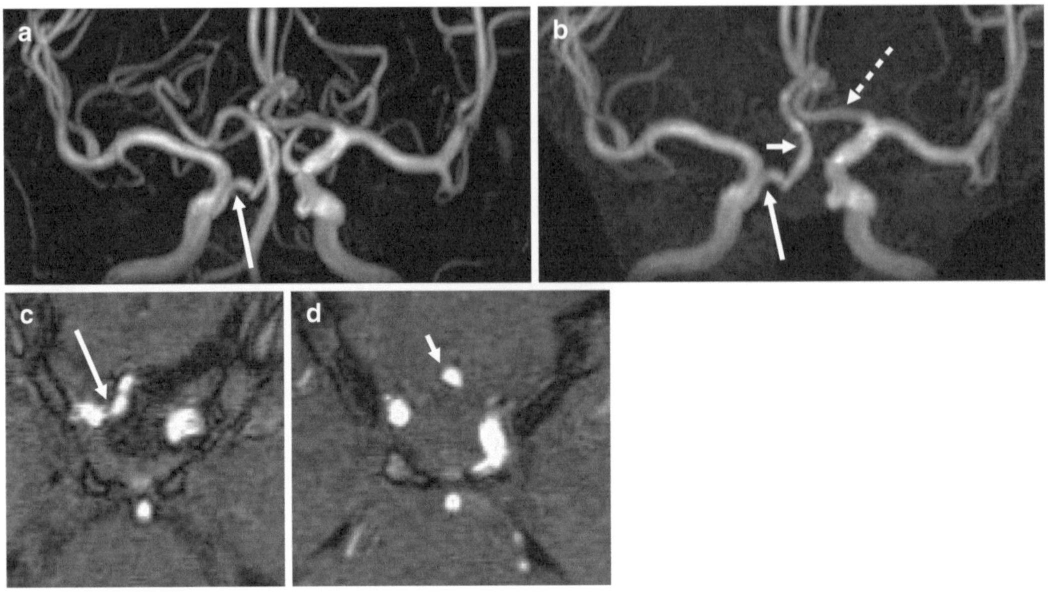

Fig. 9.5 (**a**) A-P projection of MR angiography, (**b**) partial MIP image, and (**c**, **d**) MR angiographic source images show an anomalous artery arising from the medial wall of the ophthalmic segment of the right ICA (*long arrows*) and running cranially through the space between the optic nerves (*short arrows*). A contralateral A1 is present (*dotted arrow*), but there is no ipsilateral A1, indicative of a type 2 carotid-ACA anastomosis. A small aneurysm is seen at the paraclinoid segment of the left ICA

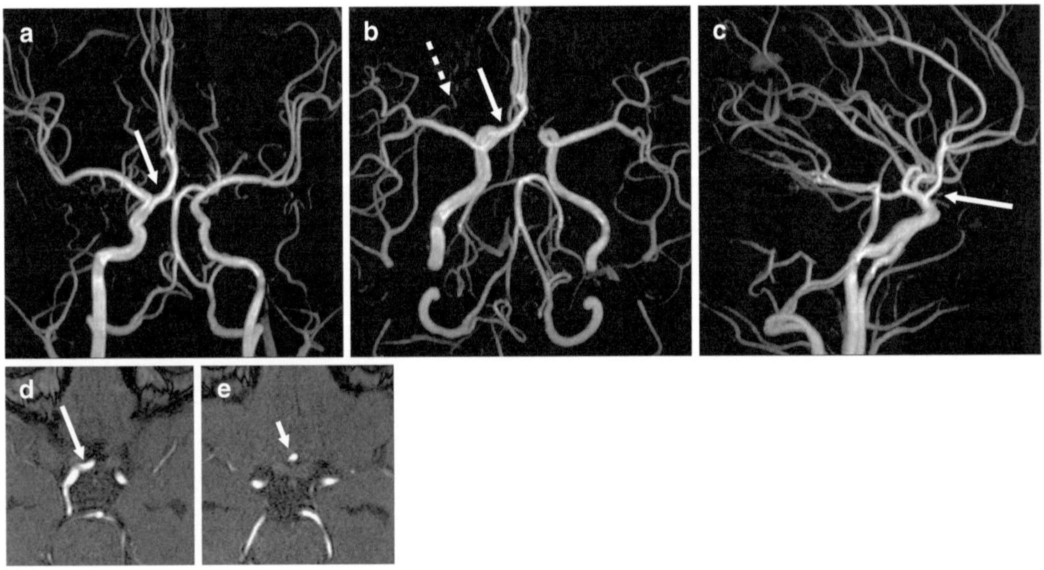

Fig. 9.6 (**a**) A-P, (**b**) AI-PS, and (**c**) lateral projections of MR angiography and (**d**, **e**) source images show an anomalous artery arising from the medial wall of the ophthalmic segment of the right ICA (*long arrows*) and running cranially through the space between the optic nerves (*short arrow*). Finally, this artery continues to the azygos ACA (Sect. 9.7). The bilateral A1s are absent, indicative of a type 3 carotid-ACA anastomosis. The right OphA arises from the MMA (*dotted arrow*) (Sect. 6.3)

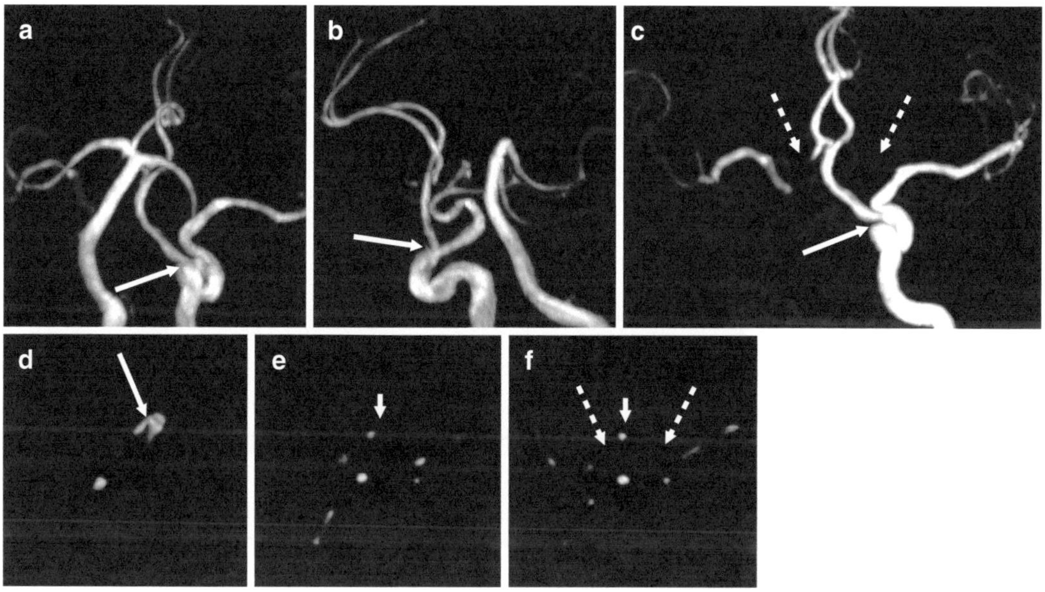

Fig. 9.7 (**a**) A-P and (**b**) lateral projections of MR angiography, (**c**) partial MIP image, and (**d–f**) MR angiographic source images show an anomalous artery arising from the medial wall of the ophthalmic segment of the left ICA (*long arrows*) and running cranially through the space between the optic nerves (*short arrows*). The bilateral A1s are present but small in caliber (*dotted arrows*), indicative of a type 1 carotid-ACA anastomosis. With the exception of the terminal segment, the right ICA is occluded

9.3 Persistent Primitive Olfactory Artery (PPOA)

Rarely, the proximal segment of the ACA courses extremely anteroinferiorly, makes a hairpin turn, and connects posterosuperiorly to the normal A2 segment. Its prevalence on MR angiography was reported to be 0.14%, with no laterality in frequency and rare bilaterality [13].

Embryologically, the rostral division of the primitive ICA constitutes the primitive olfactory artery, which terminates in the nasal fossa. The secondary branch of the primitive olfactory artery is the medial olfactory artery, which constitutes the future ACA [14]. The primitive olfactory artery usually regresses during early gestation, but when it persists, this anomalous ACA, called persistent primitive olfactory artery (PPOA), is formed.

PPOA is classified into 5 types (Fig. 9.11) [15]. Type 1 is most common and has the typical appearance of a hairpin turn (Fig. 9.12). In some patients, an aneurysm is seen at the hairpin turn, probably due to hemodynamic stress (Fig. 9.13). Types 2 and 3 are rare and connect to the ethmoidal artery. Because the ethmoidal artery is small in caliber, the detection of this variation using routine MR angiography is difficult (Fig. 9.14) [16]. Type 4 is rare and connects to the accessory MCA instead of the distal ACA (Fig. 9.15) [17]. Type 5 is rare and runs superiorly and connects to the A3 segment of the ACA without a hairpin turn (Fig. 9.16) [15]. Type 1 also occurs in association with A2 variation (Fig. 9.17) [18].

PPOA is clinically significant because its presence increases the risk of aneurysm formation at the hairpin turn. Surgery in the anterior cranial fossa and suprasellar region may be dangerous.

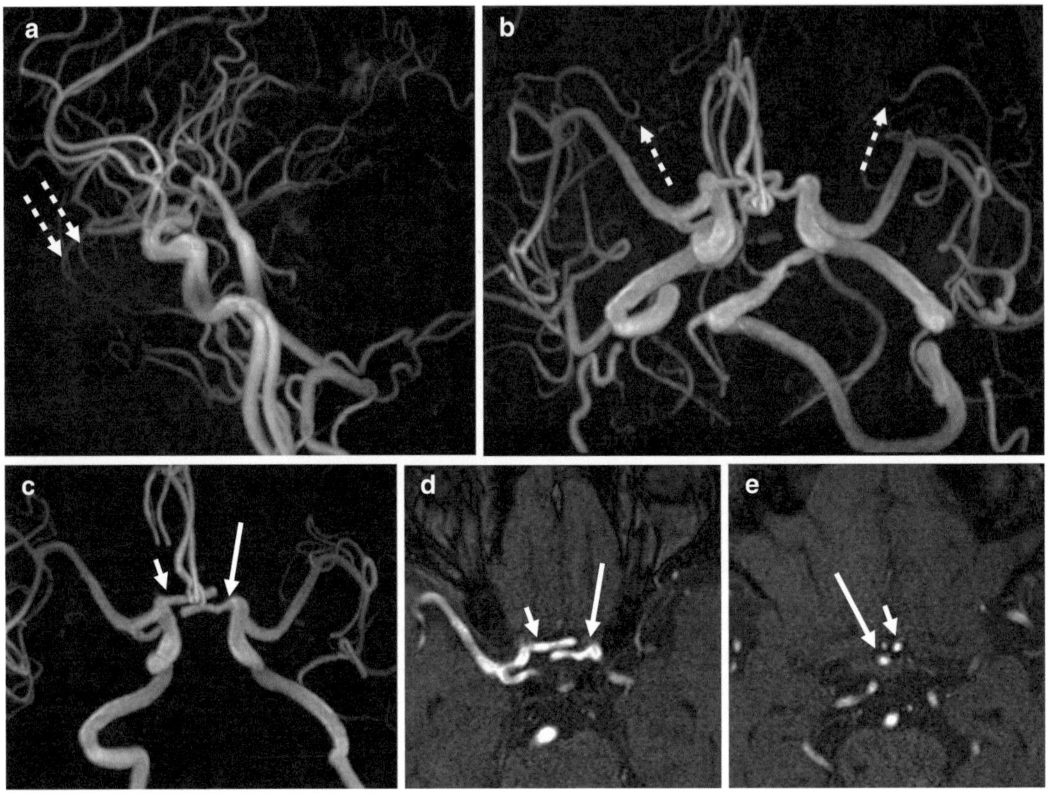

Fig. 9.8 (**a**) Lateral and (**b**) I-S projections of MR angiography, (**c**) partial MIP image, and (**c–e**) MR angiographic source images show the bilateral OphAs arising from the MMAs (*dotted arrows*). Anomalous arteries arise from the medial wall of the ophthalmic segment of the bilateral ICAs (*short and long arrows*) and run cranially through the space between the optic nerves. The bilateral A1s are absent, indicative of bilateral type 3 carotid-ACA anastomoses

9.4 Duplicate Origin of the ACA

Duplicate origin of the ACA results from the fusion of two arteries that arise from the terminal segment of the ICA to form the A1 segment of the ACA (Fig. 9.18) [19]. This variation is rare and differs from the ACA arising from the fenestration of the terminal ICA (Fig. 9.19).

9.5 Fenestration of the ACA

ACA fenestrations are mainly seen at the distal A1 segment (Fig. 9.20), A1-A2 junction (Fig. 9.21), and proximal A2 segment (Fig. 9.22). Its prevalence on MR angiography was reported to be 1.2% [2]. However, using catheter angiography, its prevalence was reported to be only 0.058% [20]. Because the two fenestrated A1 branches are usually divided horizontally, these vessels are superimposed on conventional 2-dimensional angiographic images. In contrast, MR angiographic images are made from 3-dimensional data. Thus, the superimposition of vessels can be easily identified. It is rarely seen bilaterally (Fig. 9.23). An aneurysm rarely occurs at the proximal end of the fenestration (Fig. 9.24) [21].

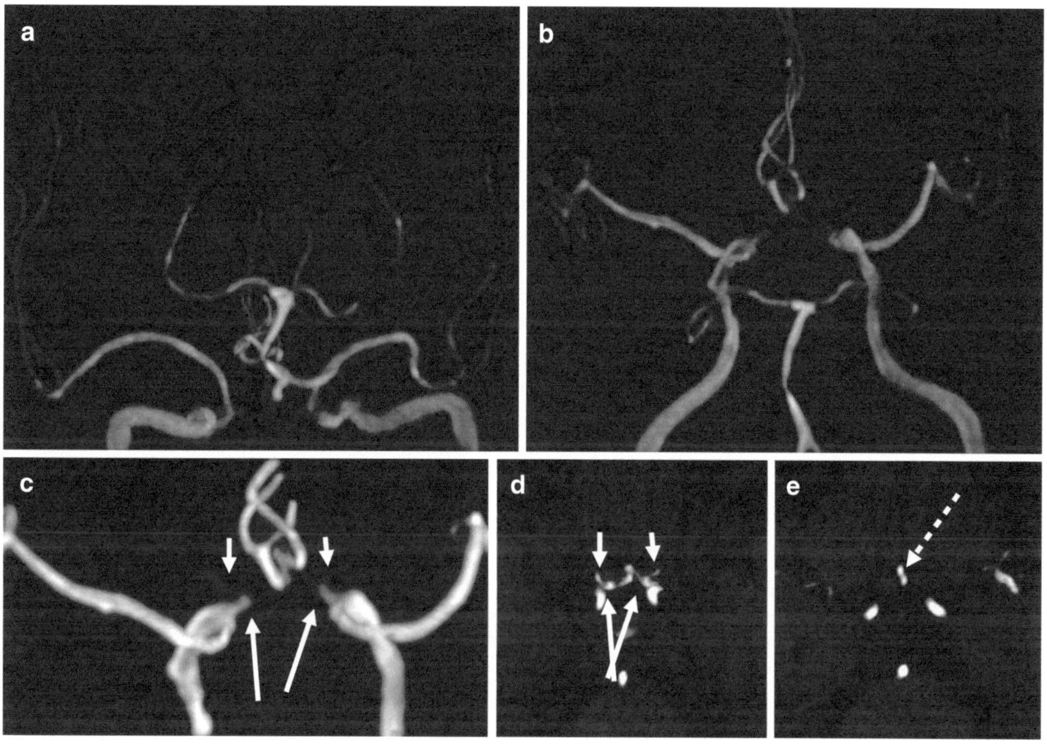

Fig. 9.9 (**a**) AS-PI and (**b**) AI-PS projections of MR angiography, (**c**) partial MIP image, and (**d**, **e**) MR angiographic source images show anomalous arteries arising from the medial wall of the ophthalmic segment of the bilateral ICAs (*long arrows*) and running cranially through the space between the optic nerves (*dotted arrow*). The bilateral OphAs arise from the anomalous arteries (*short arrows*). The bilateral A1s are absent, indicative of bilateral type 3 carotid-ACA anastomoses

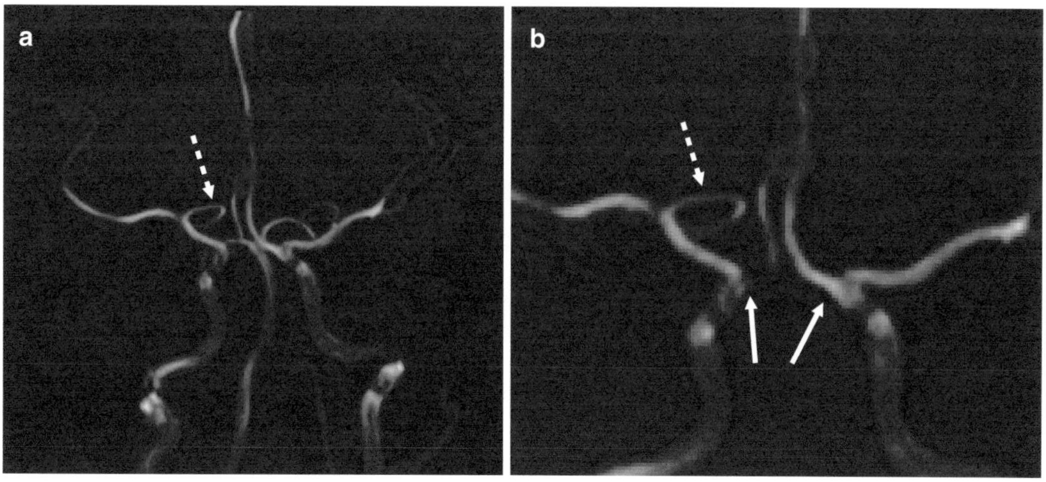

Fig. 9.10 (**a**) A-P projection of MR angiography and (**b**) partial MIP image show bilateral carotid-ACA anastomoses (*long arrows*). The left A1 is absent. The right A1 is present, but it only supplies an accessory MCA (*dotted arrows*) (Sect. 8.2). (Courtesy of Dr. Kanehiro Hasuo)

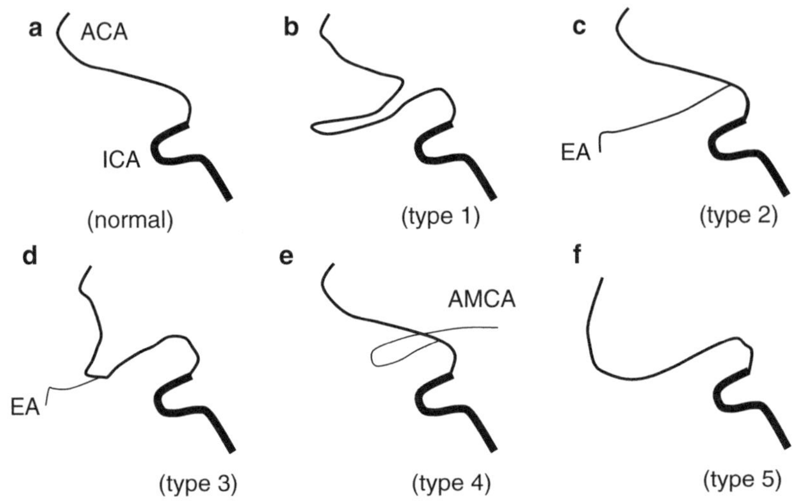

Fig. 9.11 Schematic illustration of five types of PPOA (left lateral projection). (Modified from [15]). *ACA* anterior cerebral artery, *AMCA* accessory middle cerebral artery, *EA* ethmoidal artery, *ICA* internal carotid artery

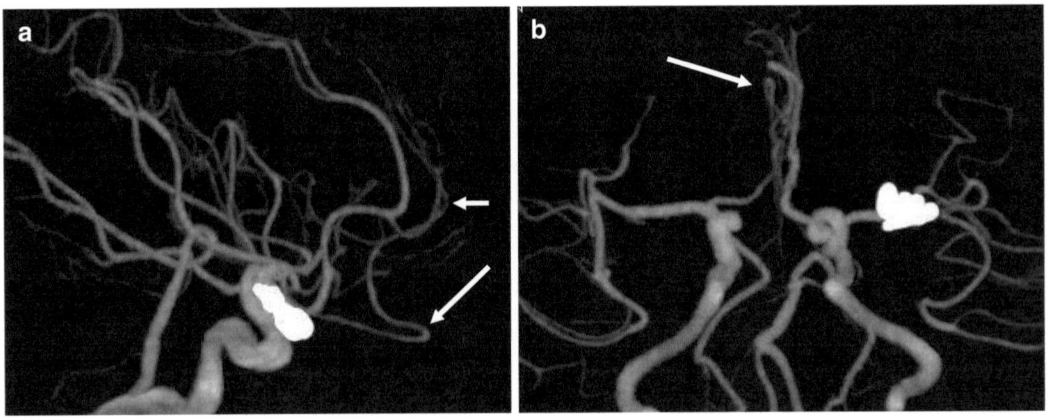

Fig. 9.12 (**a**) Lateral and (**b**) I-S projections of CT angiography show the right ACA taking an anteroinferior course and making a hairpin turn (*long arrows*), indicative of a type 1 PPOA. This artery supplies the right callosomarginal artery (*short arrow*). This patient previously underwent clipping of a left MCA aneurysm

9.6 Distal A1 Duplication

The distal A1 segment of the ACA sometimes duplicates and continues to the A2 segment separately without distal fusion, resulting in distal duplication [22]. One of the duplicated channels fuses with the contralateral ACA; thus, this variation can also be regarded as a long ACoA. In rare cases, an aneurysm can be seen at the point of duplication (Fig. 9.25).

9.7 Azygos (Unpaired) ACA

An unpaired A2 segment of the ACA is called an azygos ACA. Its prevalence on MR angiography was reported to be 1.3% [1] and 2.0% [2]. An asymmetric A2 segment, called a bihemispheric ACA (Sect. 9.8) should not be classified as an azygos ACA. However, because of the low spatial resolution of MR angiography, some of the contralateral tiny A2 segment may not be identi-

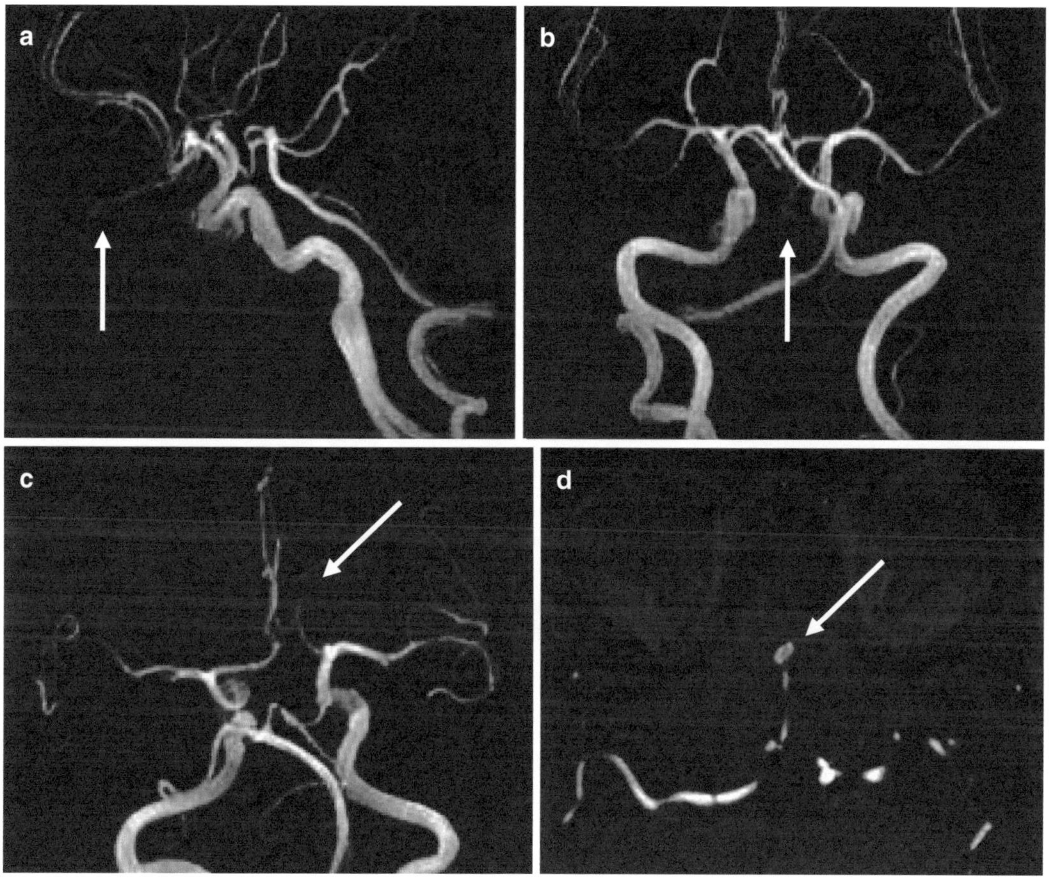

Fig. 9.13 (**a**) Lateral, (**b**) A-P, and (**c**) I-S projections of MR angiography and (**d**) MR angiographic source image show the left ACA taking an anteroinferior course and making a hairpin turn, indicative of a type 1 PPOA. An aneurysm is seen at the hairpin turn (*arrows*)

fied. Using catheter angiography, the prevalence of azygos ACA was reported to be only 0.2% [23]. Because the ACoA is absent, no aneurysm occurs at the ACA-ACoA junction. However, an aneurysm is frequently seen at the end of the unpaired A2 segment, probably due to hemodynamic stress (Fig. 9.26).

9.8 Bihemispheric (Asymmetric) ACA

As mentioned above, an asymmetric A2 segment of the ACA should not be confused with an unpaired A2 (Sect. 9.7). The larger artery usually supplies the bilateral pericallosal arteries and the ipsilateral callosomarginal artery. In contrast, the smaller artery supplies only the ipsilateral callosomarginal artery or its branches. An aneurysm is frequently seen at the A2-A3 junction of the larger artery, probably due to hemodynamic stress (Fig. 9.27) [24].

9.9 Triple ACA (Accessory ACA)

The anomalous branch arising from the ACoA is called an accessory ACA or a median artery of the corpus callosum. In patients with this variation, there is a third A2 segment, resulting in triple ACAs. Its prevalence on MR angiography was reported to be 1.3% [1] and 3.0% [2]. The

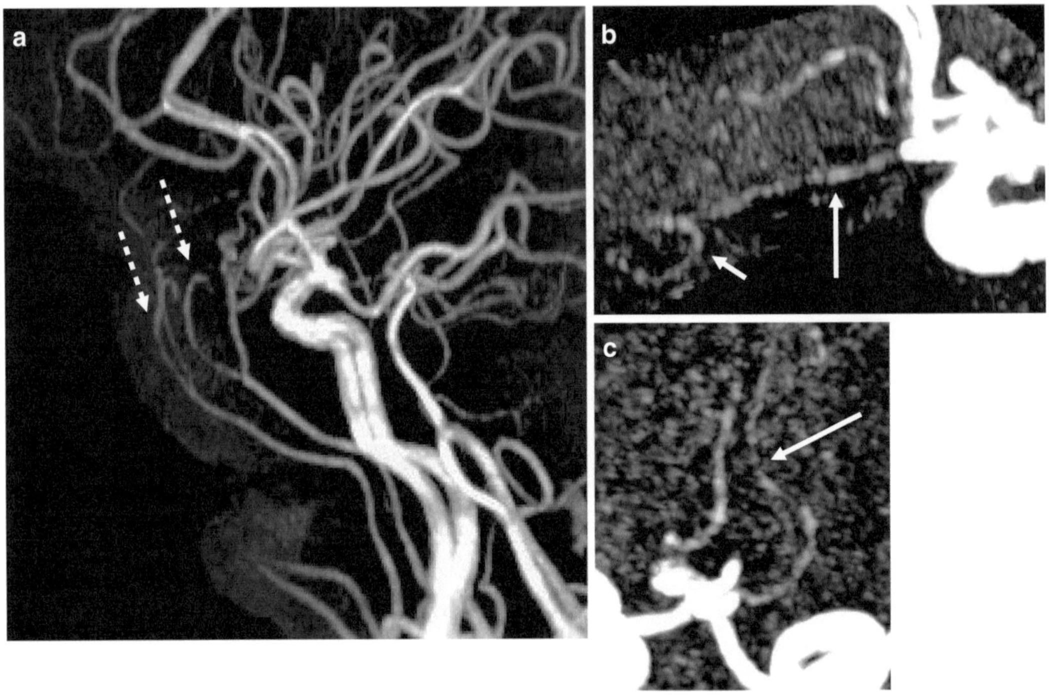

Fig. 9.14 (**a**) Lateral projection of MR angiography shows bilateral OphAs arising from the MMAs (*dotted arrows*) (Sect. 6.3). (**b**) Lateral and (**c**) I-S projections of the partial MIP images show a small artery arising from the left A1-A2 junction and taking an anteroinferior course (*long arrows*). This artery connects to the ethmoidal artery (*short arrow*), indicative of a type 2 PPOA

accessory ACA usually continues to the bilateral pericallosal arteries and the other two arteries continue to the ipsilateral callosomarginal artery (Fig. 9.28). Triple ACAs were seen in 19.4% of patients with ACoA aneurysms, which is an extremely high prevalence [25].

Rarely, there is a fourth A2 segment, resulting in quadruple ACAs (Fig. 9.29).

9.10 ACoA Duplication, Partial Duplication, and True Fenestration

Variations of the ACA-ACoA complex are common and are classified into several types (Fig. 9.30). Most are duplicated ACoAs (Fig. 9.31) and partially duplicated ACoAs (Fig. 9.32). Double partial duplications are also seen (Fig. 9.33). These variations are confused with true fenestration of the ACoA (Fig. 9.34) [26]. The majority of previously reported ACoA fenestrations are duplications or partial duplications of the ACoA. These ACoA variations can be considered as an important morphological risk factor for aneurysm rupture [27].

The ACA-ACoA junction is the most common site of cerebral aneurysms. These ACoA variations may be misinterpreted as a tiny aneurysm on MR angiography because of its low spatial resolution. Using three-dimensional rotational cerebral angiography, both ACoA variations and aneurysms can be identified clearly [28].

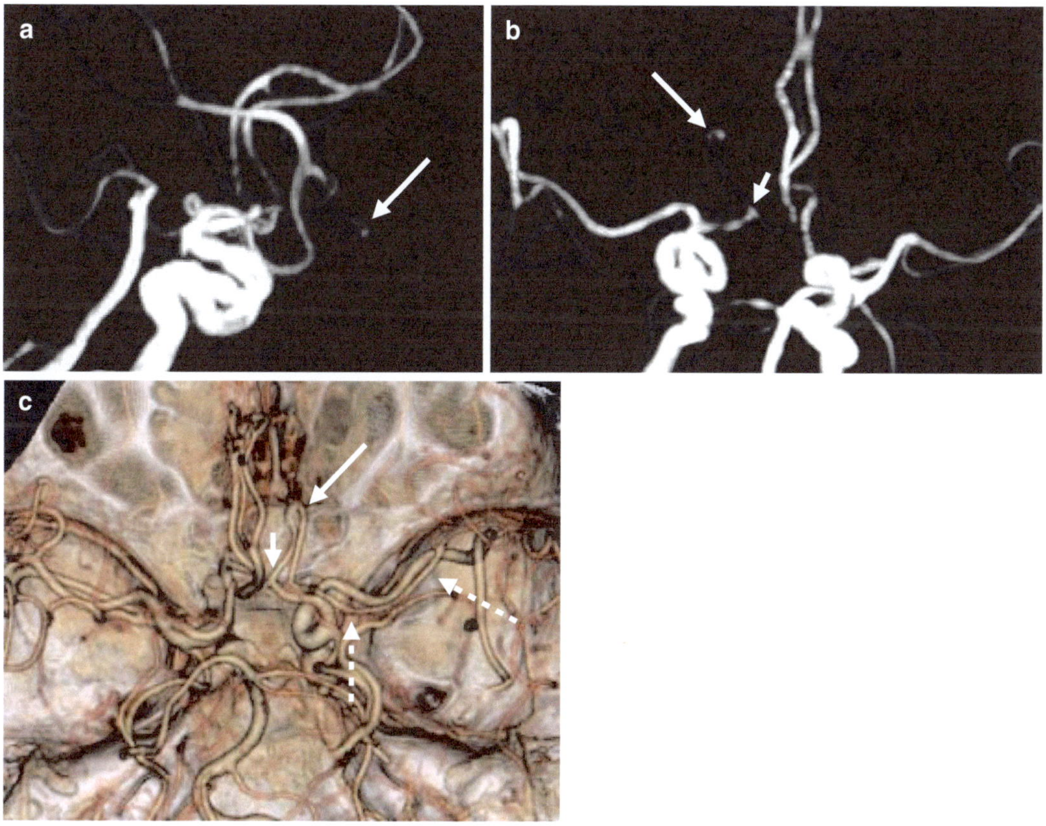

Fig. 9.15 (**a**) Lateral, (**b**) I-S, and (**c**) S-I projections of CT angiography show an anomalous artery arising from the A1 segment of the right ACA (*short arrows*) and taking an anteroinferior course. After making a hairpin turn (*long arrows*), it connects to the right accessory MCA (*dotted arrows*), indicative of a type 4 PPOA

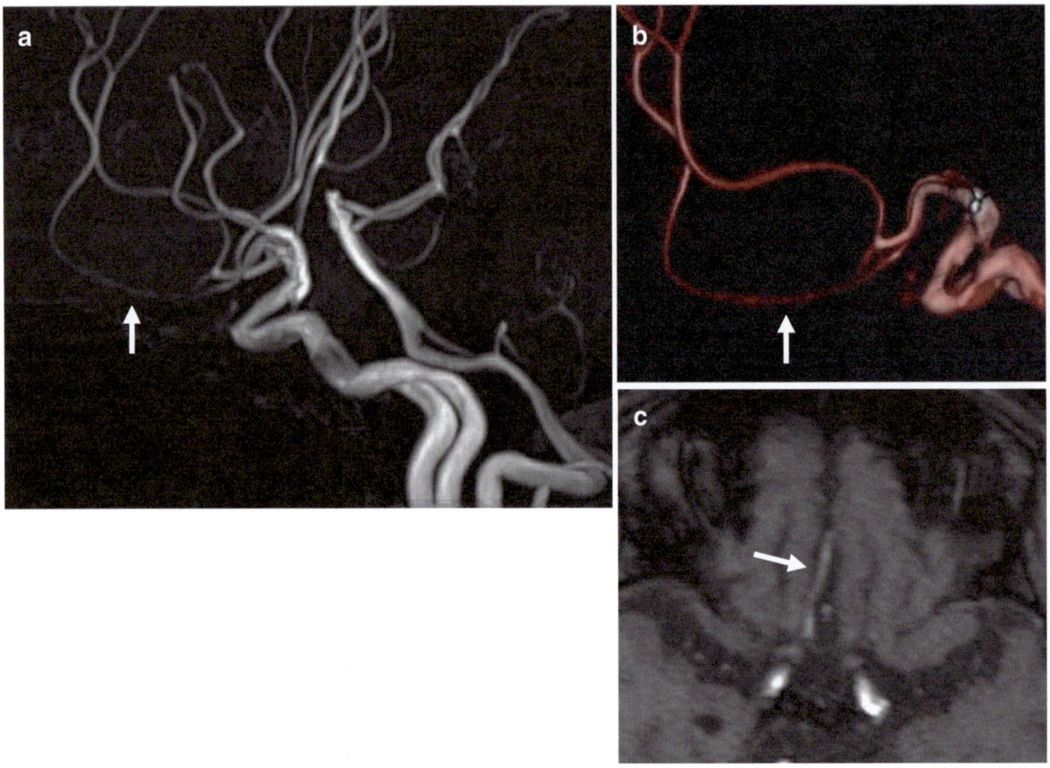

Fig. 9.16 (**a**) Lateral projection of MR angiography, (**b**) partial VR image, and (**c**) MR angiographic source image show the right ACA taking an anteroinferior course (*arrows*). This artery runs superiorly and connects to the A3 segment without a hairpin turn, indicative of a type 5 PPOA

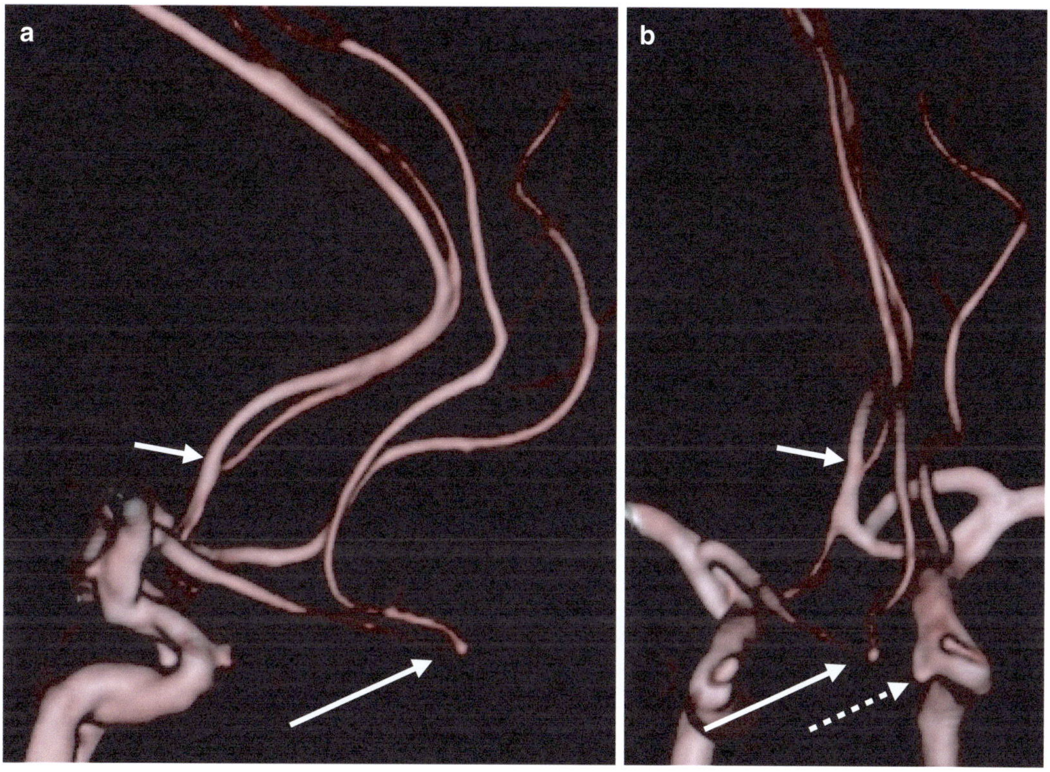

Fig. 9.17 (**a**) Lateral and (**b**) slightly RAO projections of a partial VR MR image show type 1 right PPOA (*long arrows*) continuing to the right callosomarginal artery. The accessory ACA bifurcates soon (*short arrows*) (Sect. 9.9). There is a small aneurysm at the paraclinoid left ICA (*dotted arrow*)

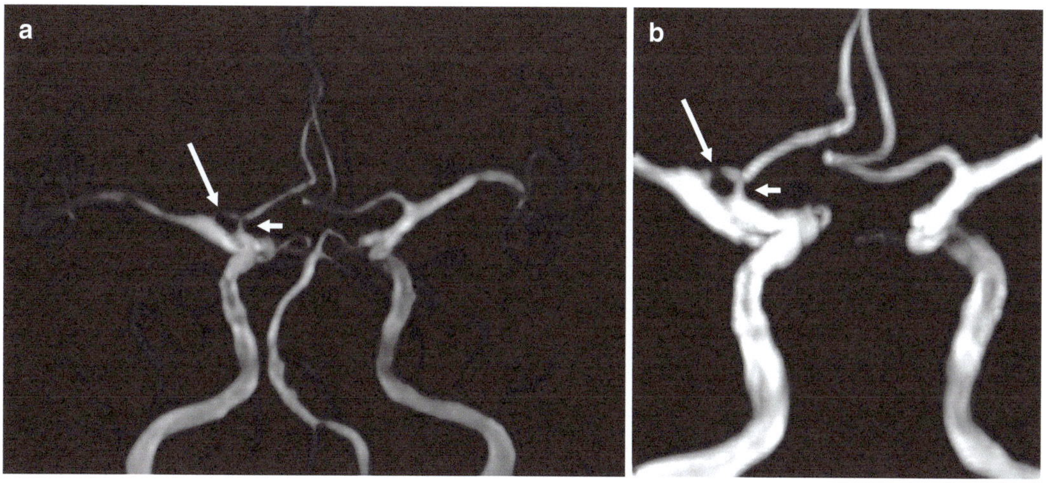

Fig. 9.18 (**a**) A-P projection of MR angiography and (**b**) partial MIP image show two small arteries arising from the terminal segment of the right ICA (*long and short arrows*) and fusing soon, forming an A1 segment with an arterial ring. The A1 segment of the right ACA is larger than both channels, suggesting that blood flow in the distally arising channel (*long arrows*) is towards the ACA, not the MCA, indicative of a duplicate origin of the ACA

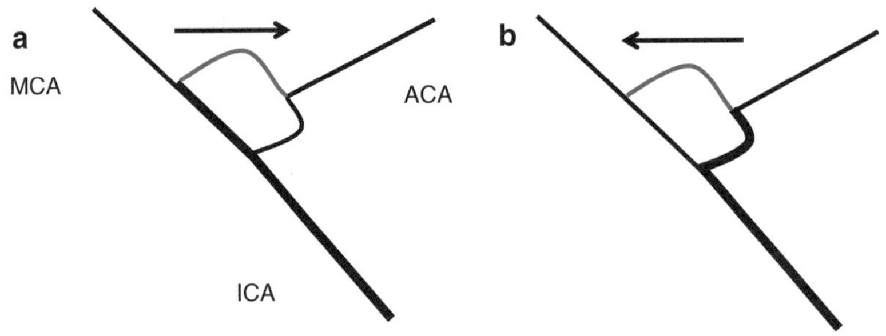

Fig. 9.19 Schematic illustration of (**a**) duplicate origin of the ACA and (**b**) ACA arising from the fenestration of the terminal ICA. The *arrows* indicate the direction of blood flow. (Modified from [19]). *ACA* anterior cerebral artery, *ICA* internal carotid artery, *MCA* middle cerebral artery

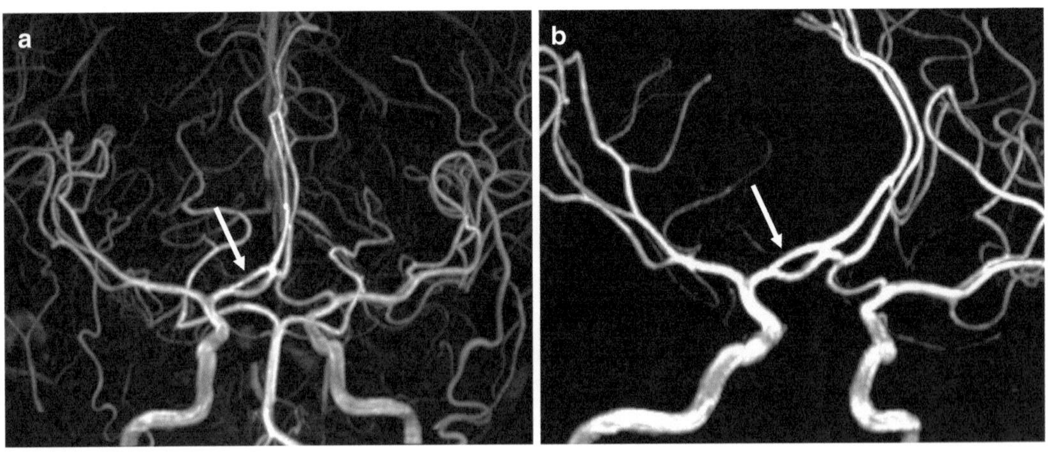

Fig. 9.20 (**a**) A-P projection of MR angiography and (**b**) partial MIP RAO projection image show a large fenestration at the distal A1 segment of the right ACA (*arrows*)

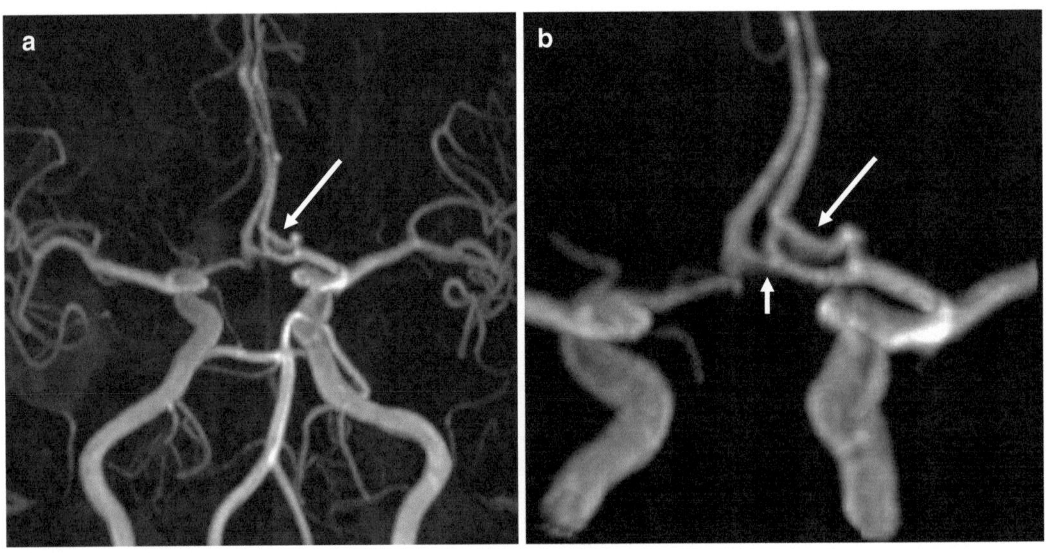

Fig. 9.21 (**a**) AI-PS projection of MR angiography and (**b**) partial MIP image show a large fenestration at the A1-A2 junction of the left ACA (*long arrows*). The *short arrow* indicates the left ACA-ACoA junction

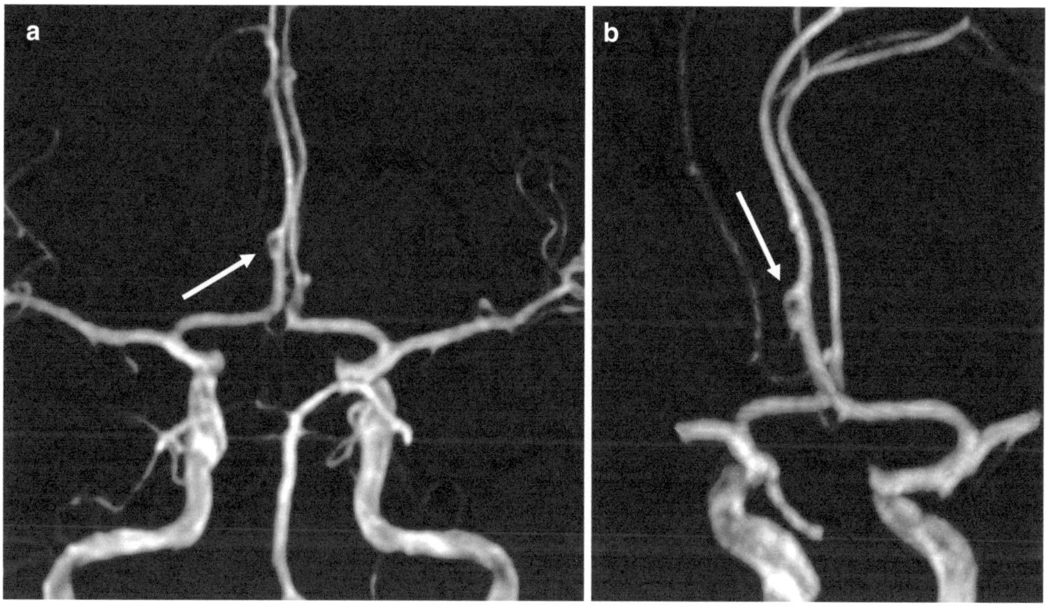

Fig. 9.22 (**a**) AI-PS projection of MR angiography and (**b**) partial MIP LAO projection image show a small fenestration at the A2 segment of the right ACA (*arrows*)

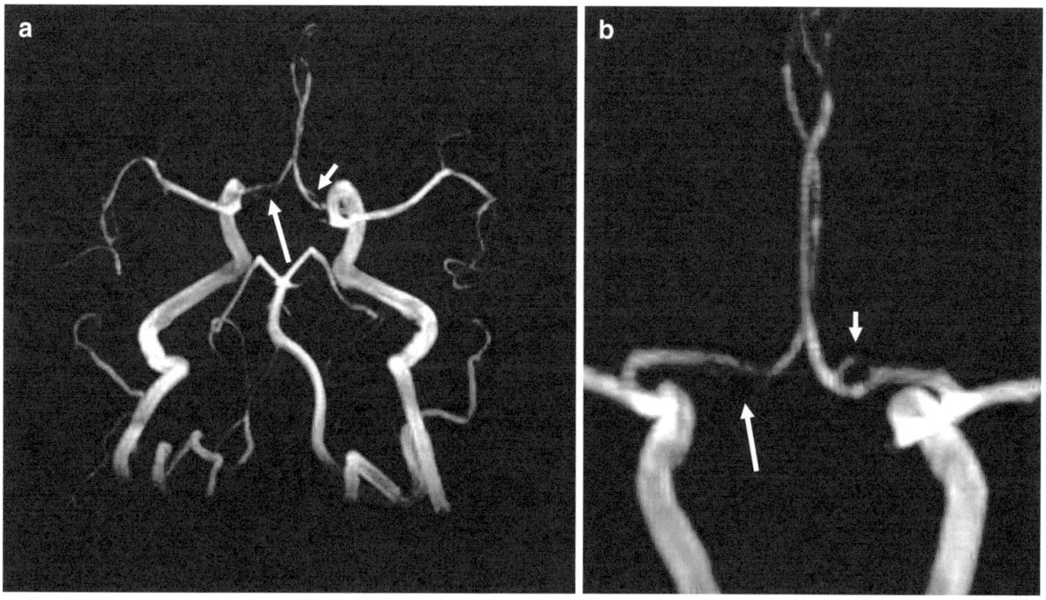

Fig. 9.23 (**a**) AI-PS projection of MR angiography and (**b**) partial MIP A-P projection image show bilateral fenestrations at the distal A1 segments (*long and short arrows*)

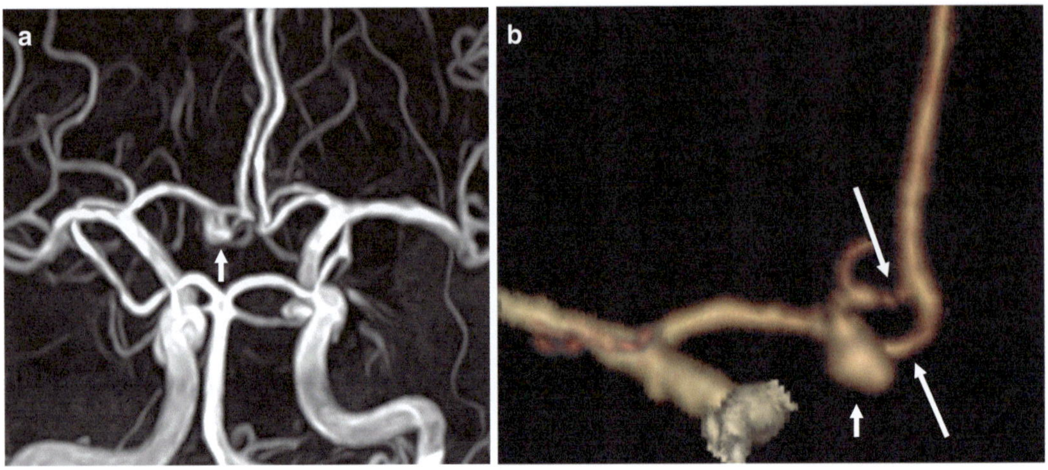

Fig. 9.24 (**a**) AI-PS projection of MR angiography and (**b**) partial VR image of CT angiography show an aneurysm at the distal A1 segment of the right ACA (*short arrows*). This aneurysm arises at the proximal end of the fenestration (*long arrows*)

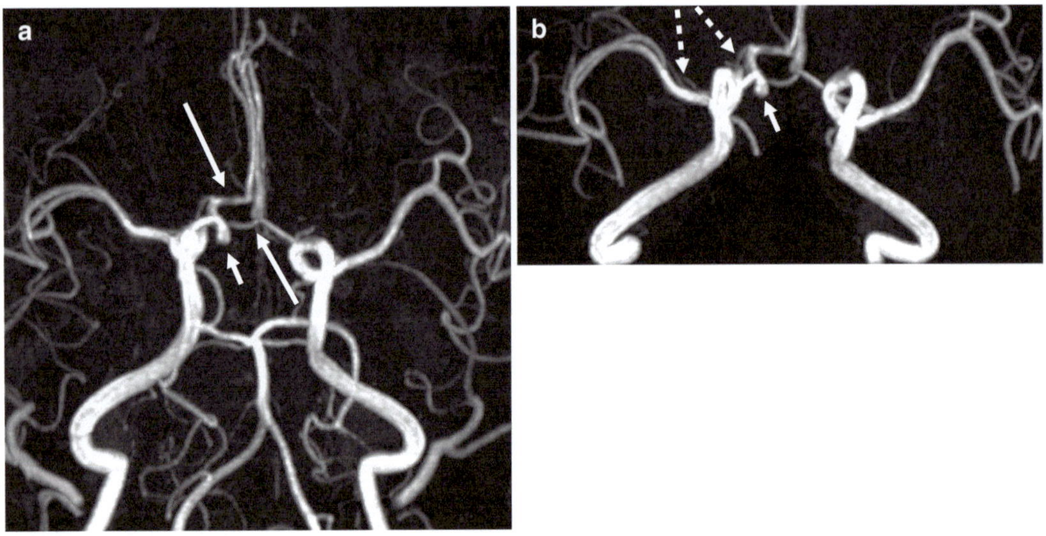

Fig. 9.25 (**a**) AI-PS projection of MR angiography and (**b**) partial MIP image show duplication at the distal A1 segment of the right ACA (*long arrows*). An aneurysm is seen at the duplicated point (*short arrows*). The right accessory MCA (Sect. 8.2.2) is also seen (*dotted arrows*)

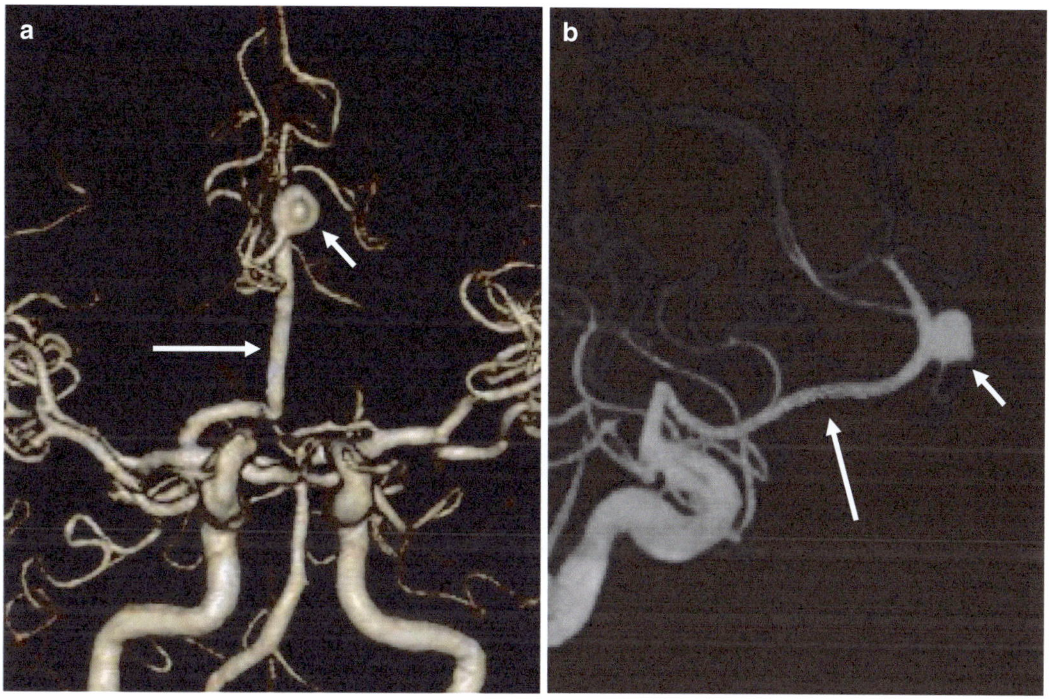

Fig. 9.26 (**a**) A-P projection of VR CT angiography and (**b**) lateral projection of MIP CT angiography show an azygos ACA (*long arrows*). At the end of the unpaired A2 segment, an aneurysm is seen (*short arrows*)

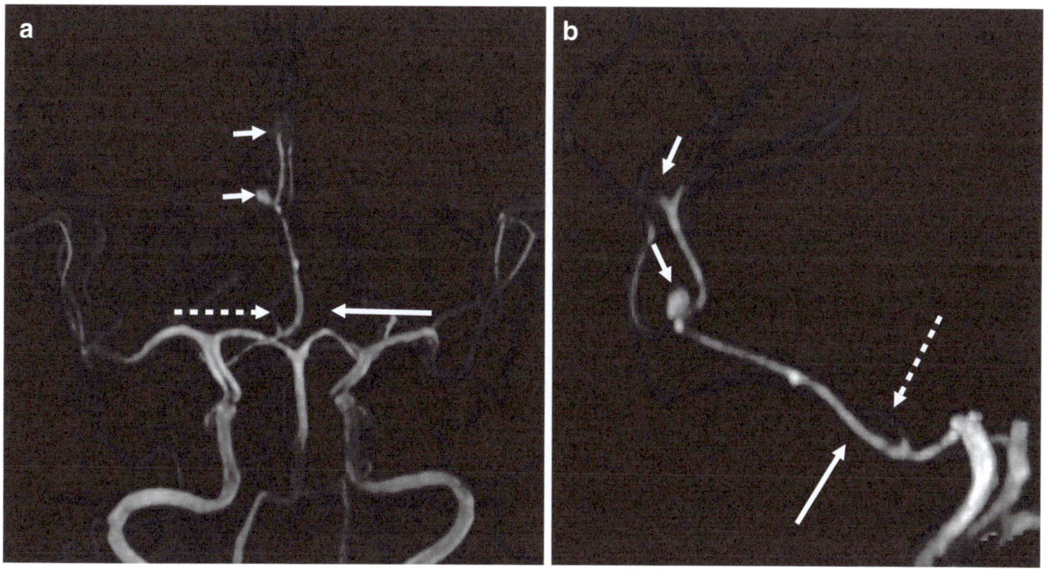

Fig. 9.27 (**a**) A-P projection of MR angiography and (**b**) partial MIP lateral image shows a large A2 segment of the left ACA (*long arrows*) and a small right A2 (*dotted arrows*), indicative of a bihemispheric ACA. Two aneurysms are seen at the distal segment of the larger artery (*short arrows*)

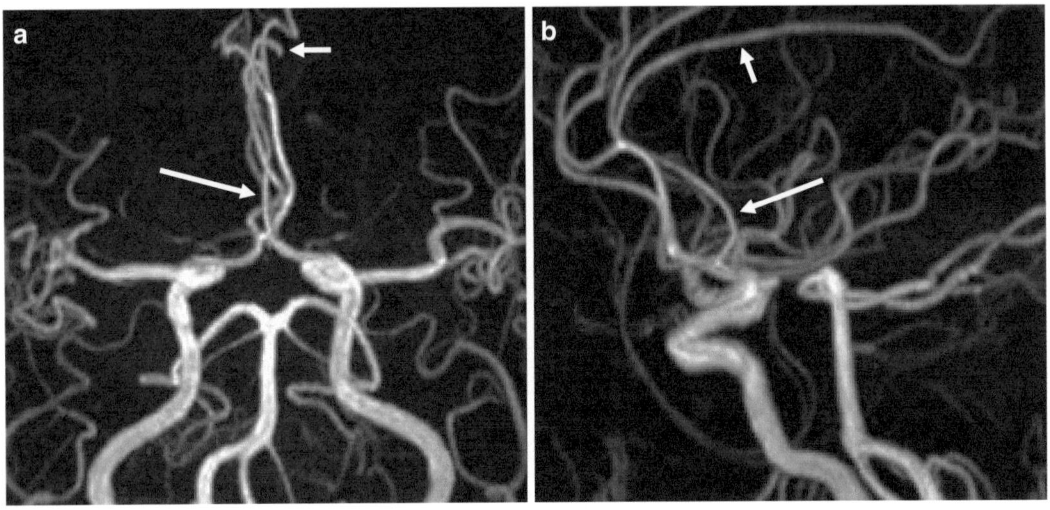

Fig. 9.28 (**a**) AI-PS and (**b**) lateral projections of MR angiography show an artery arising from the ACoA (*long arrows*), indicative of a triple ACA (accessory ACA). This third artery continues to the pericallosal artery (*short arrows*)

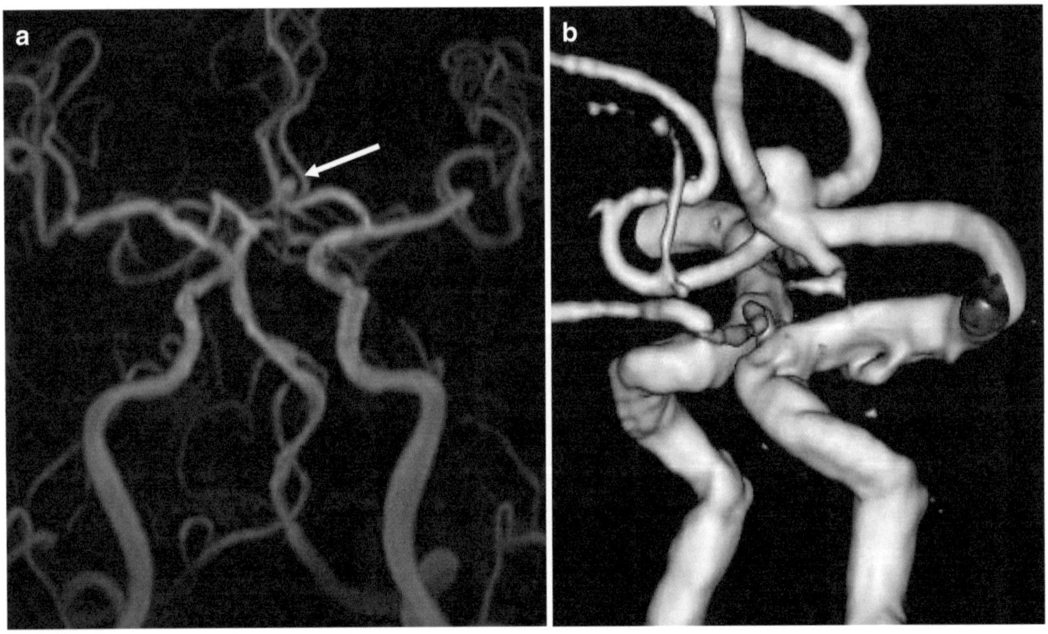

Fig. 9.29 (**a**) A-P projection of MR angiography shows an aneurysm at the ACoA (*arrow*). (**b**) Partial VR image in LAO projection shows four A2 segments, resulting in quadruple ACAs

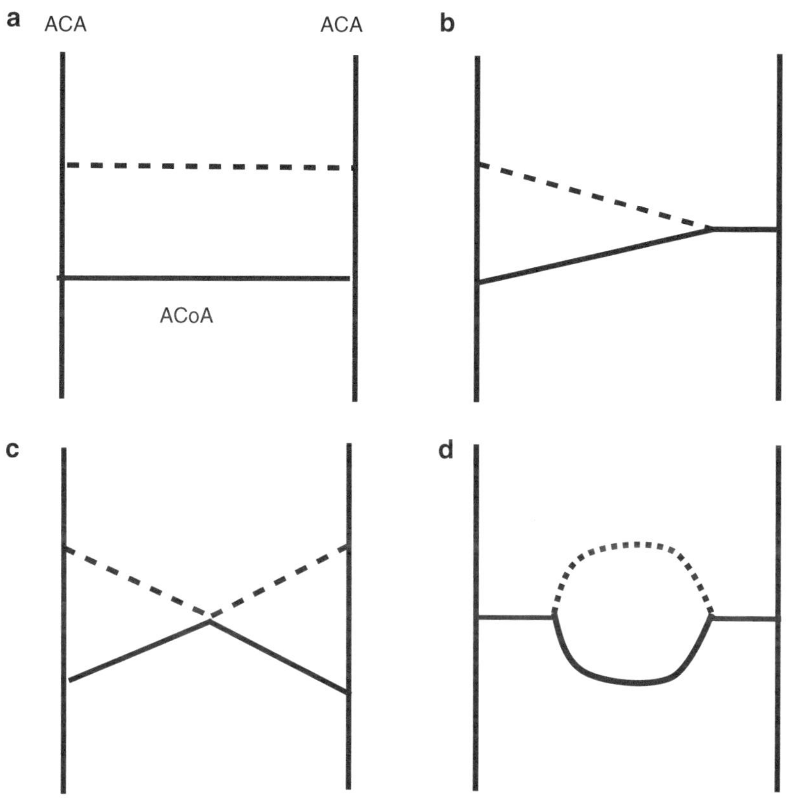

Fig. 9.30 Schematic illustration of the variations of the ACoA. (Modified from [26]). **a**: Duplication, **b**: Partial duplication, **c**: Double partial duplications, **d**: True fenestration. *ACA* anterior cerebral artery, *ACoA* anterior communicating artery

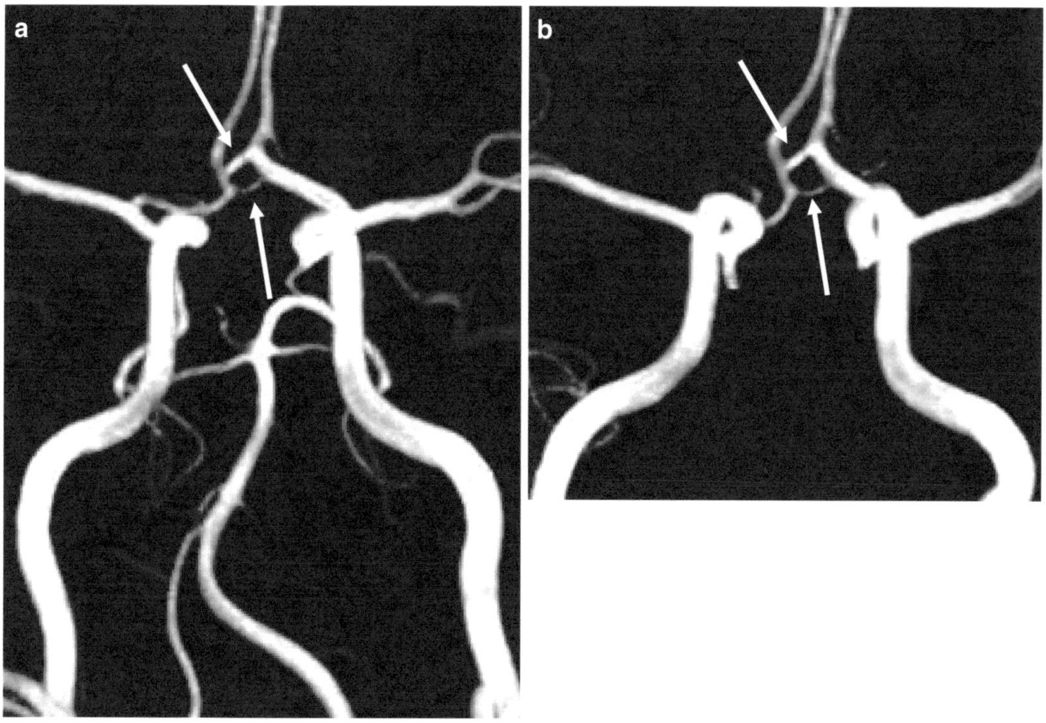

Fig. 9.31 (**a**) AI-PS projection of MR angiography and (**b**) partial MIP image show two ACoAs (*arrows*). This is a duplication, not a fenestration

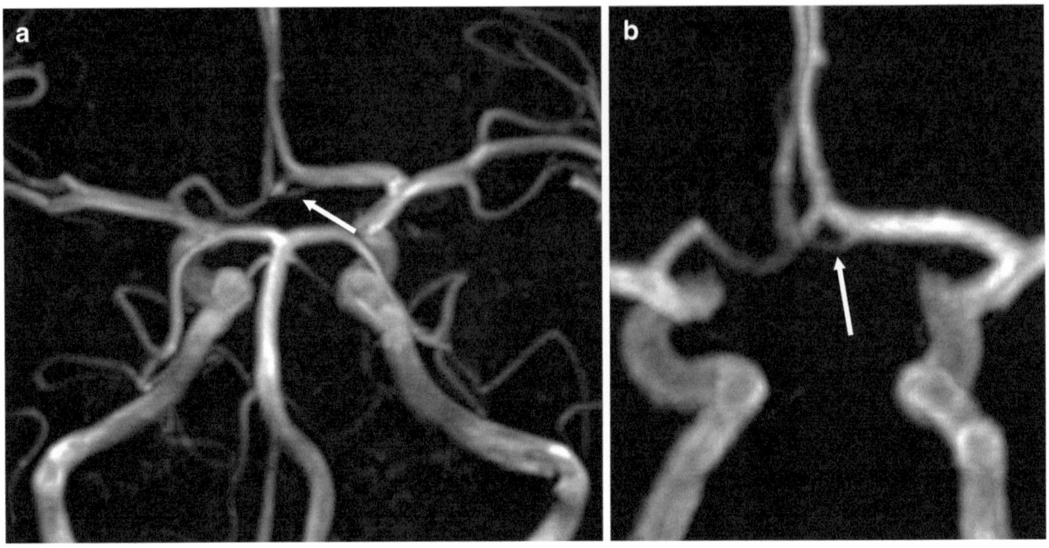

Fig. 9.32 (**a**) AI-PS projection of MR angiography and (**b**) partial MIP image show two ACoAs arising from the left ACA and fusing together with the right ACA (*arrows*). This is a partial duplication, not a fenestration

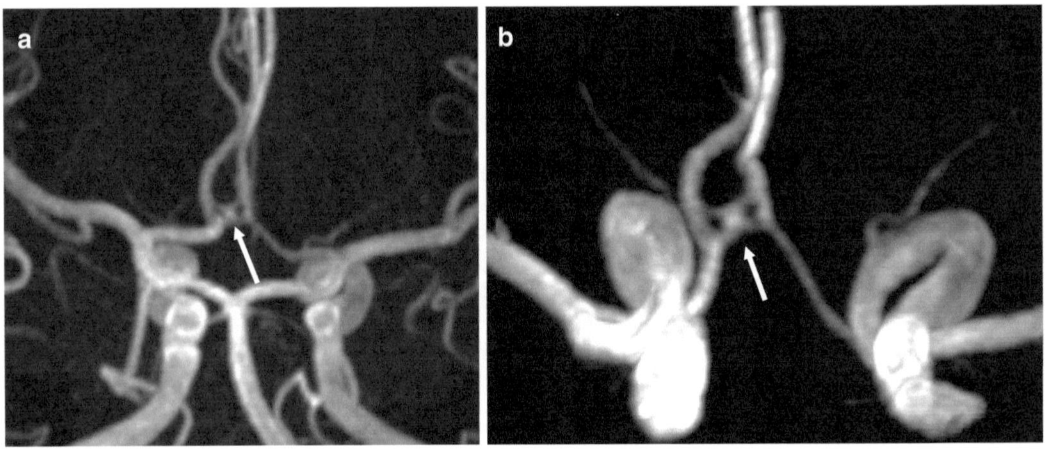

Fig. 9.33 (**a**) AI-PS projection of MR angiography and (**b**) partial MIP image show two ACoAs arising from the bilateral ACAs and fusing together at the midportion, forming two arterial rings (*arrows*). These are double partial duplications, not two fenestrations

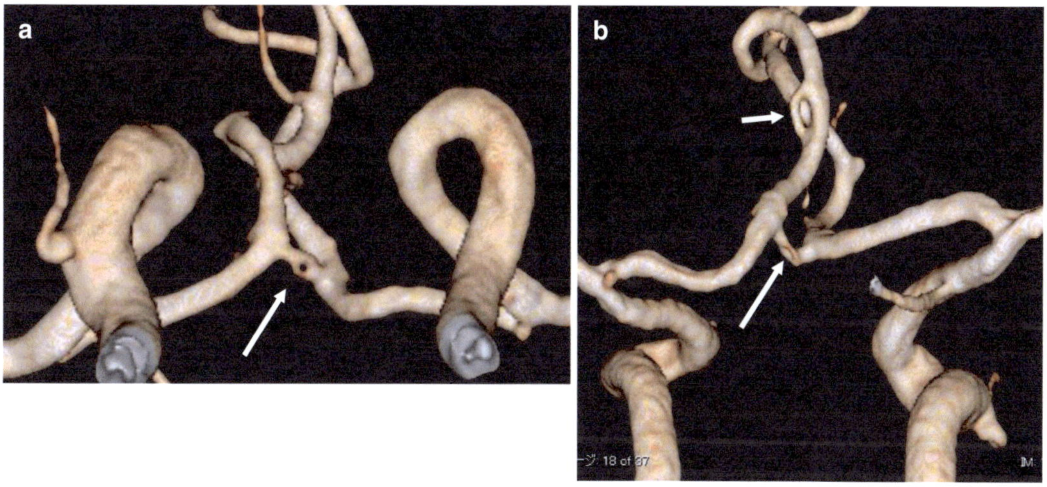

Fig. 9.34 (**a**) I-S and (**b**) P-A projections of partial VR MR angiography show a tiny true fenestration at the midportion of the ACoA (*long arrows*). There is another fenestration at the left A2 segment (*short arrow*)

References

1. Krabbe-Hartkamp MJ, van der Grond J, de Leeuw FE, de Groot JC, Algra A, Hillen B, Breteler MM, Mali WP. Circle of Willis: morphologic variation on three-dimensional time-of-flight MR angiograms. Radiology. 1998;207:103–11.
2. Uchino A, Nomiyama K, Takase Y, Kudo S. Anterior cerebral artery variations detected by MR angiography. Neuroradiology. 2006;48:647–52.
3. Yamaguchi K, Uchino A, Sawada A, Takase Y, Kuroda Y, Kudo S. Bilateral anterior cerebral artery territory infarction associated with unilateral hypoplasia of the A1 segment: report of two cases. Radiat Med. 2007;22:422–5.
4. Uchino A, Sawada A, Takase Y, Imaizumi T, Egashira R, Matsuo M, Kudo S. Carotid-anterior cerebral artery anastomosis: MR angiographic features and literature review. Clin Imaging. 2004;28:377–80.
5. Uchino A, Saito N, Okada Y, Inoue K. Carotid-anterior cerebral artery anastomosis on MR angiography: a university hospital-based study. Neuroradiology. 2012;54:13–8.
6. Wong ST, Yuen SC, Fok KF, Yam KY, Fong D. (2008) Infraoptic anterior cerebral artery: review, report of two cases and an anatomical classification. Acta Neurochir. (Wien) 2008;150:1087–96.
7. Okano N, Uchino A, Saito N, Maruyama H. Left carotid-anterior cerebral artery anastomosis diagnosed by MR angiography: a case report. Surg Radiol Anat. 2015;37:311–3.
8. Uchino A, Saito N, Yamane F. Bilateral carotid-anterior cerebral artery anastomoses associated with bilateral ophthalmic arteries arising from the middle meningeal arteries diagnosed by magnetic resonance angiography: a case report. Surg Radiol Anat. 2017;39:1289–92.
9. Uchino A, Saito N, Tanahashi N. Bilateral carotid-anterior cerebral artery anastomoses associated with bilateral ophthalmic arteries arising from the anastomotic arteries diagnosed by magnetic resonance angiography: a case report. Surg Radiol Anat. 2018;40:721–5.
10. Matsuura K, Uchino A, Saito N, Ishida J, Suzuki T. Carotid-anterior cerebral artery (ACA) anastomosis associated with azygos ACA and ophthalmic artery arising from the middle meningeal artery: a case report. Surg Radiol Anat. 2020;42:211–4.
11. Uchino A, Saito N, Kozawa E, Masutani S. Multiple variations of the cerebral arteries associated with tetralogy of Fallot: a case report. Surg Radiol Anat. 2017;39:1161–4.
12. Hoshino E, Uchino A, Saito N, Yoshiba S. Association of tetralogy of Fallot with multiple variations of the cerebral arteries diagnosed by magnetic resonance angiography. Radiol Case Rep. 2020;15:349–52.
13. Uchino A, Saito N, Kozawa E, Mizukoshi W, Inoue K. Persistent primitive olfactory artery: MR angiographic diagnosis. Surg Radiol Anat. 2011;33:197–201.
14. Padget DH. Development of cranial arteries in human embryo. Contrib Embryol. 1948;32:205–62.

15. Uchino A, Ohno H, Ogiichi T. Persistent primitive olfactory artery without a hairpin turn. Surg Radiol Anat. 2021;43:231–4.
16. Uchino A, Baba Y. Type 2 persistent primitive olfactory artery associated with bilateral ophthalmic arteries arising from the middle meningeal arteries diagnosed by magnetic resonance angiography. Surg Radiol Anat. 2021;43:1731–3.
17. Kim MS, Lee GJ. Persistent primitive olfactory artery: CT angiographic diagnosis and literature review for classification and clinical significance. Surg Radiol Anat. 2014;36:663–7.
18. Uchino A, Mochizuki A. Persistent primitive olfactory artery associated with early bifurcated accessory anterior cerebral artery. Surg Radiol Anat. 2021;43:1731–3.
19. Uchino A, Saito N, Nagamine Y, Takao M. Duplicate origin of the anterior cerebral artery diagnosed by magnetic resonance angiography: a case report. Surg Radiol Anat. 2016;38:1239–41.
20. Sanders WP, Sorek PA, Mehta BA. Fenestration of intracranial arteries with special attention to associated aneurysms and other anomalies. AJNR Am J Neuroradiol. 1993;14:675–80.
21. Yoshida M, Ezura M, Sasaki K, Chonan M, Mino M. Endovascular repair of ruptured aneurysm arising from fenestration of the horizontal segment of the anterior cerebral artery: case report. Neurol Med Chir (Tokyo). 2012;52:924–7.
22. Paladino J, Pirker N, Gluncić V. Early bifurcation of the left A1 segment giving rise to both A2 segments and a hypoplastic right A1 segment. Acta Neurochir. 2000;142:825–6.
23. Huber P, Braun J, Hirschmann D, Agyeman JF. Incidence of berry aneurysms of the unpaired pericallosal artery: angiographic study. Neuroradiology. 1980;19:143–7.
24. Kashiwagi D, Kuroda S, Horiuchi N, Takahashi A, Asano T, Ishikawa T, Iwasaki Y. Ruptured aneurysm of bihemispheric anterior cerebral artery bifurcation: case report. No Shinkei Geka 2005;33:383–7. (In Japanese with English abstract).
25. Jalali A, Srinivasan VM, Kan P, Duckworth EAM. Association of anterior communicating artery aneurysms with triplicate A2 segment of the anterior cerebral artery. World Neurosurg. 2020;140:e234–9.
26. Uchino A, Saito N, Uehara T, Neki H, Kohyama S, Yamane F. True fenestration of the anterior communicating artery diagnosed by magnetic resonance angiography. Surg Radiol Anat. 2016;38:1095–8.
27. Choi JH, Jo KI, Kim KH, Jeon P, Yeon JY, Kim JS, Hong SC. Morphological risk factors for the rupture of anterior communicating artery aneurysms: the significance of fenestration. Neuroradiology. 2016;58:155–60.
28. de Gast AN, van Rooij WJ, Sluzewski M. Fenestrations of the anterior communicating artery: incidence on 3D angiography and relationship to aneurysms. AJNR Am J Neuroradiol. 2008;29:296–8.

10 Variations of the Vertebral Artery (VA) and Vertebrobasilar Junction (VBJ)

Abstract

This chapter includes (1) Anomalous level of entry to the transverse foramen, (2) C2 segmental type VA, (3) C3 segmental type VA, (4) Extracranial and craniovertebral junction VA fenestration, (5) Intracranial VA fenestration and VBJ arterial ring, and (6) VA termination at the posterior inferior cerebellar artery. There are 15 figures and 3 illustrations.

Before either neck surgery or posterior fossa surgery, VA variations should be identified to prevent complications.

Keywords

Fenestration · Transverse foramen · Vertebral artery · Vertebrobasilar junction

10.1 Anomalous Level of Entry to the Transverse Foramen (TF)

It is well known that VA usually enters the C6 TF. The prevalence of entrance at an abnormal level into the C7, C5, C4, C3 TF is reported to be 0.8%, 5.0%, 1.0% and 0.2%, respectively [1]. As mentioned in Sects. 1.2 and 1.3, VA origin variations are strongly correlated with variations in the level of entry to the TF [2]. In the case of direct origin of the left VA from the AA distal to the left SA (Sect. 1.2.3), the entry level is the C7 TF (Fig. 10.1). Both left VA of direct AA origin proximal to the left SA (Sect. 1.2.1) and right VA of extreme proximal right SA (Sect. 1.3.1) enter C5, C4, or C3 TF (Fig. 10.2) [3].

10.2 Anomalous Level of Entry to the Spinal Canal

10.2.1 C2 Segmental Type VA

The VA normally enters the subarachnoid space via the superior surface of the C1 posterior arch. When the VA enters the spinal canal via the C1/2 intervertebral space, this anomalous course of the VA is called a C2 segmental type VA [4] or persistent first intersegmental artery [5]. The latter name seems inadequate, because the first intersegmental artery persists and forms a normal VA. Lasjaunias et al. [6] proposed an embryological explanation for this variation (Fig. 10.3). Its prevalence on MR angiography was reported to be 3.2% [7]. CT angiography is better than MR angiography for the detailed observation of this variation, because the bony structure can be seen simultaneously (Fig. 10.4). This variation is relatively frequently observed bilaterally. However, because of its symmetric fashion, the bilateral type may be easily overlooked (Fig. 10.5).

To avoid complications during surgery at the craniovertebral junction, this common VA varia-

A. Uchino, *Atlas of the Supraaortic Craniocervical Arterial Variations*,
https://doi.org/10.1007/978-981-16-6803-6_10

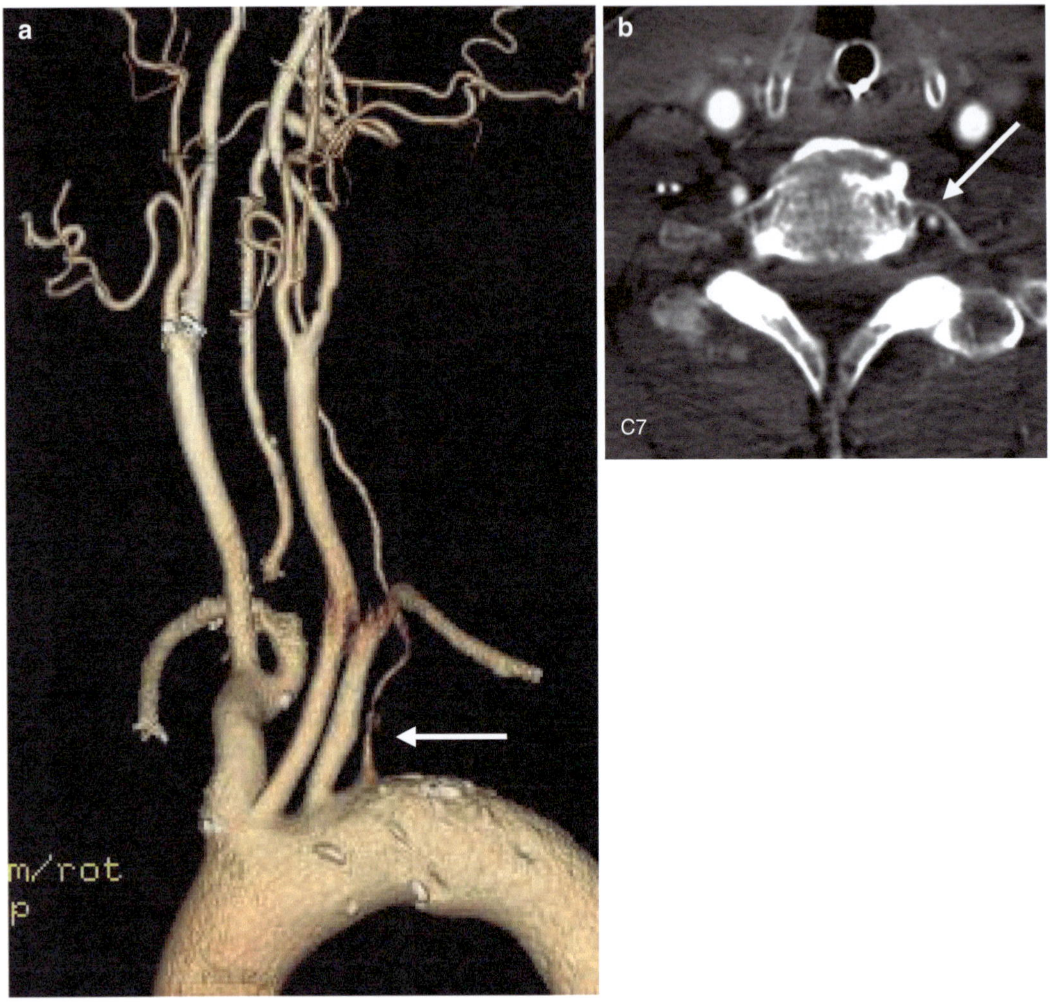

Fig. 10.1 (**a**) LAO projection of CT angiography shows the left VA arising from the AA distal to the left SA (*arrow*). (**b**) CT angiographic source image at the level of C7 vertebral body shows the left VA in the left TF (arrow)

tion should be correctly identified preoperatively. The C1/2 lateral puncture procedure is also dangerous in this variation. Compression myelopathy may result when the variation is bilateral (Fig. 10.6) [5].

10.2.2 C3 Segmental Type VA

Extremely rarely, the VA enters the spinal canal via the intervertebral foramen of the C2/3 level (Figs. 10.7 and 10.8). This is referred to as a C3 segmental type VA (Fig. 10.9) [8]. In patients with a C3 segmental type VA, the unique VA in the spinal canal may compress the spinal cord (Fig. 10.7).

10.3 VA Fenestration and Arterial Ring

10.3.1 Extracranial and Craniovertebral Junction VA Fenestration

Fenestrations can be seen at all 4 segments of the VA. The V1 segment extends from the origin of the artery to the entrance into the transverse fora-

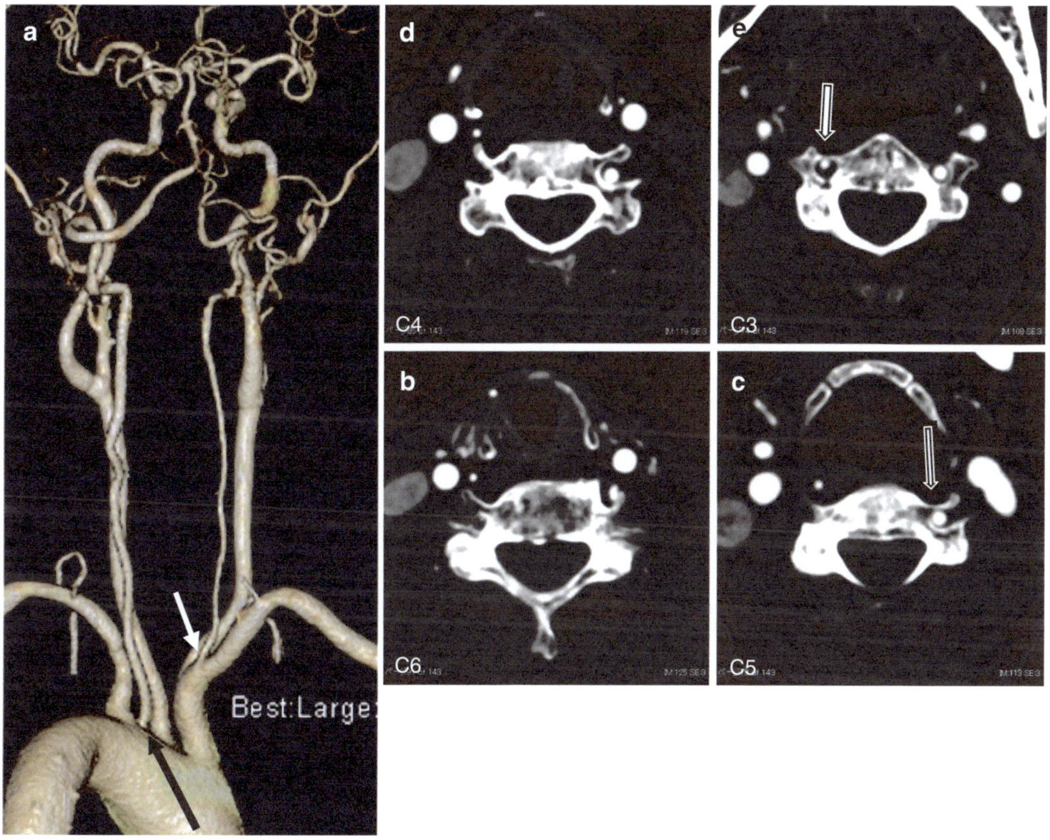

Fig. 10.2 (**a**) P-A projection of CT angiography shows the left VA arising from the AA proximal to the left SA (*long arrow*). The right VA arises from the extreme proximal right SA (*short arrow*). (**b–e**) CT angiographic source images at the levels of C6-C3 show the left VA entering the C5 TF (*long arrow*) and the right VA entering the C3 TF (*short arrow*)

men (Fig. 10.10). The V2 segment runs in the transverse foramen from the entry level to the C2 (Fig. 10.11). The V3 segment extends from the C2 to the foramen magnum (Fig. 10.12). The V4 segment takes an intradural course to connect to the basilar artery.

At the craniovertebral junction, from distal V3 to proximal V4, a large fenestration can be seen relatively frequently (Fig. 10.13). Its prevalence on MR angiography was reported to be 0.9% [7]. As mentioned above (Sect. 10.2.1), the first intersegmental artery persists normally. When both the first and the second intersegmental arteries persist, a large fenestration (arterial ring) of the VA forms at the craniovertebral junction (Fig. 10.14) [6].

10.3.2 Intracranial VA Fenestration and VBJ Arterial Ring

Fenestrations are relatively frequently seen at the V4 segment of the VA. The prevalence on MR angiography was reported to be 0.54% [9]. Fenestration of this segment is usually large, with the PICA frequently arising from this site

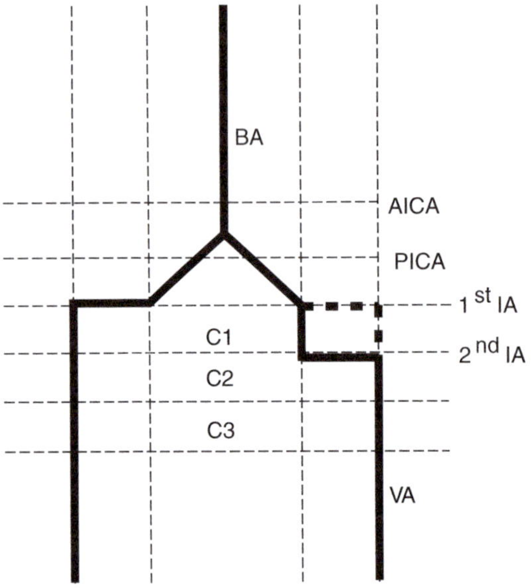

Fig. 10.3 Schematic illustration of a C2 segmental type VA. (Modified from [6]) Normally, the first intersegmental artery persists. When the first intersegmental artery regresses and the second intersegmental artery persists, a C2 segmental type VA is formed. *AICA* anterior inferior cerebellar artery, *BA* basilar artery, *IA* intersegmental artery, *PICA* posterior inferior cerebellar artery, *VA* vertebral artery

(Fig. 10.15) [10]. Thus, duplication may be better than fenestration for the name of this VA variation [11]. At the terminal segment of the VA, from the origin of the PICA to the VBJ, a small fenestration rarely can be seen (Fig. 10.16). Rarely, a triangular-shaped arterial ring is seen at the VBJ (Fig. 10.17). This is not true fenestration, rather it is premedullary duplication [11], and its prevalence on MR angiography was reported to be 0.18% [9]. The prevalence of V4 segment fenestration in patients with arteriovenous malformation was reported to be high [12].

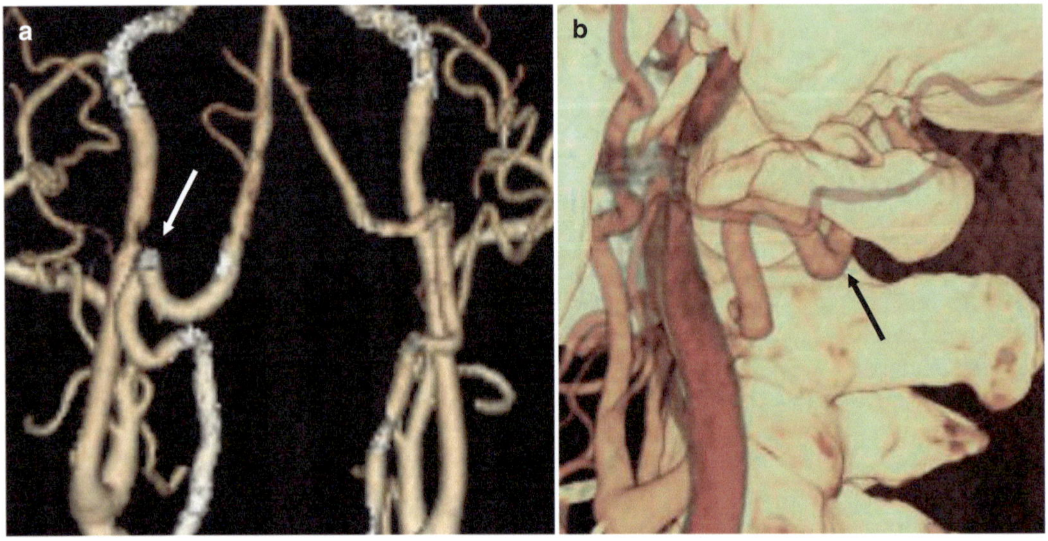

Fig. 10.4 (**a**) P-A projection of CT angiography shows the short V3 segment of the left VA (*arrow*). (**b**) Lateral projection of CT angiography with a bony structure shows the left VA entering the spinal canal via the C1/2 intervertebral space (*arrow*)

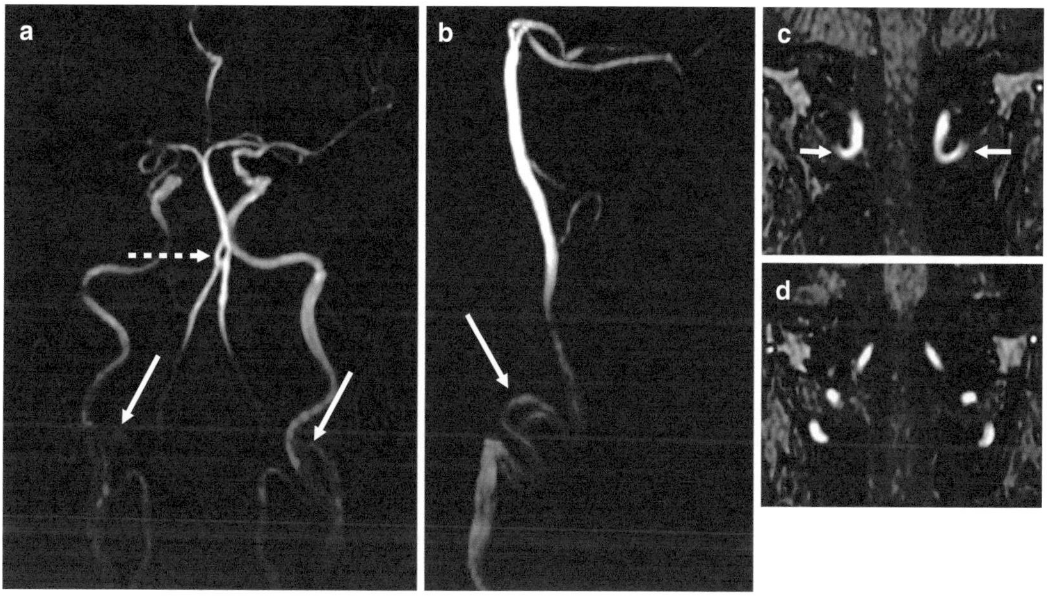

Fig. 10.5 (**a**) A-P projection of MR angiography and (**b**) partial MIP lateral image show short V3 segments of the bilateral VAs (*long arrows*). A small fenestration of the basilar artery (Sect. 11.1) is also seen (*dotted arrow*). (**c**, **d**) Coronal reformatted source images show bilateral VAs entering the spinal canal via the C1/2 intervertebral space (*short arrows*)

10.4 VA Termination at the Posterior Inferior Cerebellar Artery (PICA)

The terminal segment of the hypoplastic VA is frequently absent on MR angiography, resulting in the termination of the VA at the PICA (Fig. 10.18) [13]. There are two possibilities: congenital aplasia and acquired occlusion. Basiparallel anatomic scanning (BPAS) is useful for differentiating between these two conditions [14]. Using this technique, the occluded arterial segment can be visualized.

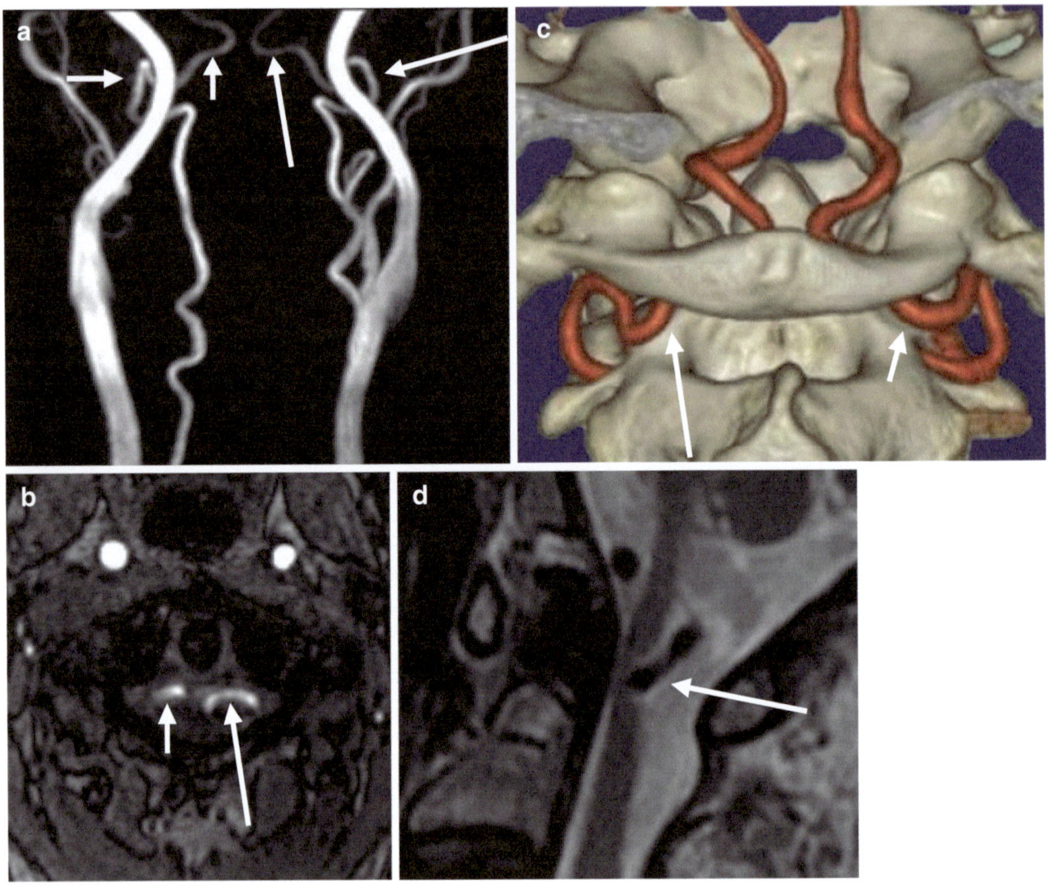

Fig. 10.6 (**a**) A-P projection of MR angiography shows the short length of the V3 segments of the bilateral VAs and a short distance between the VAs at the proximal V4 segments (*long and short arrows*). (**b**) MR angiographic source image at the level of C1 shows bilateral VAs compressing the spinal cord anteriorly (*long and short arrows*). (**c**) P-A projection of CT angiography with a bone image shows the bilateral VAs entering the spinal canal at the level of the C1/2 intervertebral space (*long and short arrows*). (**d**) T2-weighted sagittal MR imaging shows the left VA compressing the spinal cord anteriorly at the C1 level (*long arrow*). (Courtesy of Dr. Maki Umino)

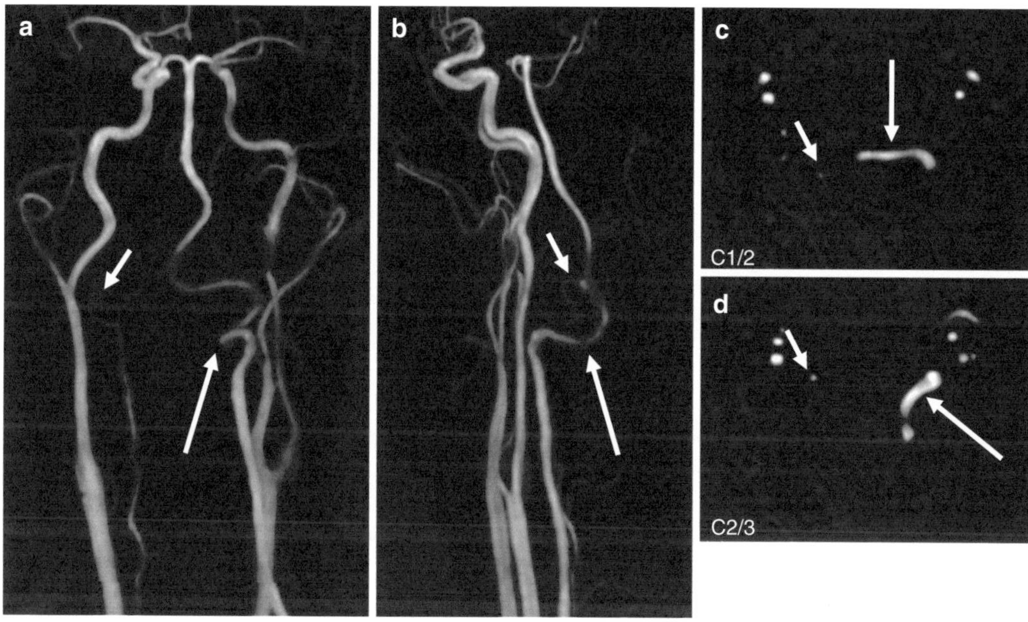

Fig. 10.7 (**a**) A-P and (**b**) lateral projections of MR angiography, (**c**, **d**) MR angiographic source images show a hyperplastic left VA entering the spinal canal via the C2/3 intervertebral space, indicative of a C3 segmental type VA (*long arrows*). The left VA in the spinal canal is compressing the spinal cord. The hypoplastic right VA enters the spinal canal via the C1/2 intervertebral foramen, indicative of a C2 segmental type VA (*short arrows*)

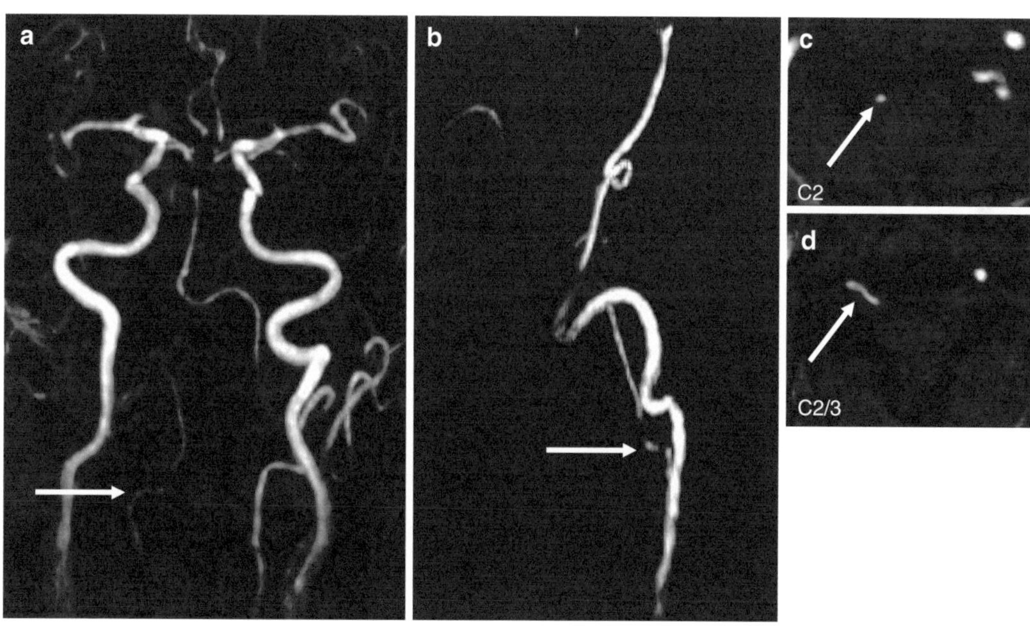

Fig. 10.8 (**a**) A-P projection of MR angiography, (**b**) partial MIP lateral image, and (**c**, **d**) MR angiographic source images show the right VA entering the spinal canal via the C2/3 intervertebral foramen (*arrows*), indicative of a C3 segmental type VA

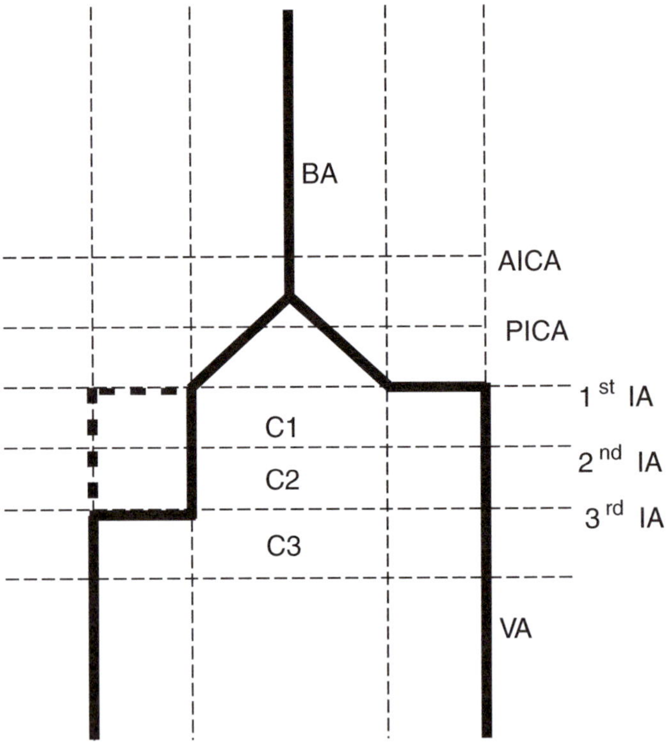

Fig. 10.9 Schematic illustration of a C3 segmental type VA. (Modified from [8]). Normally, the first intersegmental artery persists. When the first intersegmental artery regresses and the third intersegmental artery persists, a C3 segmental type VA is formed. *AICA* anterior inferior cerebellar artery, *BA* basilar artery, *IA* intersegmental artery, *PICA* posterior inferior cerebellar artery, *VA* vertebral artery

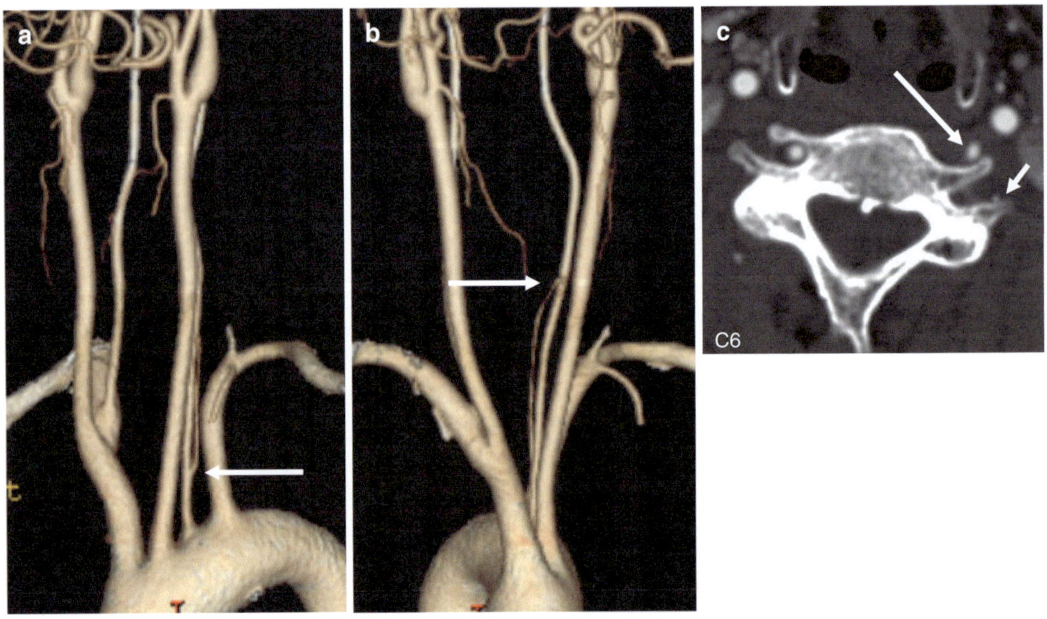

Fig. 10.10 (**a**) LAO and (**b**) P-A projections of CT angiography show the left VA arising from the AA proximal to the left SA. This artery is divided soon and fuses together, forming a large slit-like fenestration (*arrows*). (**c**) CT angiographic source image at the level of C6 shows that the smaller channel (*short arrow*) is in the TF, while the larger channel (*long arrow*) is located anteriorly

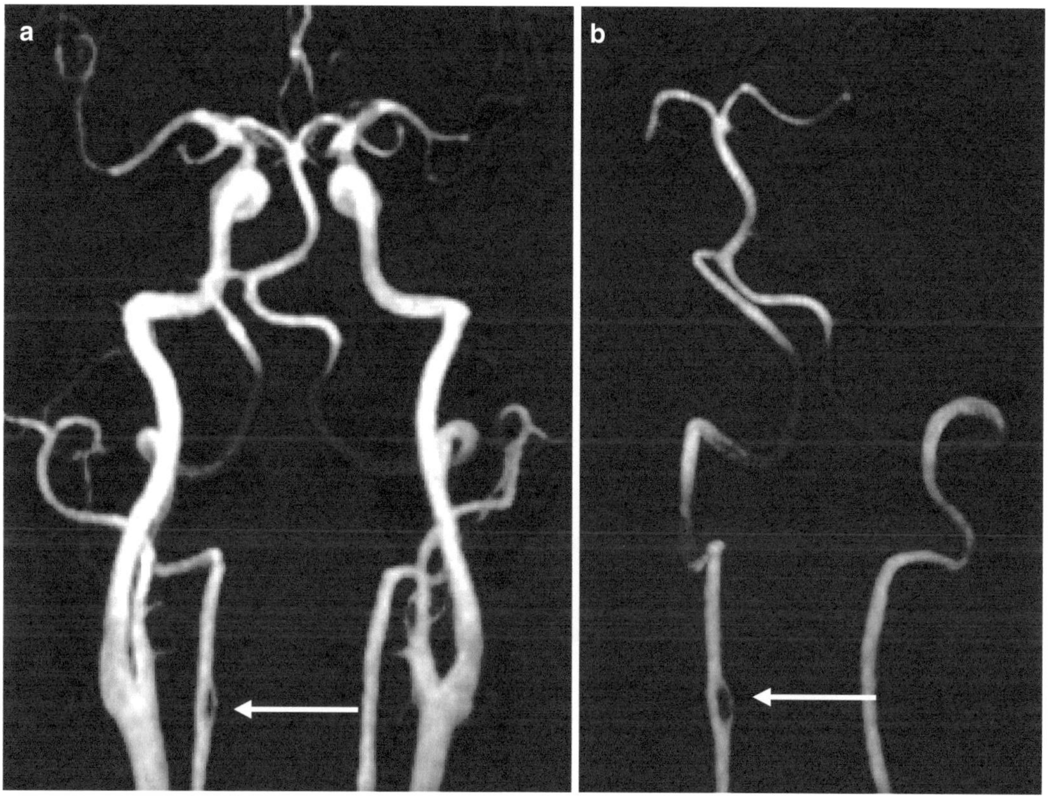

Fig. 10.11 (**a**) A-P projection of MR angiography and (**b**) partial MIP image show a small slit-like fenestration at the V2 segment of the right VA (*arrows*)

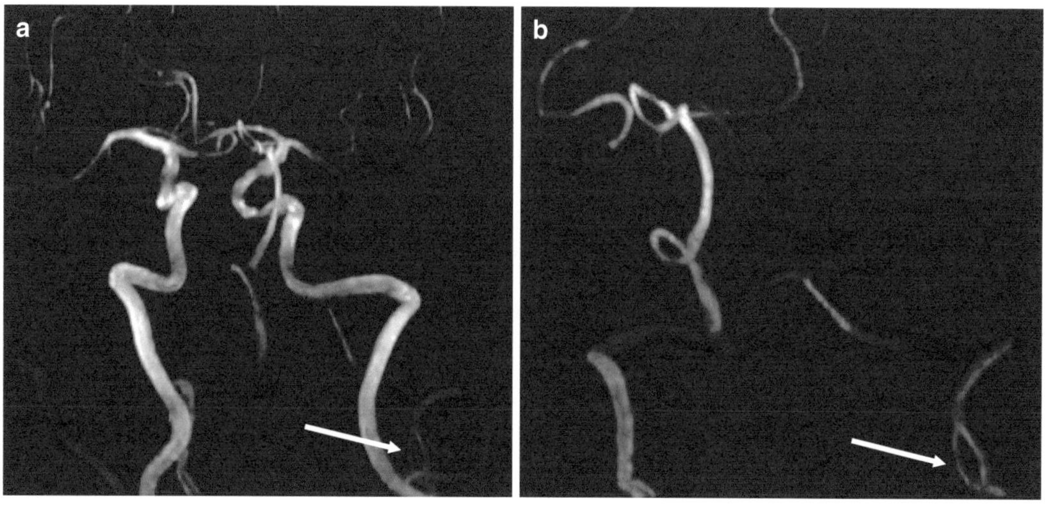

Fig. 10.12 (**a**) Slightly LAO projection of MR angiography and (**b**) partial MIP image show a small slit-like fenestration at the V3 segment of the left VA (*arrows*)

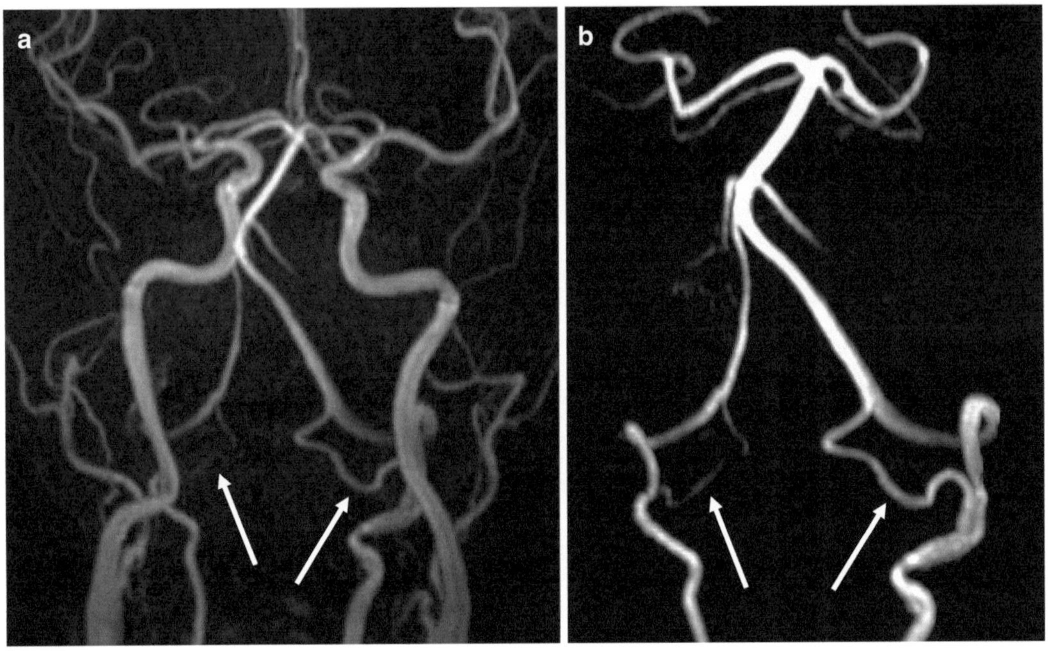

Fig. 10.13 (**a**) A-P projection of MR angiography and (**b**) partial MIP image show bilateral large VA fenestrations (arterial rings) at the C1 level (*arrows*)

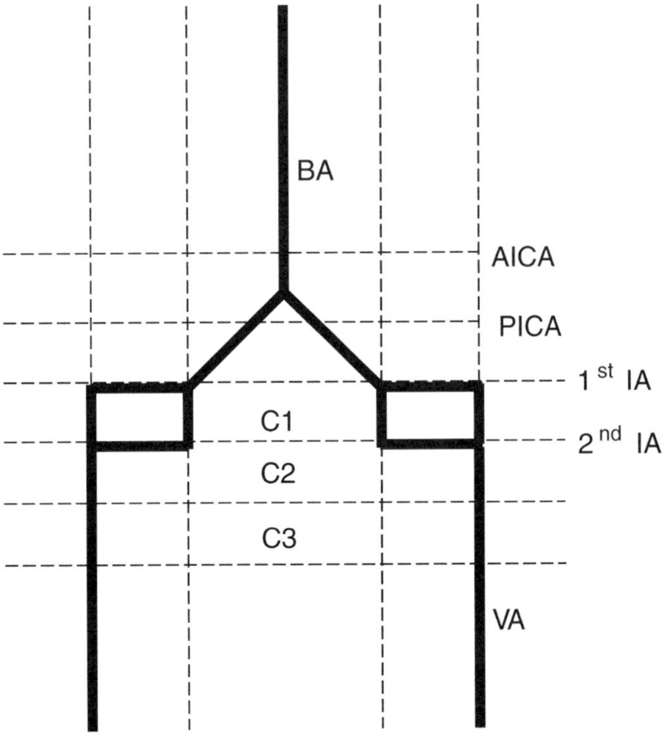

Fig. 10.14 Schematic illustration of bilateral fenestrations of the VA at the craniovertebral junction. (Modified from [6]). When both the first and the second intersegmental arteries persist, a large fenestration (arterial ring) of the VA at the craniovertebral junction is formed. *AICA* anterior inferior cerebellar artery, *BA* basilar artery, *IA* intersegmental artery, *PICA* posterior inferior cerebellar artery, *VA* vertebral artery

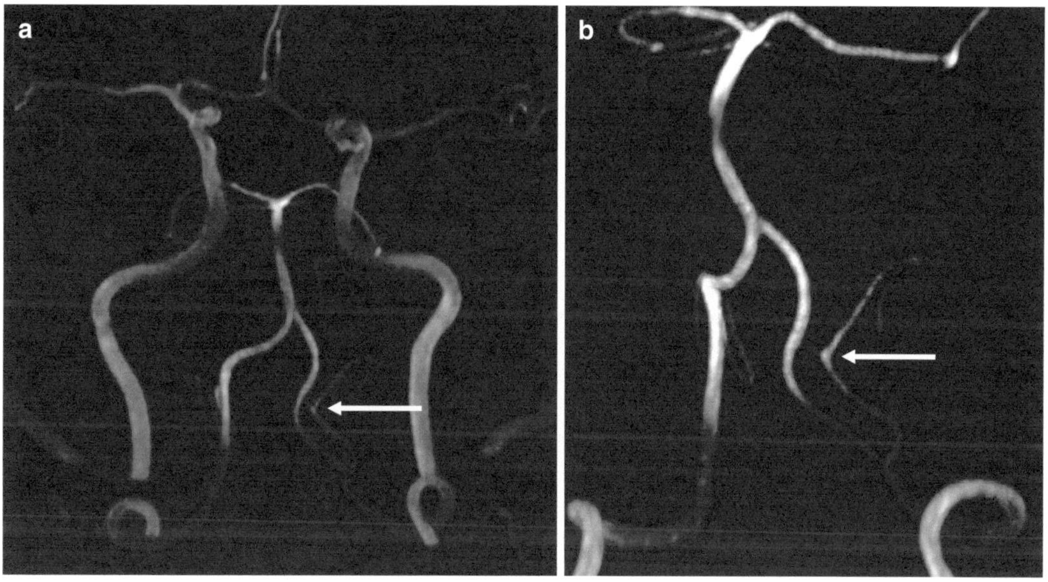

Fig. 10.15 (**a**) AI-PS projection of MR angiography and (**b**) partial MIP image show a large fenestration of the V4 segment of the left VA. The left PICA arises from the fenestrated segment (*arrows*)

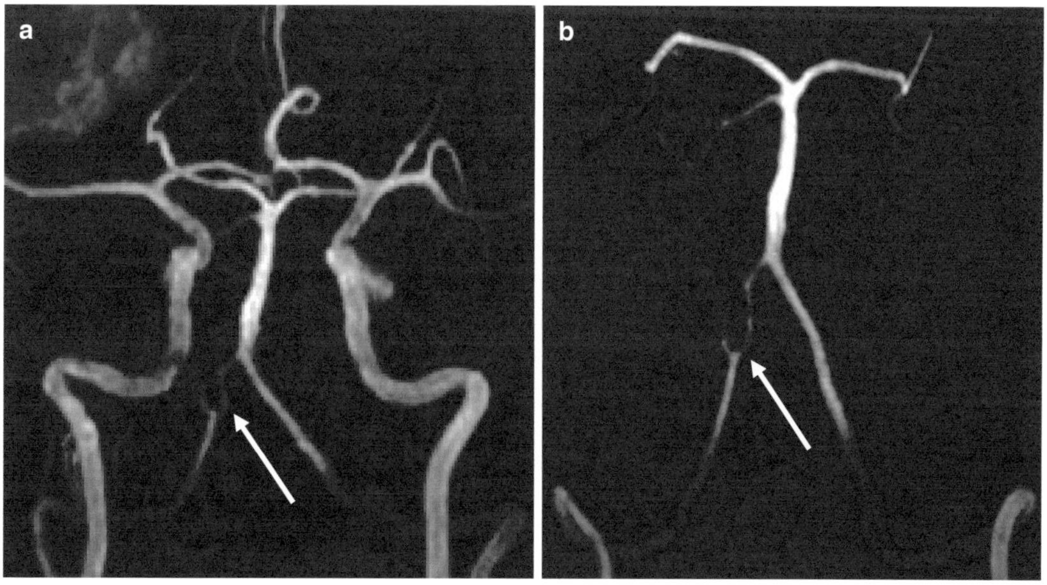

Fig. 10.16 (**a**) A-P projection of MR angiography and (**b**) partial MIP image show a small fenestration of the V4 segment of the right VA, distal to the origin of the PICA (*arrows*)

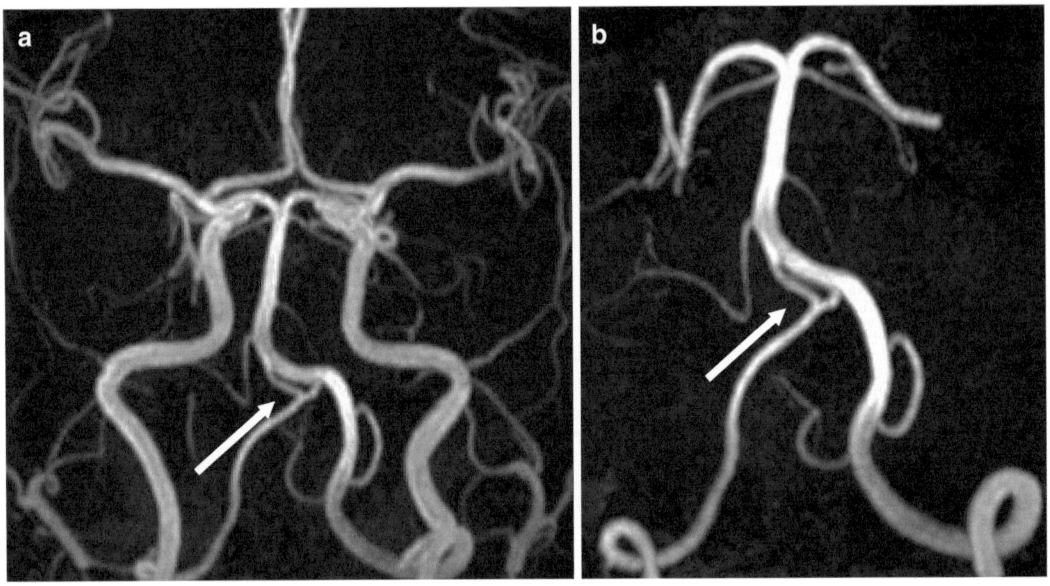

Fig. 10.17 (**a**) A-P projection of MR angiography and (**b**) partial MIP image show a small triangular-shaped arterial ring of the right VBJ (*arrows*)

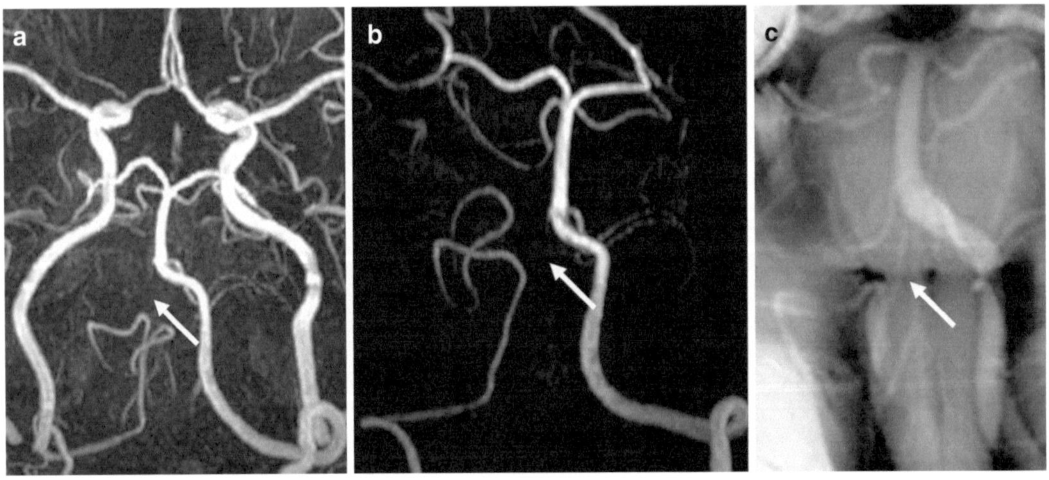

Fig. 10.18 (**a**) AI-PS projection of MR angiography and (**b**) partial MIP image show a hypoplastic right VA, and the terminal segment of the right VA is not visualized (*arrows*), indicative of a termination at the PICA. (**c**) BPAS shows a tiny artery connecting between the right VA and BA (*arrow*), which suggests acquired occlusion rather than congenital aplasia

References

1. Bruneau M, Cornelius JF, Marneffe V, Triffaux M, George B. Anatomic variations of the V2 segment of the vertebral artery. Neurosurgery. 2006;59[ONS Suppl 1]:ONS-20-4.
2. Uchino A, Saito N, Takahashi M, Okada Y, Kozawa E, Nishi N, Mizukoshi W, Nakajima R, Watanabe Y. Variations in the origin of the vertebral artery and its level of entry into the transverse foramen diagnosed by CT angiography. Neuroradiology. 2013;55:585–94.
3. Uchino A, Mochizuki A, Ishihara S. Right vertebral artery entering the third transverse foraman diagnosed by magnetic resonance angiography: a report of two cases. Surg Radiol Anat. 2021;43:455–8.
4. Yoshida T, Shiga K, Uraoka M, Yoshikawa K, Owada K, Nakagawa M. C2 segmental type of vertebral artery with recurrent embolic strokes. Cerebrovasc Dis. 2005;20:58–61.
5. Takahashi T, Tominaga T, Hassan T, Yoshimoto T. Cervical cord compression with myelopathy caused by bilateral persistence of the first intersegmental arteries: case report. Neurosurgery. 2003;53:234–7.
6. Lasjaunias P, Berenstein A, ter Brugge KG. Arterial supply to the posterior fossa central nervous system. In: Lasjaunias P, Berenstein A, ter Brugge KG, editors. Surgical neuro-angiography. Vol. 1. Clinical vascular anatomy and variations. 2nd ed. Berlin: Springer; 2001. p. 224–60.
7. Uchino A, Saito N, Watadani T, Okada Y, Kozawa E, Nishi N, Mizukoshi W, Inoue K, Nakajima R, Takahashi M. Vertebral artery variations at the C1-2 level diagnosed by magnetic resonance angiography. Neuroradiology. 2012;54:19–23.
8. Uchino A, Saito N, Uemiya N, Sonoda K. Diagnosis of a C3 segmental type of vertebral artery by magnetic resonance angiography: report of two cases. Surg Radiol Anat. 2016;38:873–6.
9. Uchino A, Saito N, Okada Y, Kozawa E, Nishi N, Mizukoshi W, Inoue K, Nakajima R, Takahashi M. Fenestrations of the intracranial vertebrobasilar system diagnosed by MR angiography. Neuroradiology. 2012;54:445–50.
10. Uchino A, Sawada A, Takase Y, Kudo S. Extreme fenestration of the right vertebral artery: magnetic resonance angiographic demonstration. Eur Radiol. 2002;12(Suppl 3):S32–4.
11. Yagi K, Satoh K, Satomi J, Nagahiro S. Primitive vertebrobasilar system associated with a ruptured aneurysm. AJNR Am J Neuroradiol. 2004;25:781–3.
12. Uchino A, Kato A, Abe M, Kudo S. Association of cerebral arteriovenous malformation with cerebral arterial fenestration. Eur Radiol. 2001;11:493–6.
13. Liu IW, Ho BL, Chen CF, Han K, Lin CJ, Sheng WY, Hu HH, Chao AC. Vertebral artery terminating in posterior inferior cerebellar artery: a normal variation with clinical significance. PLoS One. 2017;12:e0175264.
14. Nagahata M, Abe Y, Ono S, Hosoya T, Uno S. Surface appearance of the vertebrobasilar artery revealed on basiparallel anatomic scanning (BPAS)-MR imaging: its role for brain MR examination. AJNR Am J Neuroradiol. 2005;26:2508–13.

11 Variations of the Basilar Artery (BA)

Abstract

This chapter includes (1) BA fenestration and arterial ring, (2) Proximal BA partial duplication, (3) Partial duplication of the distal BA (Caudal fusion of BA), and (4) BA complete duplication. Various forms of fusion failure of the primitive longitudinal arteries result in BA variations. There are 12 figures.

Fenestrations frequently occur in the vertebrobasilar system, especially at the proximal segment of the BA. An aneurysms occurs at the proximal end of the fenestration, but it is extremely rarely seen.

Keywords

Basilar artery · Duplication · Fenestration

11.1 BA Fenestration and Arterial Ring

As mentioned above, the fenestrations of the intracranial arteries can be found in any of the proximal segments of the cerebral artery. Fenestrations frequently occur in the vertebrobasilar system, especially at the BA. The prevalence of BA fenestration on MR angiography was reported to be 1.0–2.1% [1–3]. Most BA fenestrations are located at the proximal segment and have a small slit-like configuration. The AICA frequently arises from the fenestrated segment (Fig. 11.1). According to Padget [5], the paired primitive longitudinal neural arteries fuse in a craniocaudal direction. This may be the reason why BA fenestration mainly occurs in the proximal segment, because BA fenestrations form when this fusion fails. One or two aneurysms occur at the proximal end of the fenestration, but the associated aneurysm is extremely rarely seen (Figs. 11.2 and 11.3). BA fenestrations rarely occur at the distal segment (Fig. 11.4). Extremely rarely, two tiny fenestrations (Fig. 11.5) and two large fenestrations (Fig. 11.6) can be seen [3]. An extremely large arterial ring of the BA (Fig. 11.7) can also be seen. This large arterial ring at the VBJ can be regarded as persistent primitive lateral vertebrobasilar anastomosis [6].

11.2 Proximal BA Partial Duplication

As mentioned above, the paired primitive longitudinal neural arteries fuse in a craniocaudal direction and form the BA [5]. If this fusion stops, fenestrations or partial duplications occur. Proximal partial duplication of the BA is relatively rare. In the case of this variation, the BA is short and the AICAs may arise from the duplicated channels (Fig. 11.8). Anastomosis between the VA and AICA can be regarded as proximal

A. Uchino, *Atlas of the Supraaortic Craniocervical Arterial Variations*,
https://doi.org/10.1007/978-981-16-6803-6_11

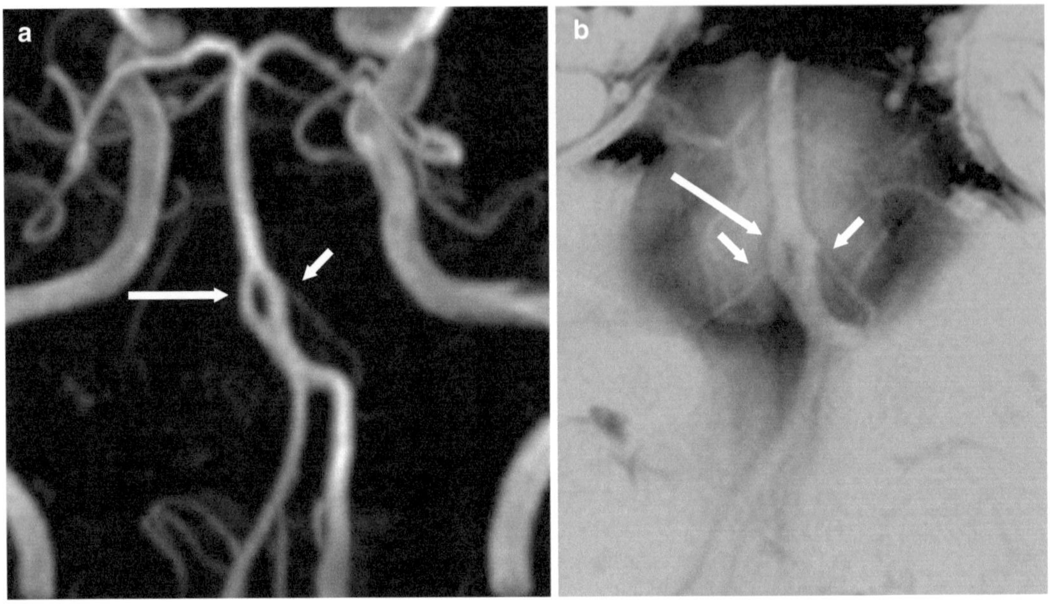

Fig. 11.1 (**a**) AI-PS projection of MR angiography and (**b**) basiparallel anatomic scanning (BPAS) [4] show a small fenestration at the proximal segment of the BA (*long arrows*). The bilateral AICAs arise from the fenestrated channels (*short arrows*)

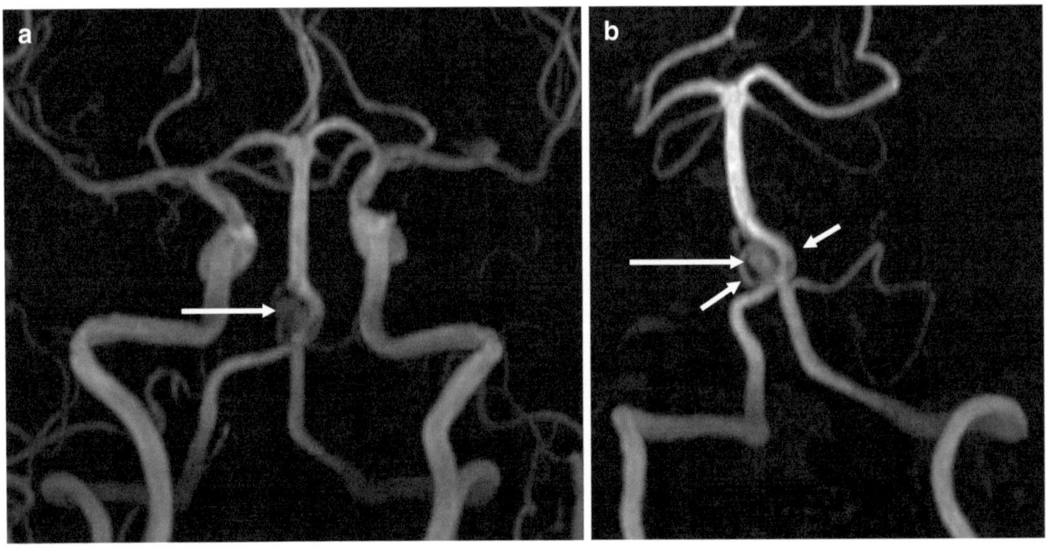

Fig. 11.2 (**a**) A-P projection of MR angiography and (**b**) partial MIP image show an aneurysm at the origin of the BA (*long arrows*). There are two channels at the proximal segment of the BA (*short arrows*), indicative of a fenestration

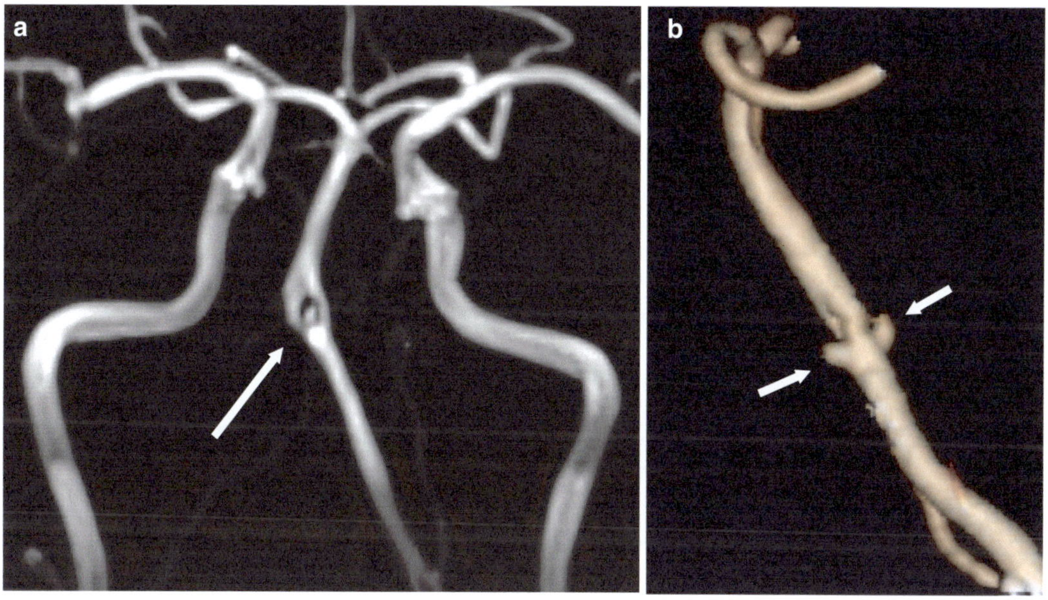

Fig. 11.3 (**a**) A-P projection of MR angiography shows a fenestration at the proximal end of the BA (*long arrow*). (**b**) Partial VR lateral image of CT angiography shows two small aneurysms arising from the proximal end of the fenestration (*short arrows*)

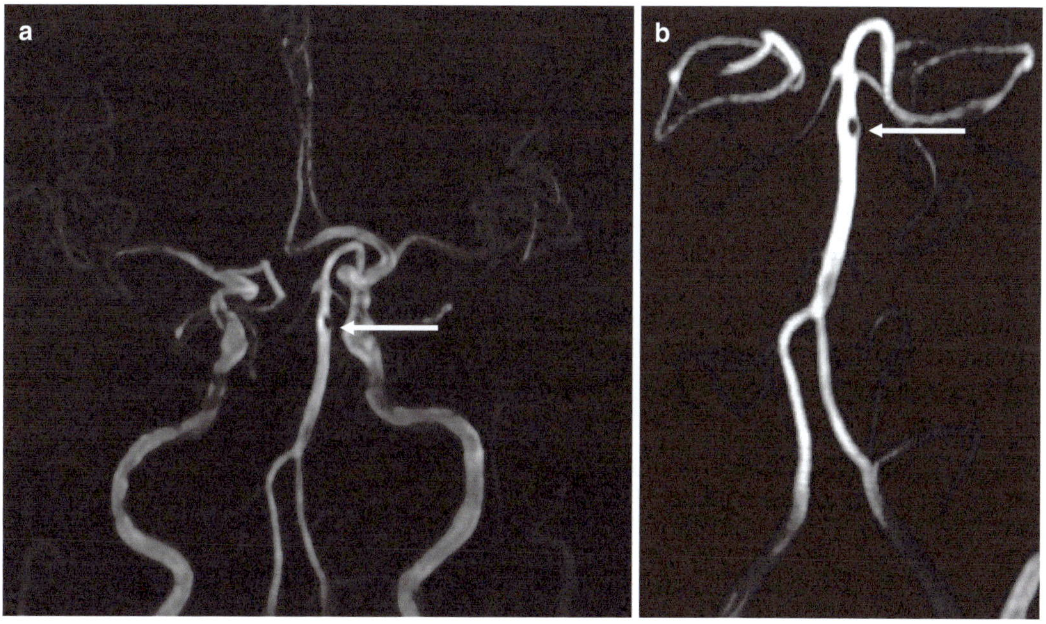

Fig. 11.4 (**a**) A-P projection of MR angiography and (**b**) partial MIP image show a tiny fenestration at the distal segment of the BA (*arrows*)

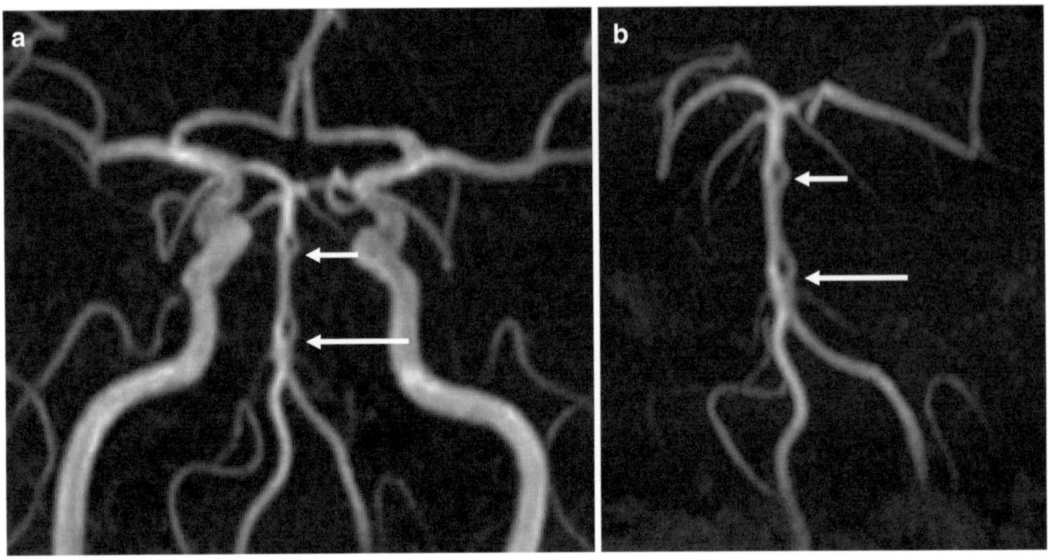

Fig. 11.5 (**a**) A-P projection of MR angiography and (**b**) partial MIP image show two small fenestrations of the BA at its proximal and distal segments (*long and short arrows*)

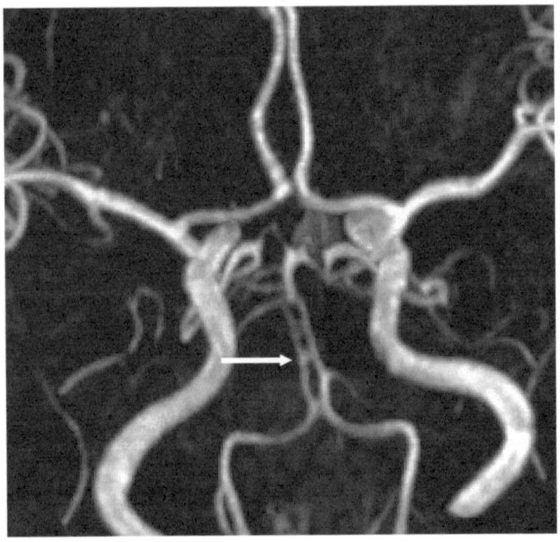

Fig. 11.6 AI-PS projection of MR angiography shows two large fenestrations of the BA (*arrow*). (Courtesy of Dr. Shinichi Kan)

BA partial duplication (Fig. 11.9) [7] and it may be formed by persistent primitive lateral vertebrobasilar anastomosis [6].

11.3 Distal BA Partial Duplication (Caudal Fusion of BA)

Fusion failure also occurs at the distal end of the BA, the symmetrical caudal fusion [8] results in partial duplication of the distal BA. In the case of this variation, the BA is short and the bilateral SCAs arise from the duplicated channels, forming a common trunk with the PCAs (Figs. 11.10 and 12.15) [9].

11.4 BA Complete Duplication

Extremely rarely, a paired BA was seen (Figs. 11.11 and 11.12). This variation was called complete duplication or extreme fenestration [10]. This extremely rare variation occurs if the paired primitive longitudinal neural arteries do not fuse entirely. This variation can be associated with other midline fusion failure, such as cleft palate and hypophyseal duplication [11].

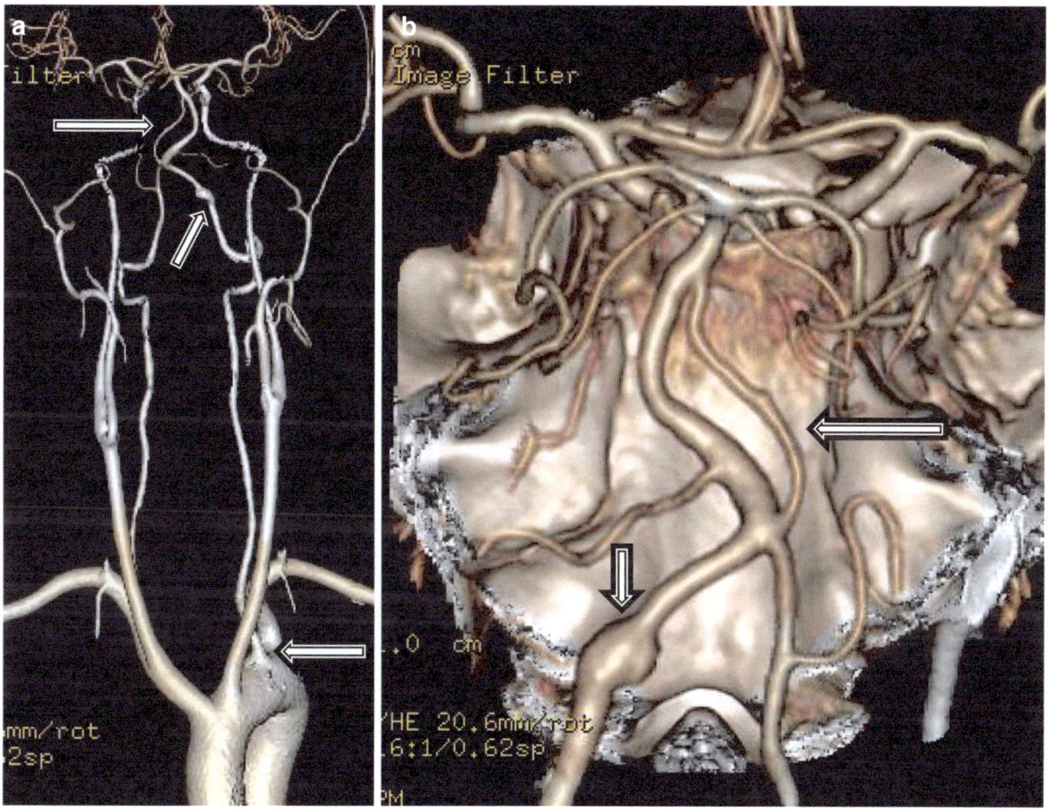

Fig. 11.7 (**a**) A-P and (**b**) S-I projections of CT angiography show an extremely large arterial ring of the BA (*long arrows*). The left VA arises from the AA proximal to the left SA (*dotted arrow*). A dissecting aneurysm is seen at the V4 segment of the left VA (*short arrows*)

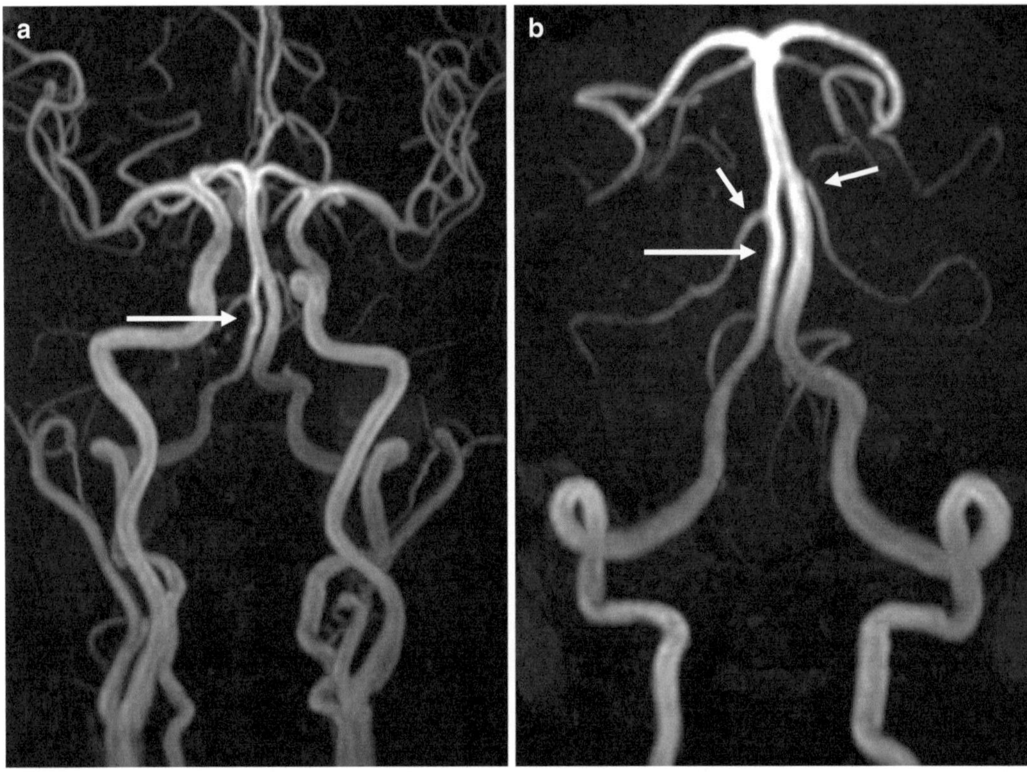

Fig. 11.8 (**a**) A-P projection of MR angiography and (**b**) partial MIP image show proximal duplication of the BA (*long arrows*). The bilateral AICAs arise from the duplicated channels (*short arrows*)

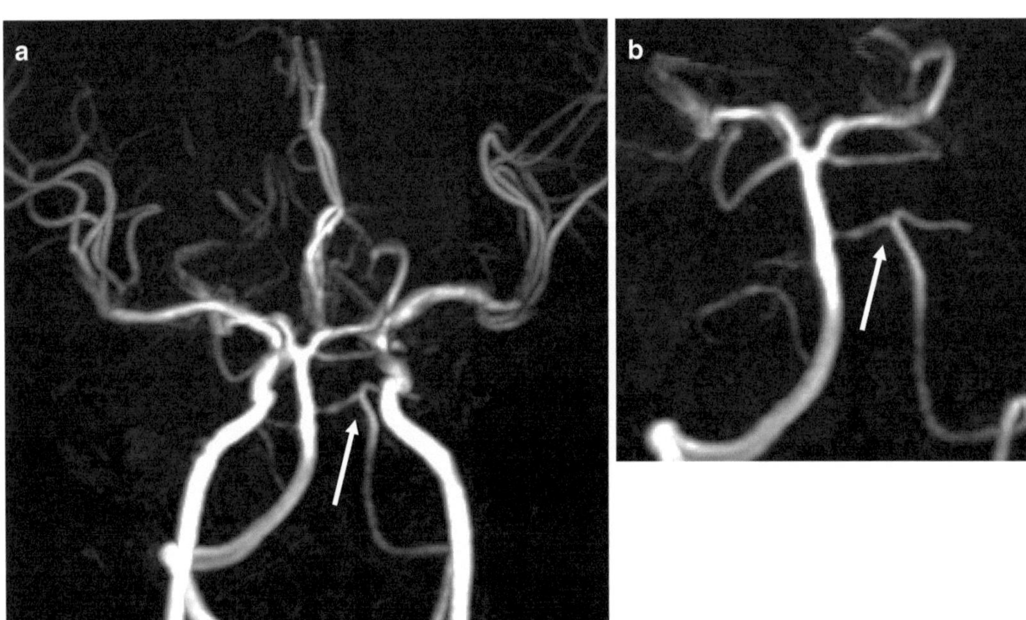

Fig. 11.9 (**a**) A-P projection of MR angiography and (**b**) partial MIP image show the left VA anastomosing with the left AICA (*arrows*) instead of the BA. This variation can be regarded as proximal partial duplication of the BA

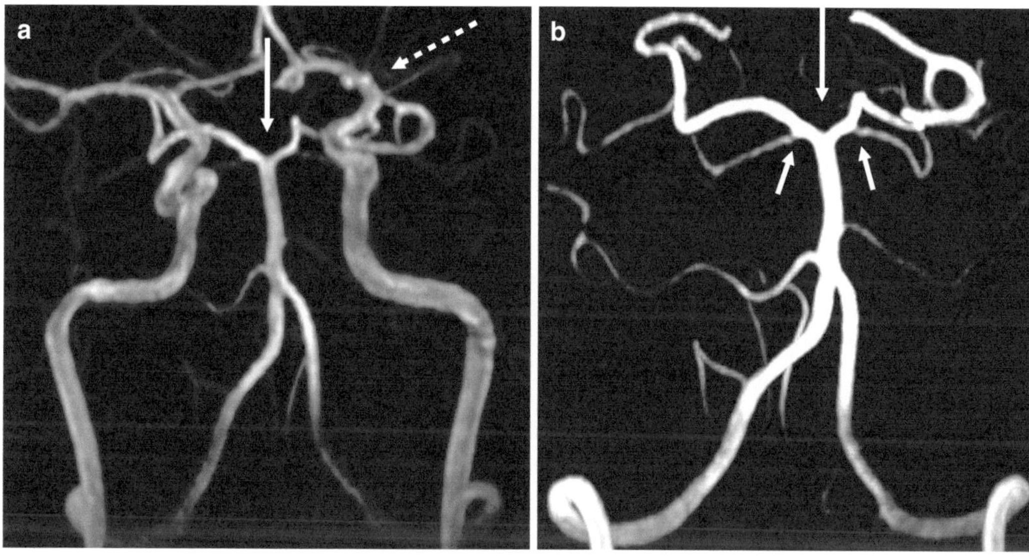

Fig. 11.10 (**a**) A-P projection of MR angiography and (**b**) partial MIP image show distal duplication of the BA (*long arrows*). The BA is short. The bilateral SCAs arise from the duplicated channels, forming a common trunk with the PCAs (*short arrows*) (Fig. 12.15). The left MCA is occluded at its origin (*dotted arrow*)

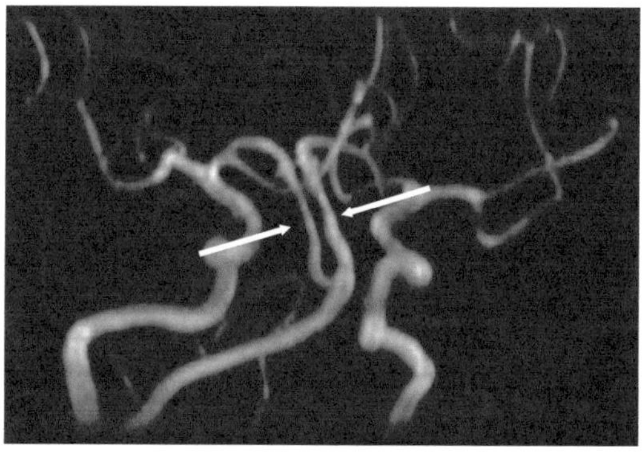

Fig. 11.11 Slightly RAO projection of MR angiography shows two BAs, indicative of a complete duplication (*arrows*). (Courtesy of Dr. Takashi Okazaki)

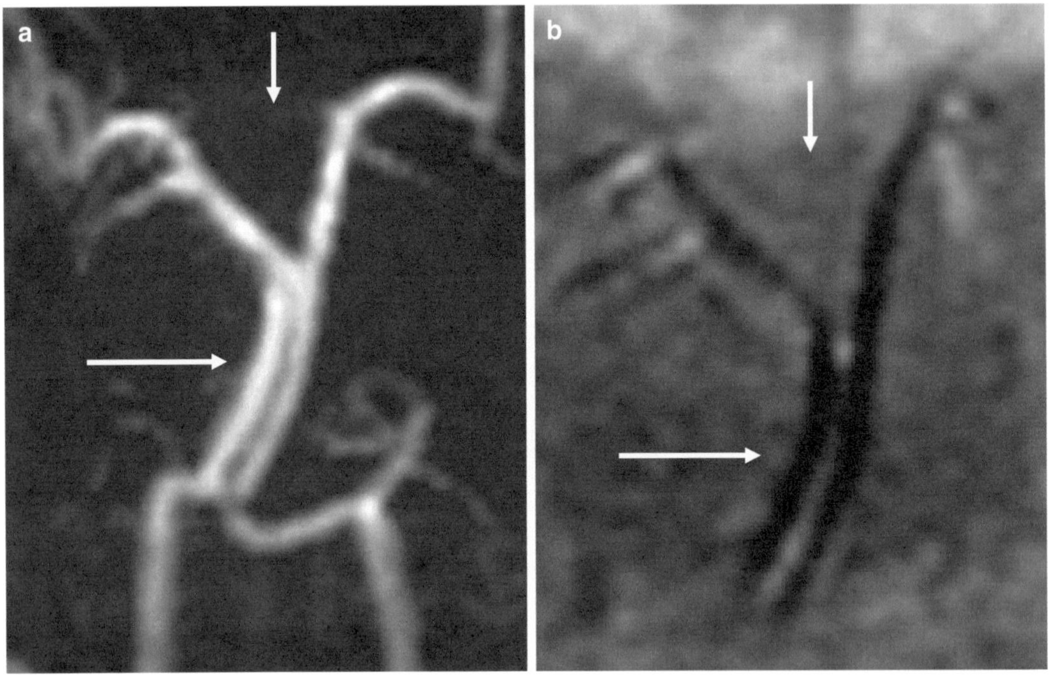

Fig. 11.12 (**a**) Partial MIP MR angiography and (**b**) coronal T1-weighted MR imaging show an extreme fenestration (*long arrows*) and a distal duplication (*short arrows*). This infant also had cleft palate, nasopharyngeal mature teratoma, and hypophyseal duplication

References

1. Tanaka M, Kikuchi Y, O'uchi T. Neuroradiological analysis of 23 cases of basilar artery fenestration based on 2280 cases of MR angiographies. Interv Neuroradiol. 2006;12(Suppl 1):39–44.
2. Uchino A, Saito N, Okada Y, Kozawa E, Nishi N, Mizukoshi W, Inoue K, Nakajima R, Takahashi M. Fenestrations of the intracranial vertebrobasilar system diagnosed by MR angiography. Neuroradiology. 2012;54:445–50.
3. Sogawa K, Kikuchi Y, O'uchi T, Tanaka M, Inoue T. Fenestrations of the basilar artery demonstrated on magnetic resonance angiograms: an analysis of 212 cases. Interv Neuroradiol. 2013;19:461–5.
4. Nagahata M, Abe Y, Ono S, Hosoya T, Uno S. Surface appearance of the vertebrobasilar artery revealed on basiparallel anatomic scanning (BPAS)-MR imaging: its role for brain MR examination. AJNR Am J Neuroradiol. 2005;26:2508–13.
5. Padget DH. The development of cranial arteries in the human embryo. Contrib Embryol. 1948;32:207–61.
6. Yagi K, Satoh K, Satomi J, Nagahiro S. Primitive vertebrobasilar system associated with a ruptured aneurysm. AJNR Am J Neuroradiol. 2004;25:781–3.
7. Hoshino E, Uchino A, Saito N, Yoshiba S. Association of tetralogy of Fallot with multiple variations of the cerebral arteries diagnosed by magnetic resonance angiography. Radiol Case Rep. 2020;15:349–52.
8. Lasjaunias P, Berenstein A, ter Brugge KG. The PCoA-P1-distal BA system. In: Lasjaunias P, Berenstein A, ter Brugge KG, editors. Surgical neuro-angiography. Vol. 1. Clinical vascular anatomy and variations. 2nd ed. Berlin Heiderberg New York: Springer-Verlag; 2001. p. 523–48.
9. Uchino A, Sawada A, Takase Y, Kudo S. Variations of the superior cerebellar artery: MR angiographic demonstration. Radiat Med. 2003;21:235–8.
10. Goldstein JH, Woodcock R, Do HM, Phillips CD, Dion JE. Complete duplication or extreme fenestration of the basilar artery. AJNR Am J Neuroradiol. 1999;20:149–50.
11. Uchino A, Sawada A, Takase Y, Fujita I, Kudo S. (2002) Extreme fenestration of the basilar artery associated with cleft palate, nasopharyngeal mature teratoma, and hypophyseal duplication. Eur Radiol. 2002;12:2087–90.

12 Variations of the Cerebellar Arteries

Abstract

This chapter includes (1) Extracranial C1/2 level origin of the posterior inferior cerebellar artery (PICA), (2) Foramen magnum level origin of the PICA, (3) Duplicate origin of the PICA, (4) Duplicated PICA, (5) Bihemispheric PICA, (6) PICA-anterior inferior cerebellar artery (AICA) anastomosis (vertebrobasilar junction large arterial ring), (7) Common trunk of the AICA-PICA (PICA or AICA aplasia), (8) Duplicated AICA and early bifurcated AICA, (9) Duplicated superior cerebellar artery (SCA) and early bifurcated SCA, and (10) SCA arising from the posterior cerebral artery. There are 13 figures and 2 illustrations.

As mentioned above (Sects. 5.1.3, 5.2.3 and 5.3), the cerebellar arteries are rarely supplied by the ICA and ascending pharyngeal artery.

Keywords

Anterior inferior cerebellar artery · Cerebellar artery · Posterior cerebral artery · Posterior inferior cerebellar artery · Superior cerebellar artery

12.1 Extracranial C1/2 Level Origin of the PICA

The PICA can arise from the extracranial V3 segment of the VA at the C1/2 level, and this type of the PICA is usually hyperplastic (Fig. 12.1). MR angiographic prevalence of this variation was reported to be 1.1% [1]. If the second intersegmental artery persists and continues to the PICA without fusion with the VA, it forms the extracranial C1/2 origin PICA. Schematic illustrations of the C2 segmental type VA (Sect. 10.2.1), VA fenestration at the craniovertebral junction (Sect. 10.3.1), and extracranial C1/2 origin of the PICA are presented in Fig. 12.2. Rarely, an aneurysm is seen at the distal segment of this type of PICA [2, 3]. Extremely rarely, the PICA arises from the lower C2 level (Fig. 12.3). It runs up and enters the C1/2 intervertebral space, the same as a C1/2 origin PICA

12.2 Foramen Magnum Level Origin of the PICA

An extradural origin of the PICA is seen in 5–20% of cases, and in the majority of cases, the PICA arises from the VA at the level of the FM [4]. The PICA of this variation is usually hyperplastic and rarely makes a caudal loop in the spinal canal (Fig. 12.4). Rarely, an aneurysm is seen at the distal segment of this type of PICA [3].

A. Uchino, *Atlas of the Supraaortic Craniocervical Arterial Variations*,
https://doi.org/10.1007/978-981-16-6803-6_12

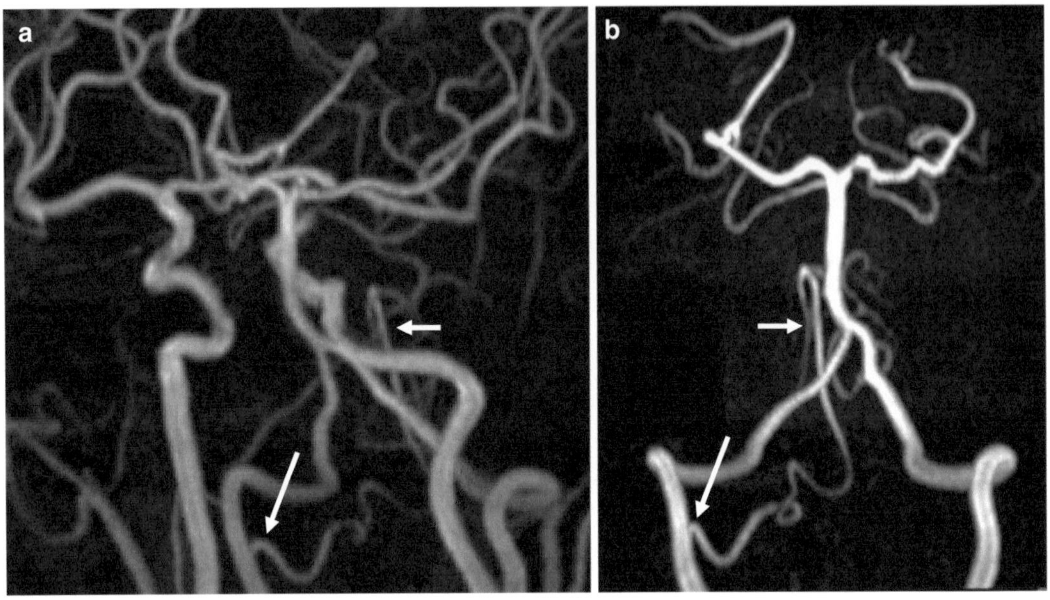

Fig. 12.1 (**a**) LAO projection of MR angiography and (**b**) partial MIP image show right PICA arising from the extracranial C1/2 level (V3 segment) of the VA (*long arrows*). This anomalous origin of the PICA is hyperplastic (*short arrows*)

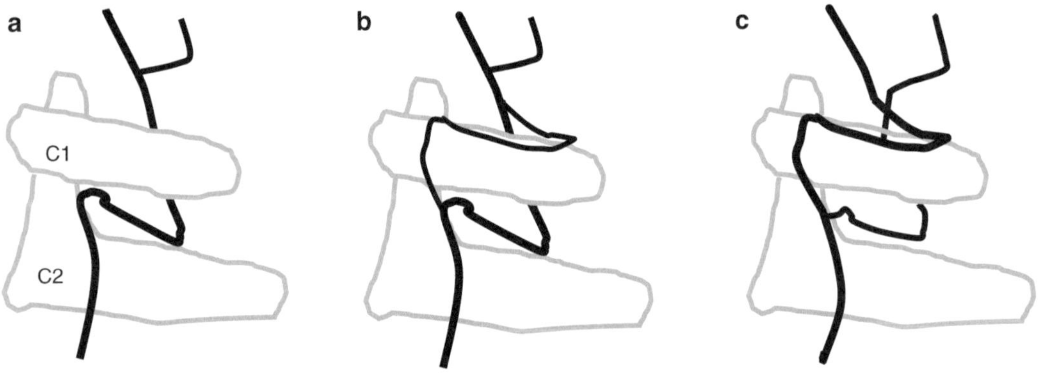

Fig. 12.2 Schematic illustrations of three types of VA variations at the C1/2 level (left lateral projection). (Modified from [1]). (**a**) C2 segmental type VA, (**b**) VA fenestration at the craniovertebral junction, (**c**) PICA originating from the C1/2 level VA

12.3 Duplicate Origin of the PICA

As mentioned above (Sect. 10.3.2), the PICA frequently arises from the fenestrated V4 segment of the VA. This common variation may be misdiagnosed as a duplicate origin of the PICA. In contrast, the true duplicate origin of the PICA is extremely rare (Fig. 12.5) [5–7]. These two variations should be correctly recognized based on the different directions of blood flow in the cranial channel from that in the distal segment of the VA fenestration from which the PICA arises (Fig. 12.6).

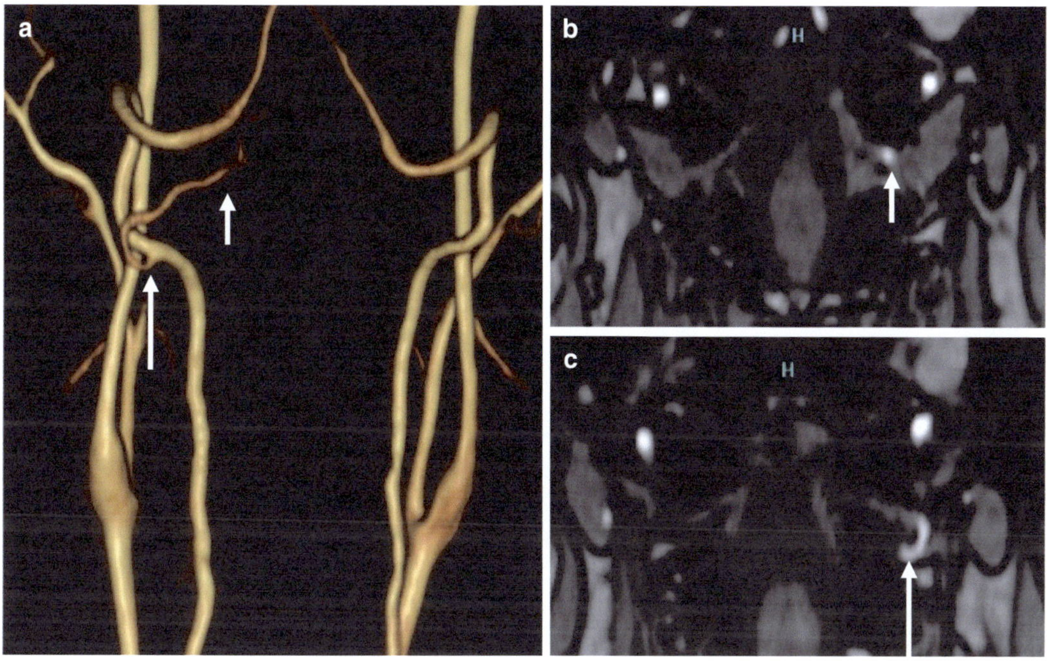

Fig. 12.3 (**a**) P-A projection of a VR image of MR angiography and (**b**, **c**) coronal reformatted source images show the left PICA arising from the lower C2 level (*long arrows*). It runs up and enters the C1/2 intervertebral space (*short arrows*)

12.4 Duplicated PICA

Rarely, two arteries arise from the V4 segment of the ipsilateral VA (Fig. 12.7). This is regarded as a duplicated PICA [8]. The distal branch supplies the territory of the AICA and there is usually no AICA, suggesting that the distal branch is the replaced AICA.

12.5 Bihemispheric PICA

Rarely, a unilateral PICA supplies both cerebellar hemispheres (Fig. 12.8). This bihemispheric type of the PICA is usually hyperplastic, and the contralateral PICA is absent or hypoplastic [9]. An aneurysm may arise at the VA-PICA junction or the distal segment of the hyperplastic PICA probably due to increased hemodynamic stress [10].

12.6 PICA-Anterior Inferior Cerebellar Artery (AICA) Anastomosis

If the PICA and AICA fuse, a large arterial ring is formed at the VBJ (Fig. 12.9). This variation can also be regarded as persistent primitive lateral vertebrobasilar anastomosis [11], from which a hyperplastic AICA arises.

12.7 Common Trunk of the AICA-PICA (PICA or AICA Aplasia)

The SCAs are constantly observed bilaterally. However, the ipsilateral PICA or AICA is frequently absent (Fig. 12.10). In patients with an absent PICA or AICA, the ipsilateral AICA or PICA, respectively, is hyperplastic to overcome the lack of blood supply. The hyperplastic AICA

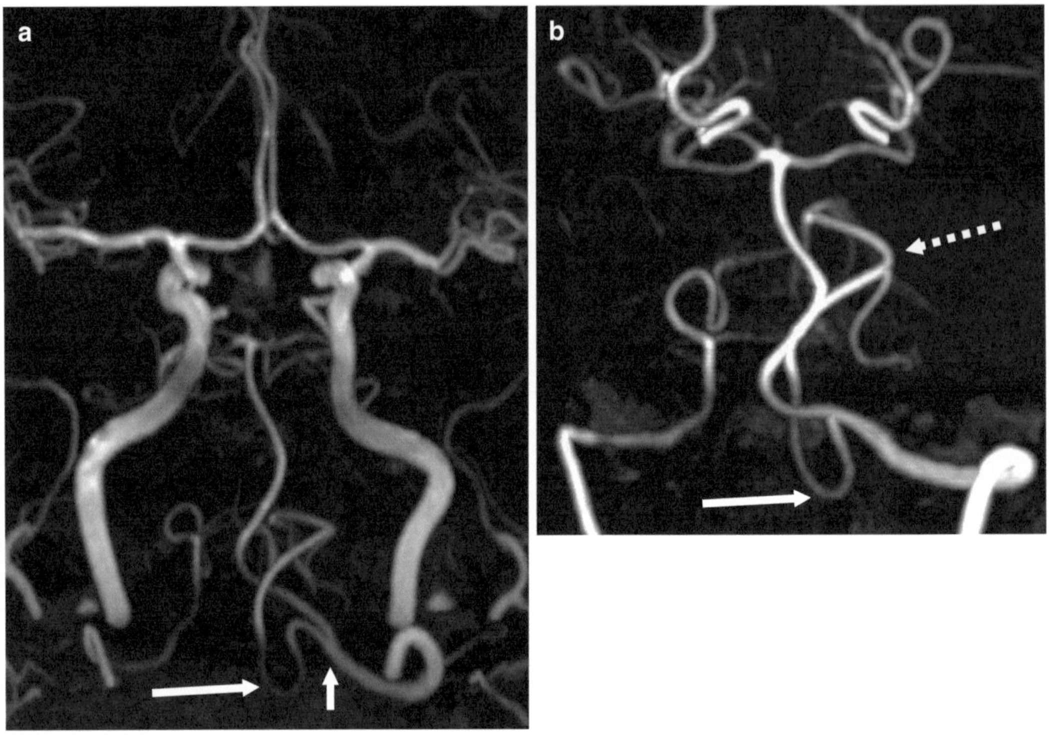

Fig. 12.4 (**a**) AI-PS projection of MR angiography and (**b**) partial MIP image show the left PICA arising from the VA at the level of the FM (*short arrow*). This low-origin PICA makes a caudal loop at the level of the FM (*long arrows*). This artery is hyperplastic (*dotted arrow*)

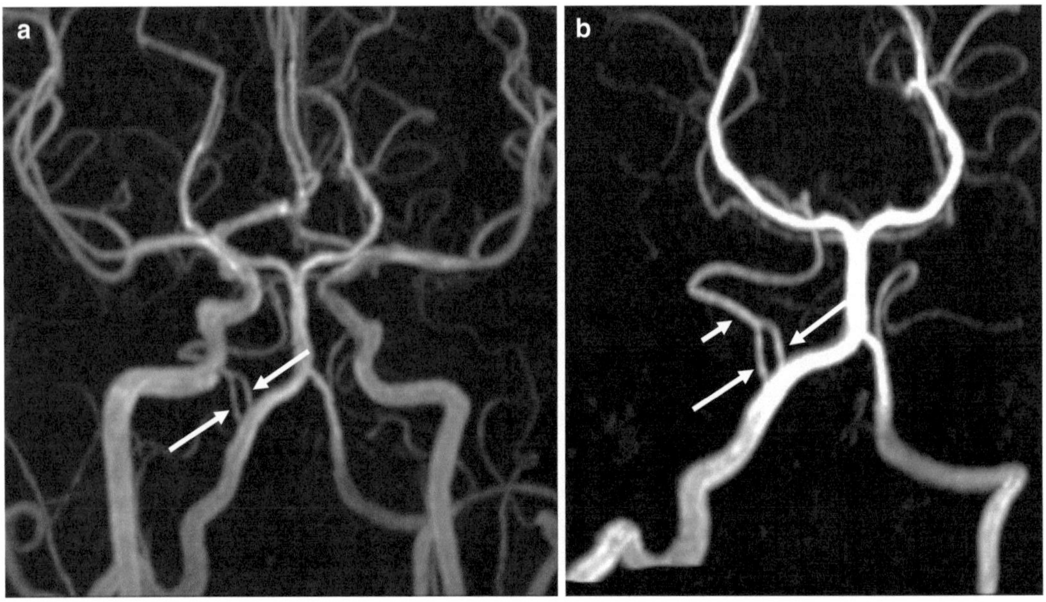

Fig. 12.5 (**a**) A-P projection of MR angiography and (**b**) partial MIP image show two arteries arising from the right VA (*long arrows*) and fusing together soon to form a PICA trunk (*short arrow*). The PICA trunk is larger than the two proximal arteries, indicative of a duplicate origin of the PICA, not a VA fenestration

or PICA can be regarded as a common trunk of the AICA-PICA, and its prevalence of catheter angiography was reported to be 22.1% per hemisphere; thus, the frequency is extremely high [12].

12.8 Duplicated AICA, Early Bifurcated AICA

Two arteries frequently arise from the proximal BA. This variation is regarded as a duplicated AICA. Its anatomic prevalence was reported to be 26% among 50 AICAs [8]. The prevalence on catheter angiography was recently reported to be 10.4% per hemisphere [12]. The ipsilateral PICA is usually absent or hypoplastic (Fig. 12.11). Thus, the proximally arising AICA supplies the territory of the PICA.

The hyperplastic AICA rarely bifurcates soon [13]. The caudal branch supplies the territory of the PICA (Fig. 12.12).

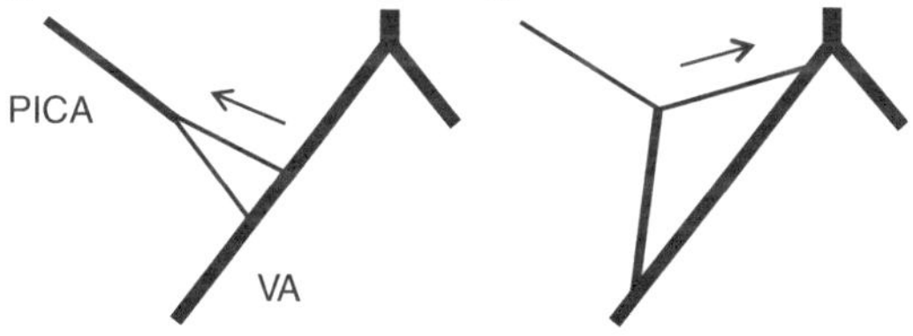

Fig. 12.6 Schematic illustrations of (**a**) duplicate origin of the PICA and (**b**) PICA arising from VA fenestration. (Modified from [7]). The *arrows* indicate the directions of blood flow. *PICA*, posterior inferior cerebellar artery; *VA*, vertebral artery

12.9 Duplicated Superior Cerebellar Artery (SCA), Early Bifurcated SCA

Two SCAs relatively frequently arise from the terminal segment of the BA, and this variation is sometimes seen bilaterally (Fig. 12.13). Its microsurgical anatomic prevalence was reported to be 14% [14]. Using a 1.5 tesla scanner, the prevalence on MR angiography was reported to be 9.6% [15], which is lower in comparison to the anatomic study, probably due to the low spatial resolution of MR angiography.

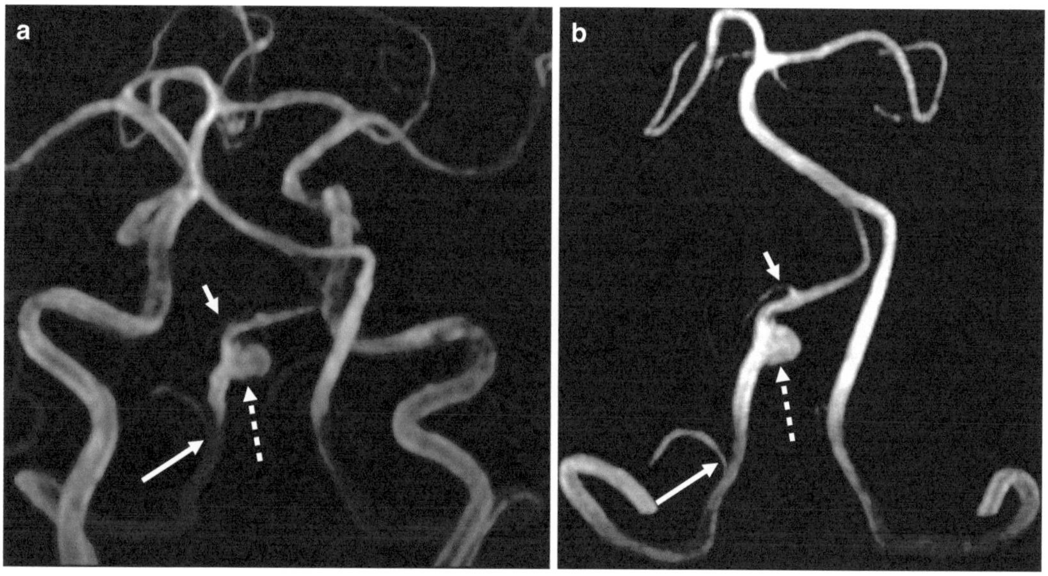

Fig. 12.7 (**a**) A-P projection of MR angiography and (**b**) partial MIP image show two arteries arising from the V4 segment of the right VA, indicative of a duplicated PICA (*long and short arrows*). A dissecting aneurysm of the VA is seen between the two arteries (*dotted arrow*)

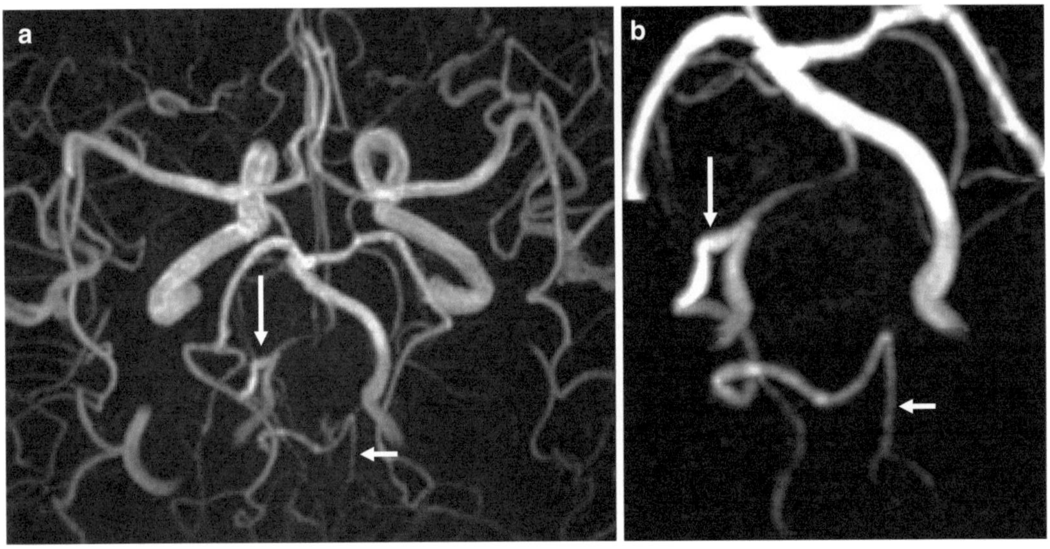

Fig. 12.8 (**a**) I-S projection of MR angiography and (**b**) partial MIP image show a hyperplastic right PICA (*long arrows*). This artery crosses the midline and supplies the distal segment of the left PICA, indicative of a bihemispheric PICA (*short arrows*)

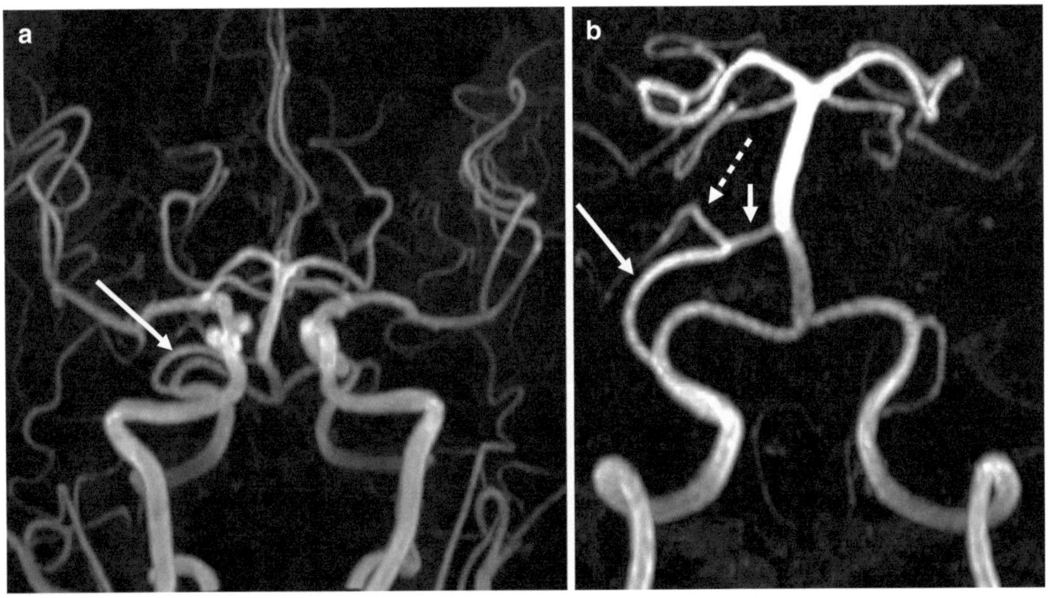

Fig. 12.9 (**a**) AS-PI projection of MR angiography and (**b**) partial MIP A-P image show a large arterial ring at the right side of the VBJ. The proximal segment of the lateral channel is large and long (*long arrows*). In contrast, the distal segment is small and short (*short arrow*). A hyperplastic right AICA arises from the lateral channel (*dotted arrow*), suggestive of the PICA-AICA anastomosis or persistent primitive lateral vertebrobasilar anastomosis

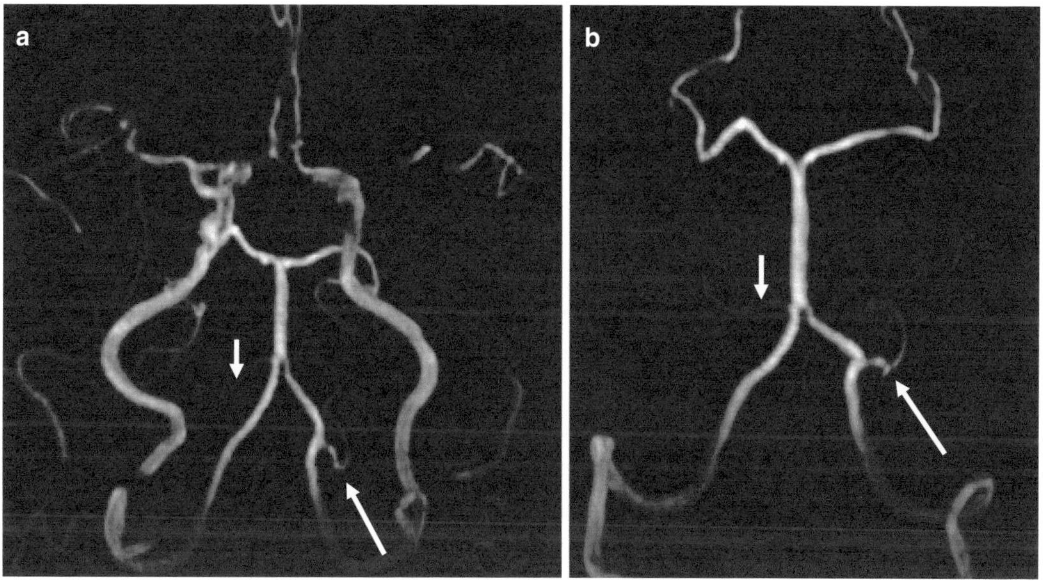

Fig. 12.10 (**a**) AI-PS projection of MR angiography and (**b**) partial MIP image show a left PICA (*long arrows*) and right AICA (*short arrows*). Neither a left AICA nor a right PICA is seen. The bilateral SCAs are observed

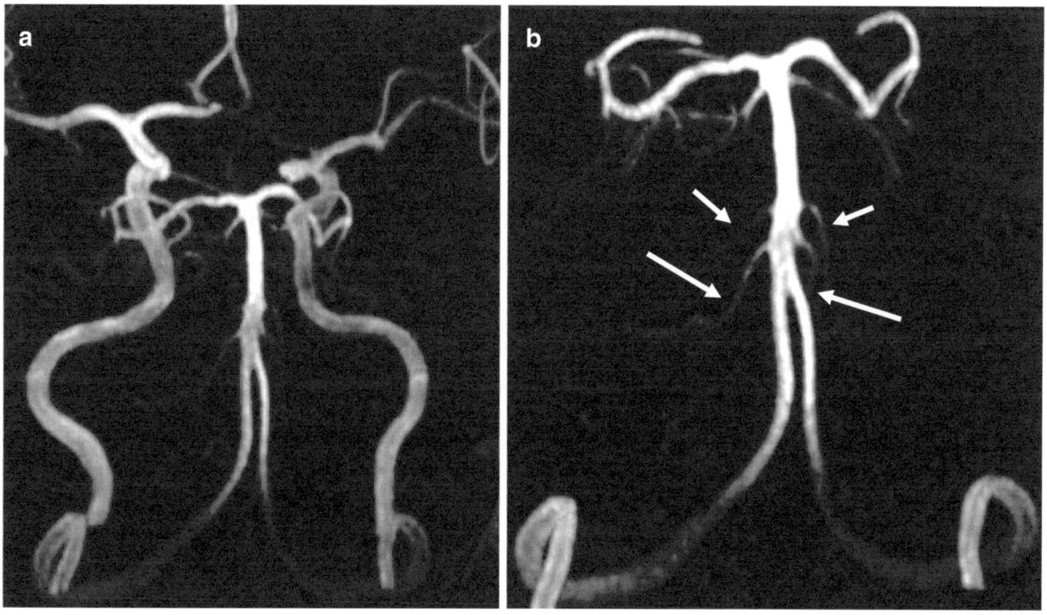

Fig. 12.11 (**a**) A-P projection of MR angiography and (**b**) partial MIP image show two AICAs arising bilaterally (*long and short arrows*). The bilateral proximally arising arteries are hyperplastic and supplying the territories of the PICAs (*long arrows*)

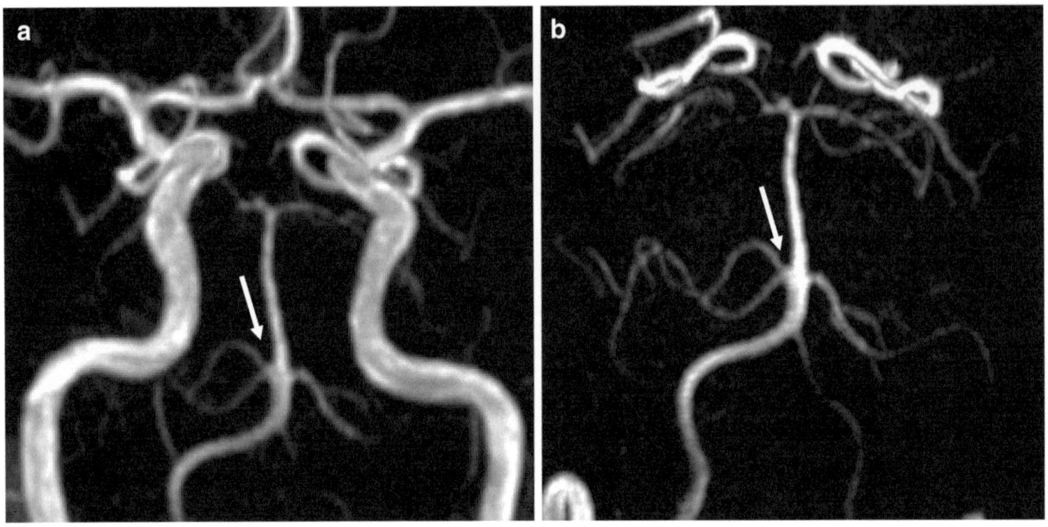

Fig. 12.12 (**a**) A-P projection of MR angiography and (**b**) partial MIP image show hyperplastic AICAs and absent PICAs bilaterally. The right AICA duplicates soon (*arrows*)

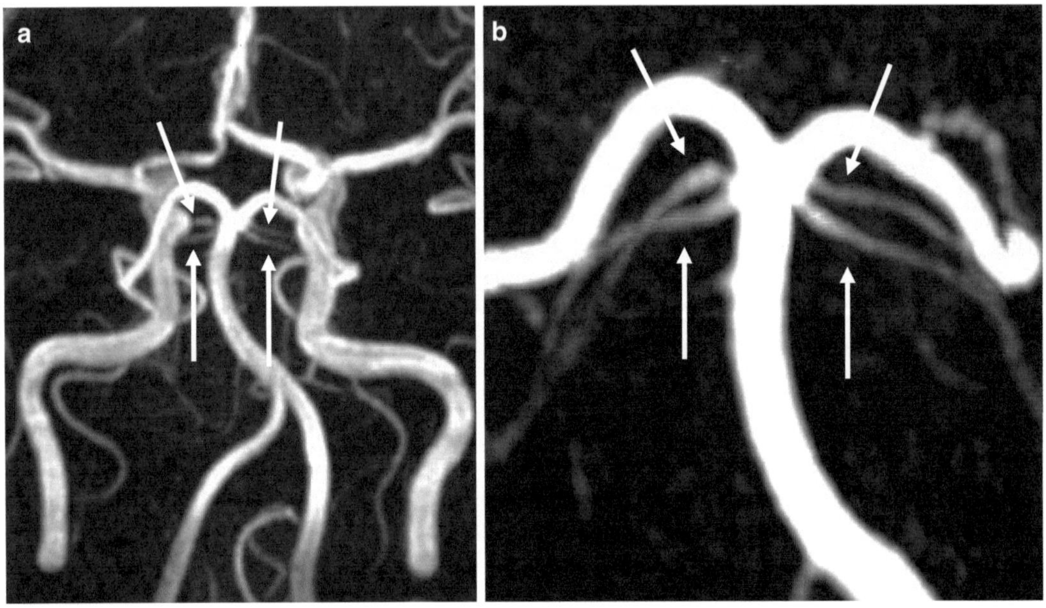

Fig. 12.13 (**a**) A-P projection of MR angiography and (**b**) partial MIP image show two SCAs arising bilaterally (*arrows*)

The SCA generally arises as a single vessel from the BA and bifurcates into two major trunks: one rostral and one caudal. This bifurcation occurs between 0.6 and 34.0 mm (average, 19 mm) [8]. When the bifurcation occurs at the proximal anterior pontomesencephalic segment, it is regarded as early bifurcation (Fig. 12.14). Its MR angiographic prevalence was reported to be 3.0% [15].

12.10 SCA Arising from the Posterior Cerebral Artery

SCA frequently arises from the P1 segment of the PCA, forming the common trunk of the PCA and SCA, and this variation is sometimes seen bilaterally (Fig. 12.15). Its microsurgical anatomic prevalence was reported to be 4% [14].

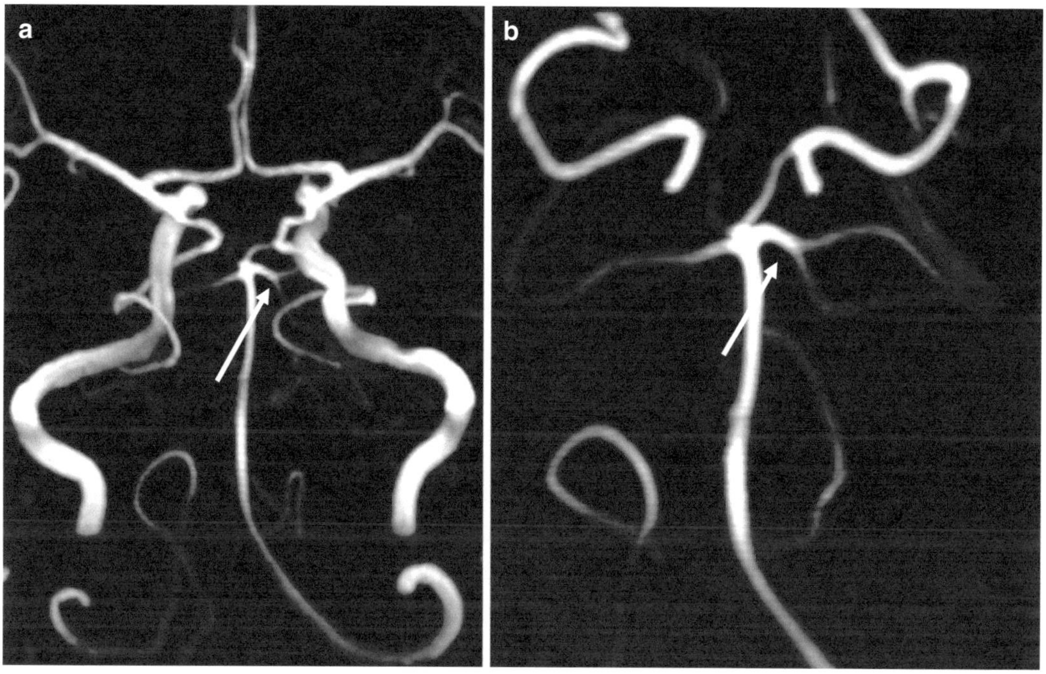

Fig. 12.14 (**a**) AI-PS projection of MR angiography and (**b**) partial MIP image show an early bifurcating left SCA (*arrows*). The distance from the origin to the bifurcation is 3 mm

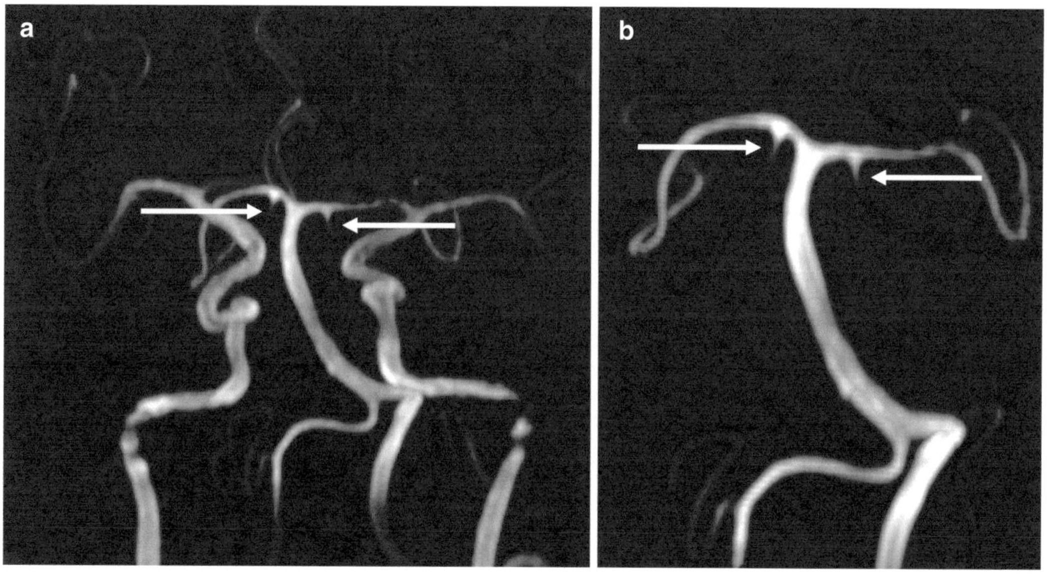

Fig. 12.15 (**a**) A-P projection of MR angiography and (**b**) partial MIP image show bilateral SCAs arising from the P1 segments of the PCAs, forming the common trunk of the PCA and SCA (*arrows*)

Using a 1.5 tesla scanner, its prevalence on MR angiography was reported to be 4.4% [15]. As mentioned above (Sect. 11.3), the bilateral type of this variation is formed by symmetric caudal fusion of the BA [16] and can also be regarded as a partial duplication of the distal BA. Rarely, an SCA arises from the duplicate origin of the PCA (Fig. 7.14).

References

1. Uchino A, Saito N, Watadani T, Okada Y, Kozawa E, Nishi N, Mizukoshi W, Inoue K, Nakajima R, Takahashi M. Vertebral artery variations at the C1-2 level diagnosed by magnetic resonance angiography. Neuroradiology. 2012;54:19–23.
2. Abe T, Kojima K, Singer RJ, Marks MP, Watanabe M, Ohtsuru K, Nishimura H, Hayabuchi N. Endovascular management of an aneurysm arising from posterior inferior cerebellar artery originated at the level of C2. Radiat Med. 1998;16:141–3.
3. Lin CF, Hsu SPC, Chen MT, Chen HH, Shih YH, Lee LS, Chen MH. Posterior inferior cerebellar artery with extracranial origin harboring an extracranial aneurysm. Surg Neurol. 2007;68(S1):64–7.
4. Fine AD, Cardoso A, Rhoton AL Jr. Microsurgical anatomy of the extracranial-extradural origin of the posterior inferior cerebellar artery. J Neurosurg. 1999;91:645–52.
5. Pasco A, Thouveny F, Papon X, Tanguy JY, Mercier P, Caron-Poitreau C, Herbreteau D. Ruptured aneurysm on a double origin of the posterior inferior cerebellar artery: a pathological entity in an anatomical variation. Report of two cases and review of the literature. J Neurosurg. 2002;96:127–31.
6. Lesley WS, Rajab MH, Case RS. Double origin of the posterior inferior cerebellar artery: association with intracranial aneurysm on catheter angiography. AJR Am J Roentgenol. 2007;189:893–7.
7. Uchino A, Saito N, Ishihara S. Double origin of the posterior inferior cerebellar artery diagnosed by MR angiography: a report of two cases. Neuroradiol J. 2015;28:187–9.
8. Rhoton AL Jr. The cerebellar arteries. Neurosurgery. 2000;47:S29–68.
9. Cullen SP, Ozanne A, Alvarez H, Lasjaunias P. The bihemispheric posterior inferior cerebellar artery. Neuroradiology. 2005;47:809–12.
10. Ogasawara Y, Kashimura H, Aso K, Saura H. Subarachnoid haemorrhage due to ruptured intracranial aneurysm arising from a vertebral artery-bihemispheric posterior inferior cerebellar artery bifurcation. J Neurosci Rural Pract. 2017;8:654–6.
11. De Caro R, Parenti A, Munari PF. Persistent primitive lateral vertebrobasilar anastomosis. Acta Neurochir (Wien). 1996;138:592–4.
12. Hou K, Li G, Luan T, Xu K, Xu B, Yu J. Anatomical study of anterior inferior cerebellar artery and its reciprocal relationship with posterior inferior cerebellar artery based on angiographic data. World Neurosurg. 2020;133:e459–72.
13. Pekcevik Y. Double origin and early bifurcation of the anterior inferior cerebellar artery diagnosed by CT angiography. Surg Radiol Anat. 2015;37:1141–3.
14. Hardy DG, Peace DA, Rhoton AL Jr. Microsurgical anatomy of the superior cerebellar artery. Neurosurgery. 1980;6:10–28.
15. Uchino A, Sawada A, Takase T, Kudo S. Variations of the superior cerebellar artery: MR angiographic demonstration. Radiat. Med. 2003;21:235–8.
16. Lasjaunias P, Berenstein A, ter Brugge KG. The PCoA-P1-distal BA system. In: Lasjaunias P, Berenstein A, ter Brugge KG, editors. Surgical neuro-angiography. Vol. 1. Clinical vascular anatomy and variations. 2nd ed. Berlin Heiderberg New York: Springer-Verlag; 2001. p. 523–48.

MIX
Papier aus verantwortungsvollen Quellen
Paper from responsible sources
FSC® C105338

If you have any concerns about our products,
you can contact us on
ProductSafety@springernature.com

In case Publisher is established outside the EU,
the EU authorized representative is:
Springer Nature Customer Service Center GmbH
Europaplatz 3, 69115 Heidelberg, Germany

Printed by Libri Plureos GmbH
in Hamburg, Germany